Good Physician, Good Plastic Surgeon

Kun Hwang

Good Physician, Good Plastic Surgeon

Springer

Kun Hwang
Department of Plastic Surgery
Armed Forces Capital Hospital
Bundang-gu, Seongnam, Korea (Republic of)

ISBN 978-981-97-1866-5   ISBN 978-981-97-1864-1 (eBook)
https://doi.org/10.1007/978-981-97-1864-1

This Springer imprint is published by the registered company Springer Nature Singapore Pte Ltd.
The registered company address is: 152 Beach Road, #21-01/04 Gateway East, Singapore 189721, Singapore

Paper in this product is recyclable.

Dedicated to my mother Kyung Sun Kim, an artist (1930–),
and my wife You Bong Song, MD, PhD (1958–).

Foreword

The noblest question in the world is: What good may I do in it?
—Ben Franklin

It was a great pleasure when Dr. Kun Hwang asked me to write the foreword for his newly prepared book on humanitarian aspects of plastic surgery. I accepted the honor and the privilege, particularly as I have always reminded my students about the importance of the global arena in the dissemination of science and technology. It is also important from an empirical standpoint that we should always remove the boundaries, particularly in the field of medicine, to allow us to be transparent and to exchange our ideas, new and old, in innovations and creativity for the best care of our patients so the outcomes become beyond our expectations. Having said that as a prelude my imagination took me back thousands of years, looking in the rearview mirror of the brave new digital world. The year was 130 BC and with the Roman Empire at its helm a silk trail was formed to connect the East with the West. The East had their silk and spices and those in the West were eager to make use of them. The trail continued to serve well in biblical times. Those moving material along the silk trail (later becoming the silk road) learned how to overcome the difficulties of the terrain, the terrorist hideouts, and the thieves and charlatans on the way. Fight some, bribe others, and avoid what can be avoided. However, today we learn of the evaluation of creativity, innovations, and advances from one of the most prestigious analysts in a publishing house, and the verdict is that there is more flow of new educational material coming from the Far East. Well, we have reopened the old road and it is now digital. The old silk trail became the silk road and now the digital information road brings us together and brings closure in spite of language barriers and geographic variation. We still have hackers, plagiarism, and terrorists, but the weapons to fight back are totally different and now totally digital. It is easier to consider that all the time we have wasted in conflicts, politics, and ideologies is now spent in cooperation and collaboration to proceed with smooth relationships, creating a new digital medical world with no boundaries.

On a final note, it is imperative to stress that plastic surgeons dedicate their lives to improving the quality of life of those who may have already had their lives saved by other professionals, and on rare occasions plastic surgeons are involved in saving lives. It is important for everyone to have the quality of life they want and deserve. This book by Dr. Hwang serves to improve the human nature of the plastic surgeon, discussing beauty and how it affects the individual, and among the elderly, it is important to respect their willingness to get involved with beauty and its pursuance. If surgeons read the book in order to learn new technics, they will be disappointed. However, those who read it to make them feel that being a plastic surgeon is being humanitarian, they will be satisfied. As plastic surgeons, we should get out of the routines of practicing technics and focus on just one aspect of plastic surgery. It is human nature that we think of plastic surgery in terms of technics and improving life, but in the book we have gone beyond that and see how other aspects of life are as important in the profession. It is beyond what we do but what we feel as humans in the global social arena.

Congratulations to the author of this nice collection who gives us that great feeling of being human after all… Bravo!

Tampa, FL, USA Mutaz B. Habal

Foreword

The last half of the twentieth century witnessed an explosion in scientific research, publishing, and specialization to an extent unparalleled in human history, and this trend has only accelerated further in the first decades of the twenty-first century with the integration of information technology into the research workflow, large-scale development and implementation of computational methods, and widespread adoption of online publishing. While, on the one hand, this tremendous growth in scientific knowledge has yielded remarkable benefits to humankind—see, for example, the rapid sequencing of the SARS-CoV-2 genome after the initial COVID-19 outbreak and the unprecedentedly fast pace of COVID-19 vaccine development, less than 20 years after the Human Genome Project was completed at enormous costs—it has also prompted concerns about hyperspecialization. Above and beyond a certain nostalgia for historical figures such as Gottfried Leibniz (1646–1716), Leonhard Euler (1707–1783), and Johann Goethe (1749–1832), whose contributions spanned several domains of science and intellectual inquiry in general, there is also a practical concern that scientific hyperspecialization may hinder scientists from productive cross-pollination across different streams of research and disincentivize "blue sky" research.

The work of Dr. Kun Hwang stands in sharp contrast to these trends. Although Dr. Hwang is a distinguished anatomist, plastic surgeon, and trauma surgeon, with extensive clinical and research experience, he vividly stands out because of his broad, erudite, and humanistic vision of what those roles entail. In a nutshell, it is precisely this vision that forms the theme of this collection of essays, which trace a path from art to anatomy and the concept of beauty, before pivoting to discuss the role of the plastic surgeon as a scientist, and then concluding with reflections on what it means to be a "good" doctor and plastic surgeon.

Just like a surgeon integrates anatomical and technical knowledge to achieve a cohesive goal, Dr. Hwang's work does not pursue humanistic erudition in isolation or its own sake, but rather harmonizes knowledge and reflection in many domains towards the goal of excellence (as memorably discussed in Chap. 2's essay on the Greek concept of *aretê*) in the role of a plastic surgeon. Dr. Hwang views this role not merely as that of a technician, but rather as one requiring the harmonious combination of technical skills with a deep aesthetic commitment and an awareness of how the operations performed by plastic surgeon's touch upon the deep, age-old desires of humankind for beauty and longevity.

Thus, the 13 articles presented in Chap. 11 ("How to become a 'good' plastic surgeon?") form the capstone of this collection. In some of these essays, Dr. Hwang explores themes that are relatively widely recognized as important attributes of a plastic surgeon—such as imagination, observational and deductive reasoning abilities, creativity, and skillfulness—although always from unexpected and thought-provoking angles. In other essays, though, Dr. Hwang discusses themes that are less commonplace, such as the virtues of originality and the experience that comes with age. Another memorable article develops an analogy between plastic surgeons and actors, concluding with the statement that "As actors exist only in the memory of the audience, I believe that surgeons exist only in the postoperative results of their patients." Finally, the last essays in this chapter focus on the idea that a plastic surgeon must first and foremost be a good doctor, specifically mentioning the virtues of honesty and empathy.

Although any of the essays in this collection could, in principle, be read and enjoyed in isolation, their arrangement is no coincidence. The reader is best positioned to appreciate the full force of Dr. Hwang's vision of the role of a plastic surgeon, as articulated in Chap. 11, after having the opportunity to read and reflect upon the previous chapters. These chapters root this vision in a carefully interwoven network of human intellectual and scientific enterprise, aesthetic expression, and spiritual pursuits, drawing upon the work of artists, writers, and scientists from settings as disparate as Renaissance Europe, the Soviet Union, and premodern East Asia, with remarkable fluency and lucidity of interpretation. In a sense, Dr. Hwang's vision of a plastic surgeon grows out of these strands of human experience much like how a tall tree in the Amazonian rainforest grows out of the intricate ecosystem surrounding it.

One of the most powerful aspects of Dr. Hwang's work is its bidirectionality. It is not simply that Dr. Hwang uses his extensive knowledge of art, literature, and science to explore themes related to plastic surgery, but also that his reflections on humanistic topics, informed by his technical expertise and eye as a surgeon, shed powerful and thought-provoking light on the works of art and literature in question. As such, this collection testifies to the compelling vision of the Renaissance man, reflecting a vision of human excellence that blends the abstract and the hands-on, or the arts and the sciences, rather than a narrower view in which practice is subordinated to theory or vice versa, or in which one domain of human intellectual inquiry establishes hegemony over the other.

Finally, though, I would like to conclude in simpler terms. This is a collection of essays to which any reader could return again and again, always learning something new or finding a novel lens through which to view matters. This may seem like a straightforward compliment, but as in many cases of apparent simplicity, it in fact reflects the depth and mastery of Dr. Hwang's achievements. With that, I would like to invite the reader to jump in.

Compecs, Inc.
Seoul, South Korea

Chromophore Communications,
Berkeley, CA, USA

Andrew Dombrowski

Acknowledgments

I thank Hun Kim, PhD, for his help in classifying the published editorials. The illustrations were made by Hye Won Hu, MFA, medical illustrator.

Contents

About the Author

Kun Hwang, MD, PhD graduated from Seoul National University, Republic of Korea. He is a Plastic Surgeon at Armed Forces Capital Hospital, Republic of Korea. He has more than 500 peer-reviewed international publications. Dr. Hwang was the President of the Korean Cleft Palate-Craniofacial Association (KCPCA) and the Korean Society of Traumatology. He was awarded with the Medal of the Order of Science and Technology Merit from Korean Government in 2018.

1 Anatomist's View of Artistic Works

1.1 Adam's Apple and Airway Obstruction

I enjoy action movies like the James Bond (007) series, because many famous landmarks are filmed in them. The title of the 14th film in the 007 series was "A View to a Kill" (1985, starring Roger Moore). While watching this movie, I enjoyed the depiction of several places in France, especially the Château de Chantilly. This castle has a very beautiful garden and the Musée Condé.

Among the many collections of the museum, a drawing in a book intrigued me. A naked man is holding his neck with both hands. He seems to be suffering from asphyxia. A naked woman with an apple in her right hand is looking at him. Between the man and woman, a snake is slithering up a tree. The name of the book is *Abstract of the Bible, Revelation* (Chantilly, Condé Museum, 0028, printed in 1378) (Fig. 1.1).

This drawing was made very early, in 1378, well before the publication of Milton's *Paradise Lost* in 1667, which reads:

> Of man's first disobedience, and the fruit
> Of that forbidden tree, whose mortal taste
> Brought death into the world, and all our woe,
> With loss of Eden, till one greater man
> Restore us, and regain the blissful seat,
> Sing Heav'nly Muse…

Among the many paintings of Adam and Eve, this one is unique, because it expresses the suffering face of Adam as he experiences asphyxia caused by eating an apple. This leads to an intriguing question: why do people believe that the fruit was an apple and use the term "Adam's apple" for the thyroid cartilage? In Genesis 3:5, Vulgate, Satan says, "You will be like God, knowing good and evil (*Eritis sicut Deus, scientes bonum et malum*)." The Latin word *malum* has several meanings: evil, disaster, and apple. It seems that in this context, *malum* was understood as an apple.

As trauma surgeons, we frequently encounter patients who suffer from airway obstructions, like Adam in the above-described picture, especially in cases of facial injuries.

Airway obstruction due to a foreign body often can be easily treated; if the foreign body is removed, the patency of the airway can be restored. Airway obstruction caused by trauma, however, may lead to hypoxic brain damage. In acute upper airway obstruction, an evaluation should be conducted immediately. The necessary airway equipment should be made available at the time of evaluation.

In trauma patients, since the tongue has fallen backwards toward the posterior pharynx and blocks the airway, we can lift the tongue and clear the airway by hyperextending the head and pulling up the chin. Additionally, gentle pressure behind the jaw lifts the mandible and maintains airway patency. If this maneuver cannot restore the airway, tracheostomy should be performed following the relevant guidelines, especially in children [1].

K. Hwang, *Good Physician, Good Plastic Surgeon*, https://doi.org/10.1007/978-981-97-1864-1_1

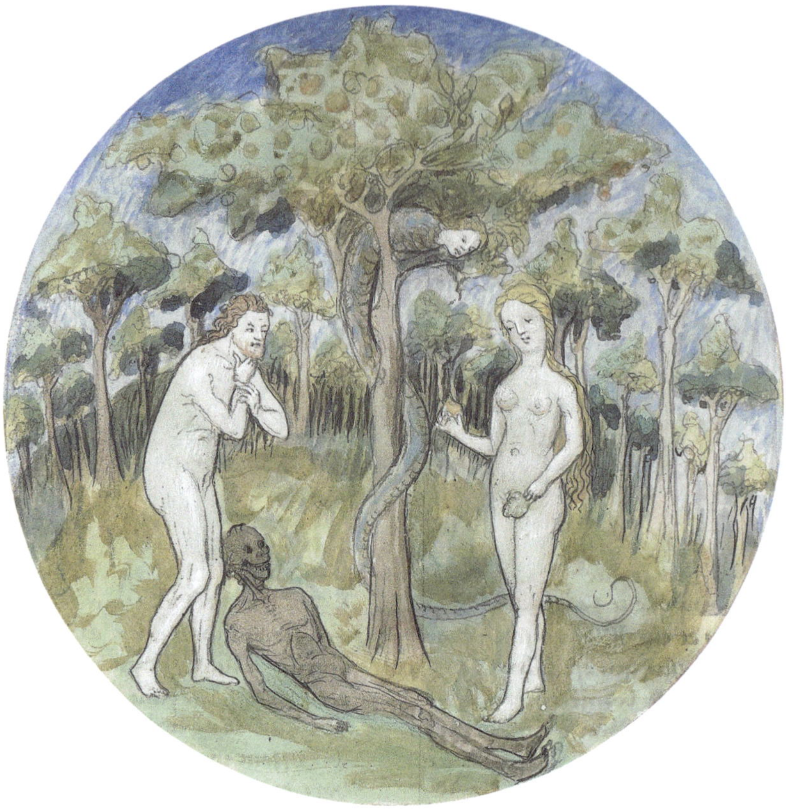

Fig. 1.1 *Abstract of the Bible, Revelation*. Adam suffers from asphyxia caused by eating a piece of an apple

In trauma patients, airway management is challenging beyond the placement of an endotracheal tube, and the outcomes depend upon the provider's ability to anticipate difficulty [2]. Among the types of facial trauma, panfacial fractures are caused by high-energy trauma and potentially result in upper airway obstruction, which needs a rapid diagnosis to save the patient's life [3].

With appropriate training, percutaneous cricothyrotomy can be easily performed as part of prehospital care [4]. Recently, four cases of prehospital surgical airway cannulation on the battlefield demonstrated three successful uses of prehospital cricothyrotomy kits [5].

As known, in cricothyrotomy, a limited skin incision is made to the cricothyroid membrane between the thyroid and cricoid cartilages, in the midline just beneath the Adam's apple. Thus, Adam—the founding father of humanity, as portrayed in the Bible—gave us a landmark to maintain the airway!

1.2 Toe Deformity of a Gilt-Bronze Pensive Bodhisattva Statue

I recently visited the National Museum of Korea, where I viewed two pensive Bodhisattvas in the Room of Quiet Contemplation. Among the two gilt-bronze statues, one was familiar to me, since I previously wrote about Bodhisattvas' face, which has a hint of a smile that exhibits a sense of serene concentration and gives the viewer the impression of an aura of deep thought [6]. In Buddhism, any person who is on the path toward Buddhahood (the condition and rank of a Buddha, awakened one) is called a "Bodhisattva." This time I focused on the cross-leg sitting and bare right foot, where I observed hyperextension of the first metatarsophalangeal joint and flexion of the interphalangeal joint of the pensive Bodhisattva (National Treasure 83, Fig. 1.2).

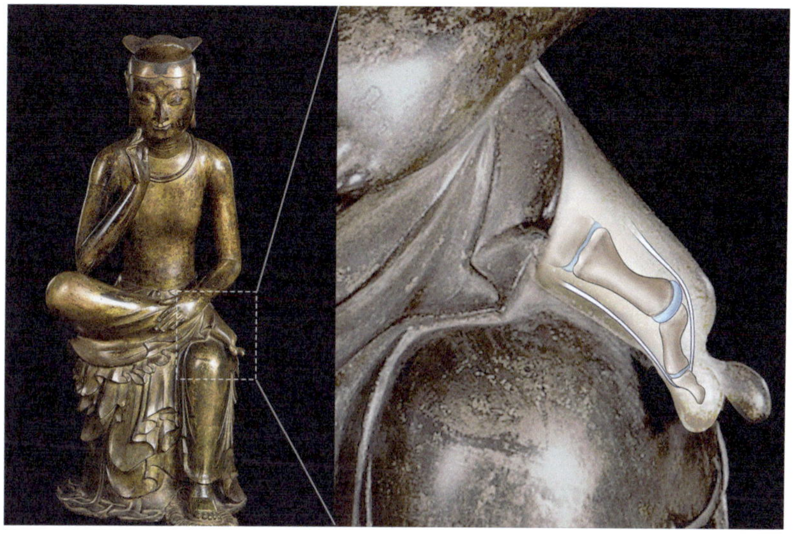

Fig. 1.2 Pensive Bodhisattva (Korean National Treasure 83). Note the hyperextension of the first metatarsophalangeal joint and flexion of the interphalangeal joint of the hallux

It is well-known that Siddhartha Gautama (Buddha, c. sixth to fifth century BC or c. fifth to fourth century BC) founded Buddhism. Before the expedition of Alexander the Great (356–323 BC) to the East, people in eastern Asia thought that transcendent beings like God could not be expressed as human figures. Thereafter, Buddhists did not make any statues of the Buddha; instead, they made stupas, which contained small crystals believed to be derived from Buddha's cremated remains. There was an approximately 500-year period when the Buddha was not represented as a figure. Later, as the Greek culture was transmitted to the East, the first statue of Buddha appeared in the Gandhara region. The resulting statues were influenced by ancient Greeks' pursuit of ideal beauty, which they perceived as arising from harmony and balance.

Buddhism was transferred to China through the Silk Road in the first century AD and then to the Three Kingdoms of Korea in the fourth to sixth century AD. The above-described pensive Bodhisattva statue was produced in the late sixth century in Shilla Kingdom.

This statue (National Treasure #83) of the pensive Bodhisattva differs from the classic contemplative pose with one leg perched up on the other knee and the fingers of one hand raised against the cheek. This pose is derived from the image of the young Indian Prince Siddhartha Gautama contemplating the nature of human life, which is quite common in Buddhist sculpture. In China, such pensive statues were most widespread in the fifth and sixth centuries, but in Korea, they were most frequently produced in the sixth and seventh centuries.

In both Korea and Japan, however, the pensive Bodhisattva is generally considered to depict the Maitreya Bodhisattva (known as the future Buddha). This iconography is thought to reflect the Sutra on the Descent of Maitreya, in which the Maitreya follows a similar path in life as that of Prince Siddhartha.

Normally, it is impossible to hyperextend the first metatarsophalangeal joint and flex the first interphalangeal joint with the remaining toes in neutral position. In a close look, a shallow groove can be seen on the medial border of the big toe and metatarsophalangeal joint. The statue definitely shows a deformity of the right big toe, known as the hallux hammertoe (hallux malleus) or claw toe.

A question then arises regarding why the artist who made this statue (600–650 AD) made a "deformed" toe in a sacred statue of the future Buddha. A likely interpretation is that the model for the statue, who was believed to be a Buddhist nun or monk, had that deformity. Then, we may ask—why did that Buddhist nun or monk have a toe deformity?

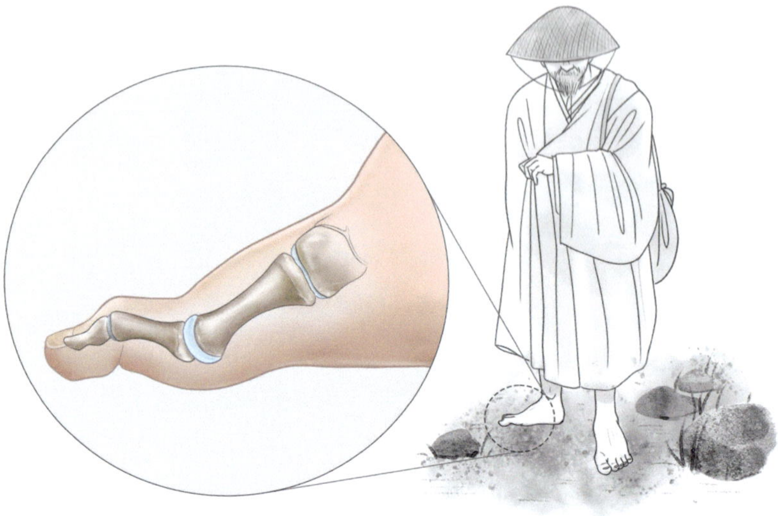

Fig. 1.3 Buddhist monks, who practiced strict asceticism, walked barefoot. This type of walking causes foot deformity (hallux hammertoe or claw toe)

A recent article could provide an answer to this question. A cross-sectional survey was conducted in combination with foot and ankle examinations of monks living in northern Thailand. In the 208 monks who were included, common foot and ankle problems were callosity (70.8%), toe deformities (18.2%), plantar fasciitis (13.4%), metatarsalgia (3.8%), and numbness (2.9%). Commonly found toe deformities included hallux valgus and claw toe. Hallux valgus was found in 14.4% of Thai monks and claw toe in 4.3%. The reasons for monks' foot deformities are as follows:

1. Thai monks usually walk without wearing shoes for long periods of time each day, causing increased pressure on the plantar surface of the foot. The push-off and heel-strike phases during barefoot walking create high pressure on the forefoot and heel, respectively.
2. Monks walk in rural areas that do not have smooth surfaces or on concrete or dirt roads. High contact pressure on the plantar aspect of the foot results in callosity.
3. Monks cease wearing shoes when they are ordained. Prior to that, their feet usually have not been accustomed to barefoot walking. Callosity and toe deformities were associated with prolonged barefoot walking over extended periods since ordainment ($P < 0.05$) [7].

Based on this article, we infer that the early seventh-century Buddhist monks, who practiced strict asceticism, walked barefoot like the Theravada monks in present-day Thailand (Fig. 1.3). Through the enigmatic smile, we also can conjecture that the Buddhist monks were happy and "awakened" despite their foot deformity caused by their barefoot training.

These deformities can now be improved by surgery. If the hallux hammertoe or claw toe is flexible, a tendon release may be helpful. If the deformity is rigid, joint fusion or arthroplasty may be needed to straighten the big toe.

1.3 Symbol of the Physician in "St. Luke Painting the Virgin"

According to the *Golden Legend* (1260), written by Blessed Jacobus de Varagine (1230–1299), Emperor Nero persecuted Christians in the aftermath of the Great Fire of Rome (AD 64). Paul, as their main leader, was arrested, tried, and condemned to death, and he awaited execution in a prison cell. Luke took a risk by visiting Paul, and in his prison cell, Luke wrote down a narrative of the conversions they performed and their missionary travels together. This text would become the "Acts of the Apostles." This narrative eventually provided encouragement to Christians in the face of possible martyrdom [8].

St. Luke, one of the four evangelists (Matthew, Mark, Luke, and John) is venerated as the patron saint of artists, physicians, bachelors, surgeons, students and butchers. His original profession was a doctor (a surgeon, as well as a physician). He was one of the first doctors of the Christian era. His symbol as an evangelist is an ox since his gospel (Gospel of St. Luke) emphasizes the priestly and sacrificial work of Jesus. The ox represents the sacrificial aspect of Jesus' ministry. Some paintings represent St. Luke as an artist painting the Virgin Mary and child (Fig. 1.4).

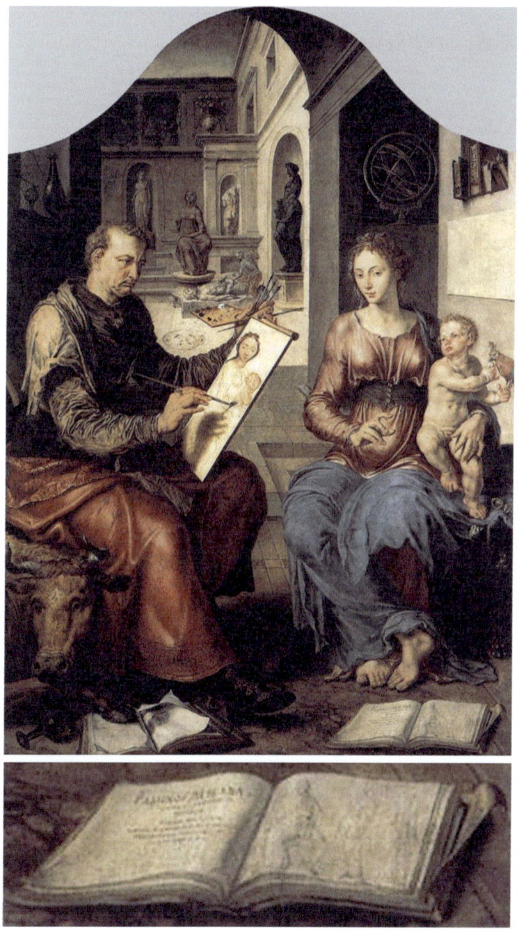

Fig. 1.4 "St. Luke Painting the Virgin" (1550–1553) drawn by Maerten van Heemskerck (1498–1574). (From public domain through https://commons.wikimedia.org/wiki/File:Maarten_van_Heemskerck_-_St_Luke_Painting_the_Virgin_-_WGA11320.jpg. Assessed 29 Jan 2022)

We are then faced with the question: what is the symbol of St. Luke as the patron saint of physicians and surgeons?

To answer this question, I searched some literature and art from the Renaissance period and found a relevant painting.

Maerten van Heemskerck (1498–1574) created a painting called "St. Luke Painting the Virgin," which is believed to have been made during 1550–1553.

In this piece, St. Luke is painting a panel supported on his lap, while other figures in the background are occupied with tasks in the artist's studio. A sculptor is putting the finishing touches on a recumbent stone figure; in the gallery in the top left, a number of people are working around a table, and the courtyard contains several pieces of sculpture. The ox and the thick volume of an opened book without letters, on which the ox is resting his foot, are definitely symbols of St. Luke as an Evangelist. The empty book will be filled and become the Gospel of Luke. In the painting, Luke is making final touches of portraits of the Virgin and the child. It is notable that the child has masculine figures. The child's forearm muscles, thigh muscles, and leg muscles are exaggerated like those of an athlete. Below the ox's leg is a glass urinal, which was used as a tool for urinalysis in that era.

In the lower right corner, a large book is open and facing the viewer. The left page, which is numbered I76, contains a text in Greek. The illustration on the right page has four figures: two human skeletons, a male nude viewed from behind, and a male figure viewed from the front, whose body appears to have been opened by frontal dissection.

According to art historians, the Greek letters are recognized as "De anatomicis administrationibus" ("On Anatomical Procedures," compiled by Galen) [9]. The alternation of the skeleton and "muscle man," with the two left-hand figures viewed from in front and the right-hand figures from behind, suggests that Heemskerck must have been acquainted with this engraving, which resembles the illustrations in Vesalius (1514–1564) drawn by Jan van Calcar (1499–1546). Giorgio Vasari, Carel van Mander, and others credit Jan van Calcar with the 11 large woodcut illustrations of anatomical studies that accompanied Andreas Vesalius's work on anatomy. The most notable of these works is the anatomical study of the human body entitled "De humani corporis fabrica libri septem" or "On the Fabric of the Human Body in Seven Books" (1543) [10].

"De humani corporis fabrica" (1543) was published just 10 years before the completion of this painting (1550–1553). In the painting, the book with Galen's guide to anatomy on one page and illustrations based on Vesalius on the other is opened towards the viewer. In fact, Galen dissected animals but never dissected a human body. It is thought that Heemskerck intended to use Galen's authority and Vesalius' new knowledge of anatomy as the symbol of the "ideal doctor" in that era.

In the Renaissance, anatomical science served as an important source of inspiration for artists. Interest in anatomy had become relatively widespread by the fifteenth century, during which artists dissected cadavers. The artists aimed to create accurate portrayals of facial expressions, positions, reflexive motions, and draped clothing. Artists' expertise primarily derives from their observations of living subjects. Instead, dissection provides a fixed model without flowing blood, which cannot be used as an animated model. Nonetheless, these artists likely learned about the anatomical origins of vivid expressions by studying the muscles lying under the skin [11].

In the present day, there are many hospitals and medical centers named after St. Luke. Moreover, numerous Christian medical doctors have "Luke" as their baptismal name. They took this name from the patron saint with the same name. What, then, will be the symbol of the ideal physician in our age?

As exemplified by the book with Galen's guide to anatomy and illustrations based on Vesalius, doctors will gain knowledge, skill, and appropriate attitudes by reviewing the old (Galen, in the painting discussed above) and learning the new (Vesalius). These will be their symbol of "authority" as good doctors.

1.4 "The Flying Eye" of a Renaissance Artist: An Anatomical View

The human eye can conjugate and focus on both near and distant objects. Conjugation requires good function of the levator palpebrae superioris, as well as the extraocular muscles or ciliary muscle. Through conjugation, artists use the law of perspective, which started in Renaissance period. The first scientific study of this phenomenon was contained in *De Pictura* (*On Painting*, published in 1450), written by Leon Battista Alberti (1404–1472) (Fig. 1.5). In his book *Ludi Rerum Mathematicarum* (*Mathematical Pastimes*, 1450–1452), he illustrated methods of measuring the natural and built environment in the perspective framework.

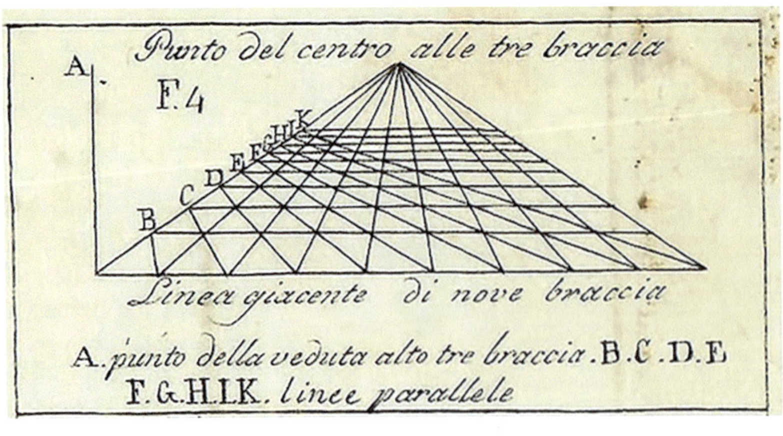

Fig. 1.5 Alberti's drawing showing the vanishing point

Alberti used the flying eye (winged eye) as his personal emblem. In Matteo de' Pasti's medallion (c. 1446–1450), the profile is on the obverse and the eye on the reverse. At the top of the eye is a pair of eagle's wings, and emanating from each corner are rays. Below is the motto "Quid Turn," meaning "What then?" or "What next?" and surrounding it, a laurel wreath (Fig. 1.6).

An Italian architect wrote that Alberti borrowed the Egyptian Horus eye, which symbolizes exactly this tireless exploration that continues even after earthly life. She interpreted the winged eye, surrounded by a bay necklace and adorned with wings, as representing an afterlife journey toward the knowledge of the true essence of nature [12].

As an anatomist, I have different opinion. In the Renaissance, anatomical science was a major source of inspiration for artists. In the period after *Anathomia* (1316) by Mundinus and before *Fabrica* (1543) by Vesalius, artists as well as anatomists dissected human cadavers. By the fifteenth century, interest had emerged in anatomy, and the artists of the period dissected cadavers. Some had a good knowledge of anatomy and applied anatomical knowledge of features, such as muscle shape and volume in their works.

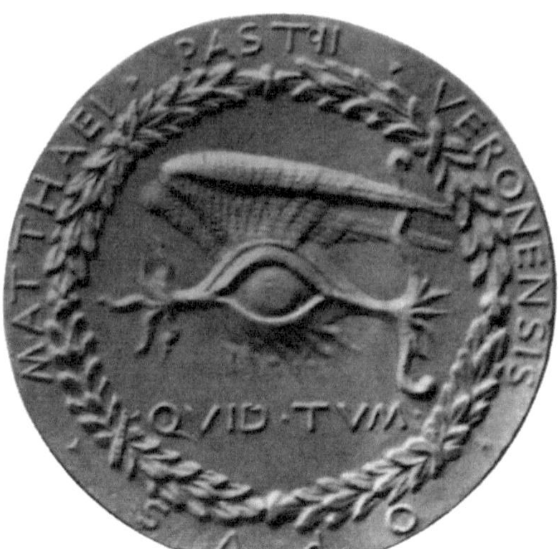

Fig. 1.6 Emblem of Alberti; the flying eye (winged eye). (*Matteo de' Pasti, National Gallery of Art, Washington, D.C. Samuel* H. *Kress Collection*)

Alberti, one of the geniuses of the fifteenth century, is also thought to have had extensive anatomical knowledge. In a close observation of Alberti's flying eye, I could see the anatomical structures represented in it. The upper and lower lid margins, as well as the tarsal plates, are carved. Medially, the medial palpebral ligament (medial canthal tendon) is attached to the medial orbital rim [13]. Laterally, the lateral palpebral ligament (lateral canthal tendon) is attached to the lateral orbital rim [14]. In the lateral view, the two wings attached to the upper tarsal plate seem to represent the eye-opening muscles: the levator palpebrae superioris and Muller's involuntary muscle [15, 16]. In the lower eyelid, the oblique stripes seem to be the capsulopalpebral fascia and arcuate expansion [17].

Artists sought to accurately portray facial expressions, positions, reflexive motions, and draped clothing. Observation of living subjects is the primary source of artists' expertise. Dissection provides a fixed model without flowing blood, which cannot be used as an animated model. It is thought that the artists of that era learned about the origins of vivid expressions from the anatomy of the muscles lying beneath the skin.

The emblem of "the flying eye" is therefore, I believe, a symbol of Alberti's profound anatomical knowledge of the human visual organ, which lay at the root of his conception of "the law of perspective."

1.5 The Missing Nose of the Virgin Mary

A man paints with his brains and not with his hands.—Michelangelo Buonarroti

I recently visited St Peter's Basilica in Vatican City, where I saw the familiar "The Pietà" (The Pity, 1498–1499) made by Michelangelo Buonarroti (1475–1564). It was located just on the right side of the entrance. Since this sculpture was protected by a very thick glass panel, I could only see a frontal view.

The reason for this protection is the damage done by a mentally disturbed geologist in 1972.

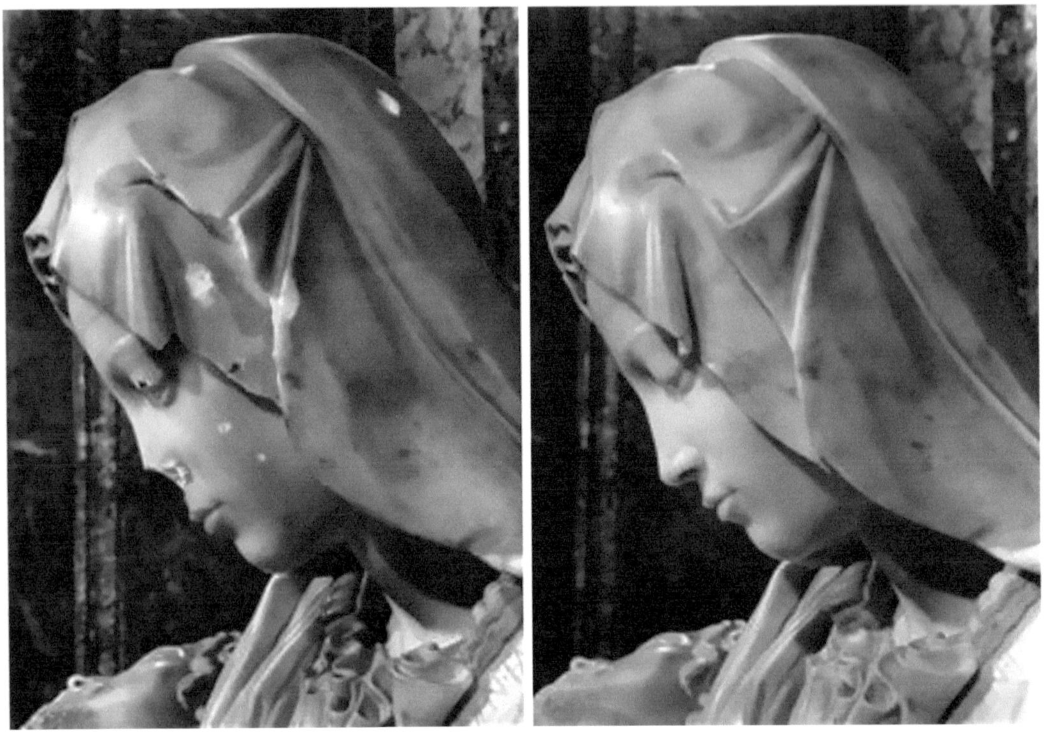

Fig. 1.7 The head of the Virgin Mary. Left: damaged (1972). Right: reconstructed from a block cut out of her back (1973)

With blows from the geologist's hammer, the Virgin Mary's elbow, one eyelid, and the most strikingly, her nose were broken (Fig. 1.7, left). Some pieces were recovered, but Mary's nose was not, and it had to be reconstructed from a block cut out of her back (Fig. 1.7, right).

I observed the Virgin Mary's restored nose with an opera glass that I carried and noted that she had nostrils, but they were very shallow, and it looked as if she only had nostril pits.

This famous work of art depicts the body of Jesus on the lap of his mother Mary after the Crucifixion. Anatomically, the nose has a three-dimensional contour with skin that covers it, a middle layer of bone and cartilage support, and an inner mucosal lining. Nasal defects require three-layer reconstruction, including resurfacing with forehead tissue; support with a septal, ear, or rib graft; and replacement of the missing lining. I prefer a scalp flap or a medial forehead flap.

When sculpting marble, it is not easy to create airways in the nose. However, it would have been possible to create airways from the nostrils to the nasal valve when restoring the missing nose. I thought that the restorer took liberties to restore it in a way that was more "rhetorical" and less "anatomical."

If the restorer had precise three-dimensional anatomical knowledge of the facial structure, the Virgin Mary would have gotten a new nose through which she could have exhaled onto her dead son.

It would be mutually beneficial if plastic surgeons and artists shared their knowledge and viewpoints.

1.6 Skinned St. Bartholomew Before (1541) and After (1556, 1562) *Fabrica* (1543)

In the Renaissance, anatomical science was a major source of inspiration for artists. By the fifteenth century, interest had emerged in anatomy as an area of research, and the artists of the period dissected cadavers.

Artists performed dissections in order to pursue divine beauty, in the belief that God created humankind in his image, whereas anatomists' goal was to gain scientific knowledge [18].

It is well known that St. Bartholomew was portrayed dressed holding a book and a knife up until the thirteenth to fourteenth centuries, alluding to the Gospel that he proclaimed and the martyrdom that he suffered.

From the Renaissance onward, the iconography of St. Bartholomew with his skin removed from his flesh was finally sanctified after Michelangelo (1541) portrayed him in such a way in the "Last Judgment" in the Vatican's Sistine Chapel. It is notable that St. Bartholomew holds his skin in his left hand. However, he himself is not skinned at all but covered with normal skin. Thereafter, the muscle underneath the skin is visualized as surface anatomy only. However, in the "Last Judgment," he holds extra skin in his hand (Fig. 1.8 upper left).

Two years after the completion of the "Last Judgment," Andreas Vesalius published his

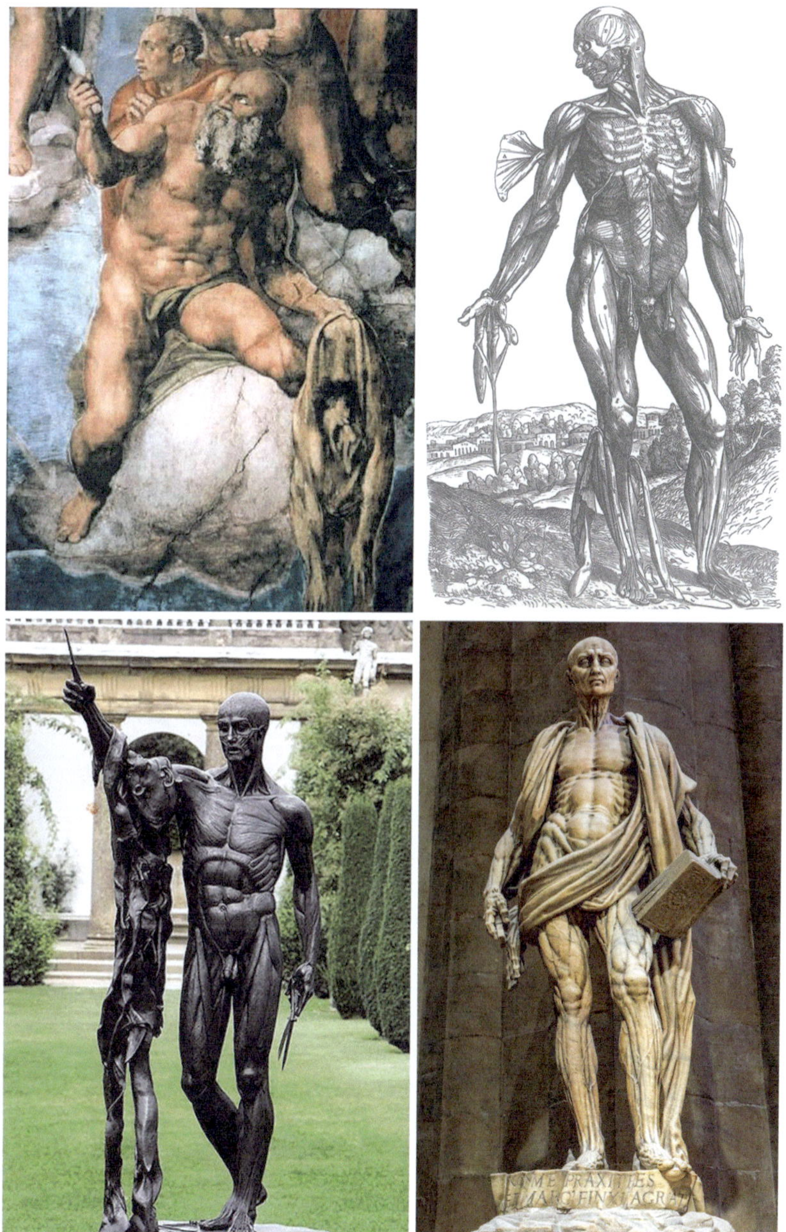

Fig. 1.8 St. Bartholomew depicted in "Last Judgment" (1541. upper left), and statues of Marco d'Agrate (lower left: bronze, 1556, lower right: marble, 1562). Dissected body in *Fabrica* (1543, upper right)

Fabrica (*De humani corporis fabrica libri septem,* 1543, Fig. 1.8 upper right).

Subsequently, 13 and 19 years after the publication of *Fabrica*, Marco d'Agrate made a bronze statue of St. Bartholomew in 1556, in front of the Certosa of Pavia (1556, Fig. 1.8 lower left), and a marble statue in the Milano Duomo (1562, Fig. 1.8 lower right), respectively.

These works of Marco d'Agrate do not show any psychological introspection or give evidence of the deep faith expressed by the martyrdom of St. Bartholomew. However, they form part of a major sixteenth-century sphere of interest: the study and presentation of human anatomy [19].

By comparing the portrayal of St. Bartholomew in Michelangelo's fresco and d'Agrate's statues, we can see the how the publication of *Fabrica* contributed to art. Artists and anatomists together produced images of the body that combined medical knowledge and an artistic vision. When illustrated anatomical texts became readily available in the seventeenth century, the general enthusiasm of artists for studying cadavers decreased.

1.7 The Cut Surface of the Neck as Depicted in Two Paintings of Judith and Holofernes

In the Renaissance, anatomical science was a major source of inspiration for artists. By the fifteenth century, interest had emerged in anatomy as an area of research and the artists of the period dissected cadavers. Artists performed dissections in order to reproduce beauty accurately, whereas the anatomists' goal was to gain scientific knowledge [18]. Artists witnessed or participated in dissections to gain a better understanding of the proportions and systems of the body.

Although detailed treatises on human proportion and beauty were published by artists and scholars such as Albrecht Dürer, the cut surface of the human body is rarely found in paintings.

The aim of this paper was to compare the cut surface of the neck depicted in two paintings of Judith and Holofernes.

Two paintings, *Judith with the Head of Holofernes* (Lucas Cranach, 1530, Jagdschloss Grunewald, Berlin) and *Judith in the Tent of Holofernes* (Johann Liss, 1628, National Gallery, London), were analyzed.

In the Bible, Judith 13:8–9 tells the story of a beautiful Jewish widow, Judith, who saves her people by murdering the Assyrian general, Holofernes. She tricks him into trusting her, but when he is drunk, she cuts off his head.

In Cranach's *Judith*, Holofernes' head is bearded and his dead eyes roll upward; the muscles and other anatomical structures in his neck are made available for our inspection. The cut surface of the neck is shown from underneath. The cervical vertebra and trachea are clearly shown. The sternocleidomastoid, trapezius, and other neck muscles are discernible. However, bleeding from the vessels is not portrayed (Fig. 1.9).

In Liss' *Judith*, Judith has cut off the head of Holofernes and looks back over her shoulder, toward the viewer. She is placing the severed head in a basket. The cut surface of the neck is shown from above. The cervical vertebra and trachea are identifiable, and blood is pumping from the carotid arteries. The muscles are discernible due to the blood (Fig. 1.10).

Mondino de Luzzi wrote *Anathomia corporis humani* in 1316. This book is considered the first example of a modern dissection manual and the first true anatomical text and remained the most widely used anatomical text for 250 years (through the sixteenth century).

Lucas Cranach (1472–1553) and Johann Liss (1597–1631) were both born in Germany.

Cranach's *Judith* (1530) was painted 5 years before *Anatomia Carpi* (1535), by Jacopo Berengario da Carpi, and 13 years before *De humani corporis fabrica* (*On the Fabric of the Human Body*), by Andreas Vesalius. It is an interesting coincidence that this *Fabrica* and the famous *De Revolutionibus Orbium Caelestium* by Nicolaus Copernicus were published in the same year (1543).

Liss' *Judith* (1628) was painted in the same year that William Harvey published *De Motu Cordis* (Fig. 1.11).

Comparing Cranach's *Judith* (1530) and Liss' *Judith* (1628), the latter portrays hemo-

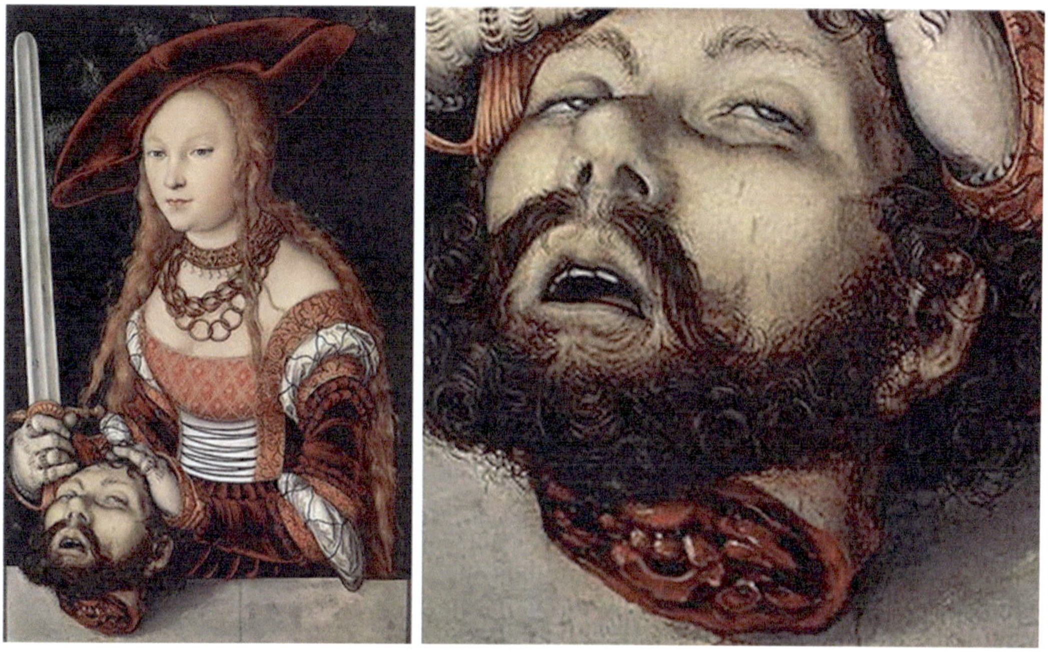

Fig. 1.9 *Judith with the Head of Holofernes* (Lucas Cranach, 1530, Jagdschloss Grunewald, Berlin)

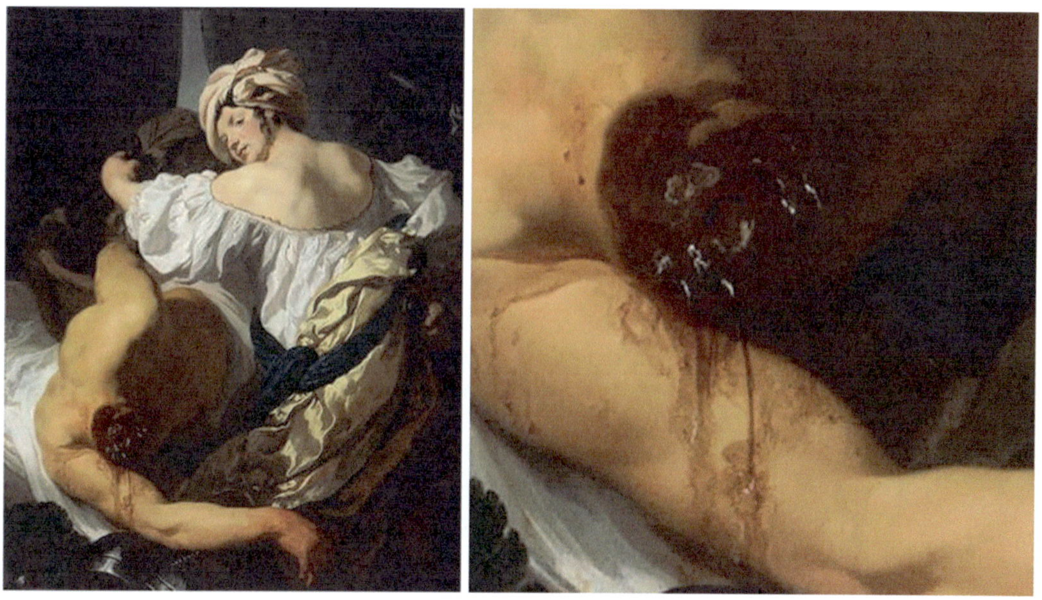

Fig. 1.10 *Judith in the Tent of Holofernes* (Johann Liss, 1628, National Gallery, London)

dynamics as well as topographical and cross-sectional anatomy. It therefore appears that over the course of one century (1530–1628), artists' anatomical and physiological knowledge improved.

For many artists in the Renaissance, to be an artist was to be an anatomist. As artists turned toward more lifelike portrayals of the human body, they needed a deeper understanding of how the structures of the body worked together.

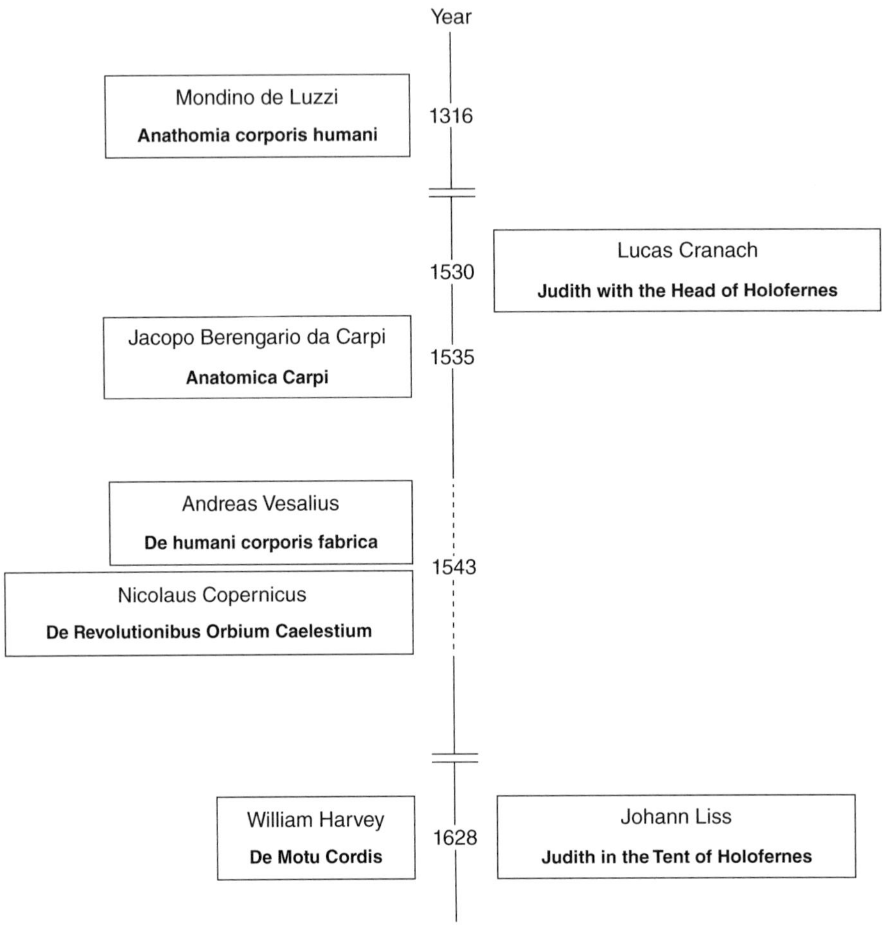

Fig. 1.11 The chronology of famous anatomy publications and the two *Judith* paintings

Artists and anatomists together produced images of the body that combined medical knowledge and an artistic vision [20]. The artists aimed to reproduce the exact surface anatomy of the human body, but the sectional depiction was very rare, and they also requested a good knowledge of the "deep" anatomy." Now, five centuries later, the main depiction of anatomy through medical imaging uses sections (CT, MRI) [21].

1.8 War Horse, Whistlejacket, and an Anatomist

During my stay in London, I had a chance to enjoy "War Horse," played at the New London Theatre located in the West End. This famous play is the story of a young boy and his beloved horse, which has been requisitioned by the army to fight in World War I. The life-sized puppet was manipulated by three puppeteers—the Head, the Heart, and the Hind—who worked together to make the character of the horse come alive on stage. The puppet was made in Cape Town, South Africa, of cane, leather, and synthetic fiber, and an aluminum-reinforced spine. With life-like accuracy, the puppeteer operators articulated the limbs of the horse and communicated its emotions (Fig. 1.12).

I was so impressed, since the skeleton and joints of the limbs as well as the spine were anatomically very similar to a real horse. In order to achieve this life-like effect, the skilled craftsmen who constructed this incredible puppet had anatomical knowledge of horses.

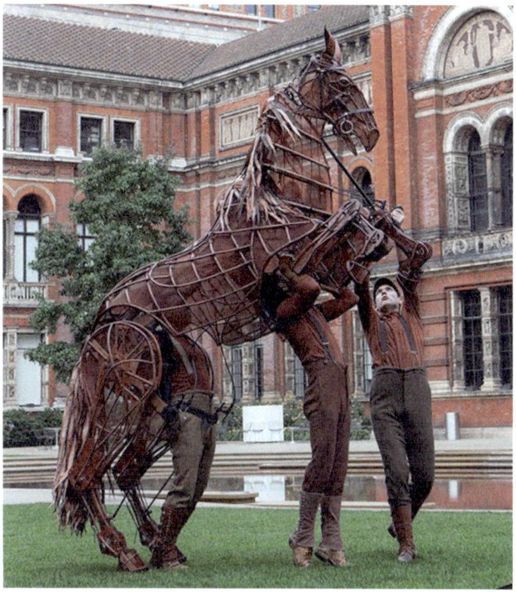

Fig. 1.12 War Horse and 3 puppeteers. (Reproduced with permission from Victoria and Albert Museum, London)

For detailing equine anatomy, Carlo Ruini's *Anatomia del Cavallo* (1618) [22] was a first, foundational text, followed by Andrew Snape's *The Anatomy of an Horse* (1683) [23]. George Stubbs published the illustrated book *The Anatomy of the Horse* (1766), which is still in print today (Fig. 1.13) [24].

Stubbs dissected horses to learn about their anatomy for his illustrations and paintings. He rented a farmhouse for study and dissection. The horses were sacrificed by cutting the jugular vein, and the blood vessels were injected with tallow. The carcass was lifted with a tackle of hooks and bars attached to the ceiling; the horse's feet were arranged on a wooden plank beneath. He removed the skin, prepared the muscles layer by layer toward the skeleton, and sketched them [25, 26].

In the National Gallery, I saw a very famous oil painting entitled "Whistlejacket" (1762) by Stubbs. The pose was typical of an equestrian portrait, although without the rider. This horse has a dynamic personality and glowing vitality (Fig. 1.14). It is obvious that Stubbs could paint horses in realistic detail, because he had great knowledge of their anatomy. He could see the muscles, bones, and joints under the skin and

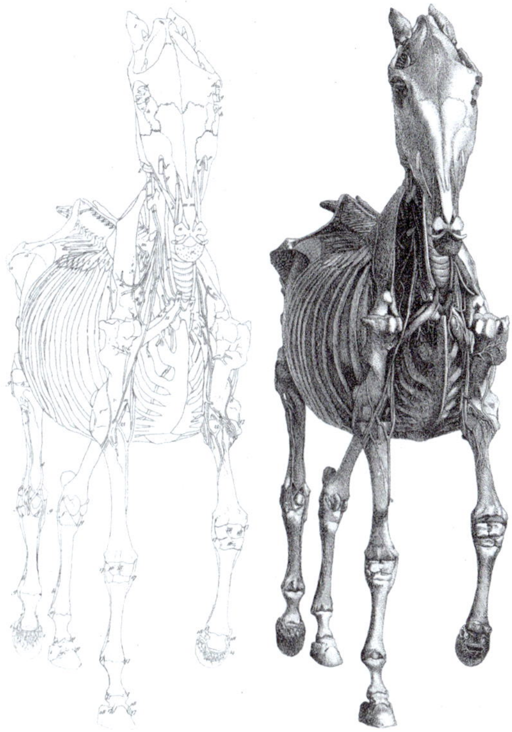

Fig. 1.13 Skeleton with reference plate from *The Anatomy of the Horse* (1766). (Reproduced with permission from The British Museum, London)

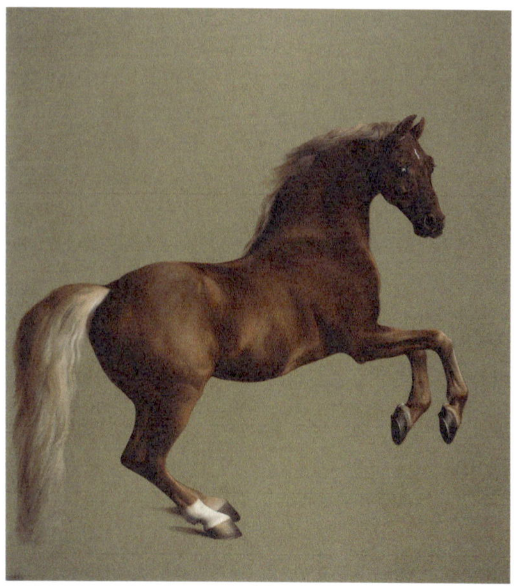

Fig. 1.14 *Whistlejacket* (1762) (oil on canvas) by George Stubbs. (Reproduced with permission from National Gallery, London)

their actions from the sketches he made during dissections.

As a plastic surgeon and a teacher in resident training program, I considered the role of anatomy for surgeons and surgical trainees. On reading the top-cited paper in the first 25 years' history of Clinical Anatomy, I realized the importance of anatomical dissection cannot be overemphasized in medical education. In that paper, 57% of the residency program directors responded that residents need a refresher in gross anatomy upon arrival, 29% thought that they were adequately prepared, whereas 14% felt they were seriously lacking. The residency programs indicated that residents need to arrive more proficient in clinical applications, general knowledge, and cross-sectional applications [27]. I was worried that about half of the anatomy departments are not consisted of training teachers of anatomy (gross anatomy, histology, embryology, and neuroanatomy) [28].

The gross anatomy is no longer a free-standing course representing anatomy-for-anatomy's-sake but rather is now strongly clinically oriented in many schools [29].

Artists need knowledge of anatomy for painting animals or human beings in realistic detail, and surgeons need precise understanding of anatomical details for successful operations. Stubbs could see the horse muscles and their actions during his dissections, and so too can surgeons recognize the critical structures, such as vessels or nerves through anatomical knowledge obtained from surgery or dissection.

Though there are many texts and atlases showing surgical and radiological anatomies for students and trainees, I do believe nothing can replace the anatomical dissection.

1.9 The Human Premaxilla and Goethe

It is safe to say that most plastic surgeons are familiar with the growth pattern of the premaxilla in bilateral cleft lip and palate patients, in whom in utero growth of the premaxilla is excessive and directed more horizontally, resulting in a protrusive premaxilla at birth [30]. Despite the common usage of the name of this bone, the origin of its nomenclature is not widely known to many plastic surgeons. I have carried out a review of publications about the premaxilla.

When Galen (131–201) was active, the premaxilla had already been observed in animals. Coiter (1573) was the first anatomist to describe this medial part of the upper jaw as a separate bone in the vertebrate skull. He also illustrated the incisive suture (*sutura incisiva*) in humans [31].

In the eighteenth century, Petrus Camper from Holland stated that a vitally important anatomical difference between humans and animals was the missing intermaxillary bone (premaxilla) in man, with this being the distinguishing feature between humans and monkeys. Contradicting this theory, Goethe (1749–1832) found the intermaxillary bone in the human skull in 1784 [32]. Goethe hoped to present this discovery through his friend Johann Merck, who was in contact with Camper and could serve as an intermediary. However, Merck delayed forwarding the manuscript and also did not forward Camper's eventual replies. Thirty-six years later, in 1820, Goethe submitted his hypothesis, but it was rejected by the leading anatomists of the time.

Last year, I visited Leipzig for research collaboration. In Leipzig, I saw the statue of Goethe (*Goethedenkmal*), which reminded me of the name of a pub (Auerbachs Keller) that appears in his *Faust*, which is set in that city. The Korean researcher accompanying me led me to the tavern and said that Goethe (1749–1832) was a regular at Auerbachs Keller as a university student from 1765 to 1768.

I saw the statues of Faust and Mephistopheles at the gate of that tavern. I also viewed a wall painting depicting the last scene of *Faust*. In the first edition of *Faust*, I observed that the midface and upper lips of Mephistopheles and Martha were retracted and the lower lip protruded like that of a cleft palate patient (Fig. 1.15).

It is therefore possible that Goethe's discovery of the premaxilla in humans, which he did not succeed in publishing, was reflected in the painting of Mephistopheles and Martha, who were portrayed with the retracted maxilla that is seen

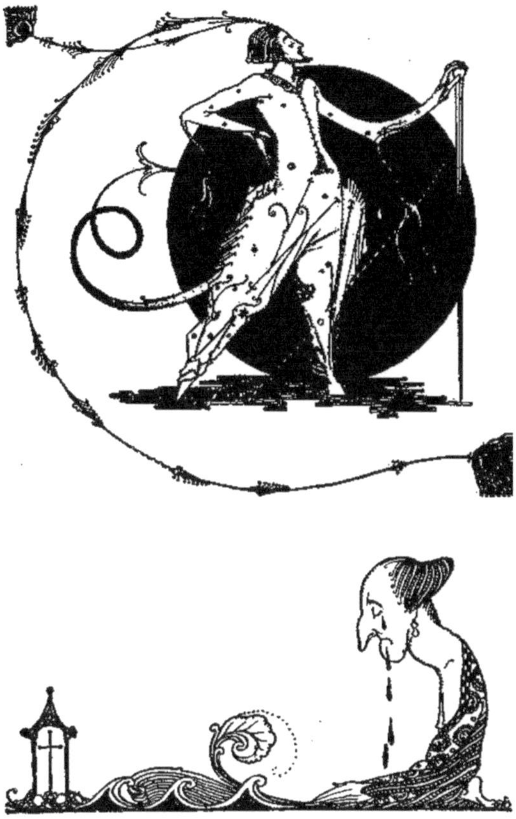

Fig. 1.15 Mephistopheles (upper) and Martha (lower) in the first edition of *Faust* (1808)

in cleft palate patients and elderly people who are losing their maxillary teeth.

References

1. Doherty C, Neal R, English C, Cooke J, Atkinson D, Bates L, et al. Multidisciplinary guidelines for the management of paediatric tracheostomy emergencies. Anaesthesia. 2018;73:1400–17.
2. Kovacs G, Sowers N. Airway management in trauma. Emerg Med Clin N Am. 2018;36:61–84.
3. Colombo LT, Mulinari-Santos G, Souza FÁ. Upper airway obstruction in a panfacial fracture. J Craniofac Surg. 2018;29:e774.
4. Hwang K, Kim HJ, Kim YC, Choi YS, Hwang SW. Manikin model with breathing tube for wire-guided percutaneous cricothyrotomy in patients applying an intermaxillary fixation. J Craniofac Surg. 2014;25:1846–8.
5. Schauer SG, April MD, Cunningham CW, Long AN, Carter R. Prehospital cricothyrotomy kits used in combat. J Spec Oper Med. 2017;17:18–20.
6. Hwang K. Enigmatic smiles for plastic surgeons. J Craniofac Surg. 2020;31(8):2120–2.
7. Vaseenon T, Wattanarojanaporn T, Intharasompan P, Theeraamphon N, Auephanviriyakul S, Phisitkul P. Foot and ankle problems in Thai monks. J Med Assoc Thail. 2015;98(1):71–6.
8. Hwang K. Importance of narratives in scientific discussion. Plast Reconstr Surg. 2021;147:1025–6.
9. Veldman IM. Maarten van Heemskerck and St. Luke's medical books. Simiolus Neth Q Hist Art. 1974;7:91–100.
10. Vasari G. Lives of the painters, sculptors, and architects (Le Vita De' Piu Eccellenti Architetti, Pittori, et scultori). Florence: Appresso I Giunti; 1568.
11. Hwang K. Artists with anatomical knowledge after Anathomia (1316) and before Fabrica (1543). J Craniofac Surg. 2021;32:350–4.
12. Proietti T. The aesthetics of proportion in Hans van der Laan and Leon Battista Alberti. Aisthesis Pratiche Linguaggi E Saperi dell'estetico. 2015;8:183–99.
13. Hwang K, Huan F, Nam YS, et al. Location and tension of the medial palpebral ligament. J Craniofac Surg. 2013;24:2119–23.
14. Hwang K, Nam YS, Kim DJ, et al. Anatomic study of the lateral palpebral raphe and lateral palpebral ligament. Ann Plast Surg. 2009;62:232–6.
15. Qin T, Chun P, Li FF, et al. Medial and lateral canthal ligaments shown in P45 sheet plastination and dissection. Indian J Ophthalmol. 2021;69:1150–4.
16. Hwang K, Huan F, Kim DJ, et al. Size of the superior palpebral involuntary muscle (Müller muscle). J Craniofac Surg. 2010;21:1626–9.
17. Hwang K, Choi HG, Nam YS, et al. Anatomy of arcuate expansion of capsulopalpebral fascia. J Craniofac Surg. 2010;21:239–42.
18. Sellmer R. Anatomy and art in renaissance. In: Whitelaw WA, editor. Proceedings of the 10th annual history of medicine days. Calgary: University of Calgary; 2001. p. 80–2.
19. Veneranda Fabbrica del Duomo di Milano. The statue of St Bartholomew in the Milan Duomo: a treaty on human anatomy sculpted in marble; between science and faith. 2018. https://www.duomomilano.it/en/article/2018/06/29/the-statue-of-st-bartholomew-in-the-milan-duomo/696e8048-5a4c-4e83-ae63-79e51cac979b/. Accessed 29 Jun 2018.
20. Science Museum. Art and anatomy. 2016. DIALOG. http://www.sciencemuseum.org.uk/broughttolife/themes/understandingthebody/anatomy. Accessed 30 Apr 2016.
21. Grignon B. Anatomy and medical imaging: a symbiotic relationship. Surg Radiol Anat. 2012;34:673–4.
22. Ruini C. Anatomia del Cavallo. Venetia: Fiorauante Prati; 1618.
23. Snape A. The anatomy of an horse. London: Miles Flesher; 1683.
24. Stubb G. The anatomy of the horse. London: J. Purser; 1766.
25. Fountain RB. George Stubbs (1724–1806) as an anatomist. Proc R Soc Med. 1968;61:639–46.

26. Vincent-Kemp R. George Stubbs and his 18th century patrons. Vet Hist. 1985;4:2–10.
27. Cottam WW. Adequacy of medical school gross anatomy education as perceived by certain postgraduate residency programs and anatomy course directors. Clin Anat. 1999;12:55–65.
28. Albertine KH. Cottam's landmark paper for clinical anatomy. Clin Anat. 2012;25:681–2.
29. Carmichael SW. Does clinical anatomy deserve another 25 years? Reflections on how clinical anatomy has changed in the past quarter century. Clin Anat. 2012;25:143–5.
30. Vargervik K. Growth characteristics of the premaxilla and orthodontic treatment principles in bilateral cleft lip and palate. Cleft Palate J. 1983;20:289–302.
31. Barteczko K, Jacob M. A re-evaluation of the premaxillary bone in humans. Anat Embryol (Berl). 2004;207:417–37.
32. Hellmich S, Hellmich J. The intermaxillary bone and Goethe's Mephistopheles. Laryngol Rhinol Otol (Stuttg). 1982;61:552–6.

2 Plastic Surgeon's View of Artistic Works

2.1 *Aretê* of Athletes, Self-discipline of Plastic Surgeons

> Areté is a word that means excellence in character and life. It is the accumulation of virtue in one's life."—Tobin Wilson (Author of *Areté Again*)

The 2021 Olympic Games were held successfully in Tokyo despite the COVID-19 pandemic. The players competed to their utmost ability in the state of *aretê*.

Aretê (ἀρετή) is a term associated with the Greek goddess of virtue and knowledge that denotes excellence in anything or of any kind (Fig. 2.1). This term may also mean "moral virtue". In Greek, *aretê* was ultimately bound up with the notion of the fulfillment of purpose or function: the act of living up to one's full potential. In the Homeric poems, *aretê* is frequently associated with bravery, but more often with effectiveness. A person with *aretê* is of the highest effectiveness; he or she uses all available faculties—strength, bravery, and wit—to achieve real results. In the Homeric world, then, *aretê* involves all of the abilities and potentialities available to humans.

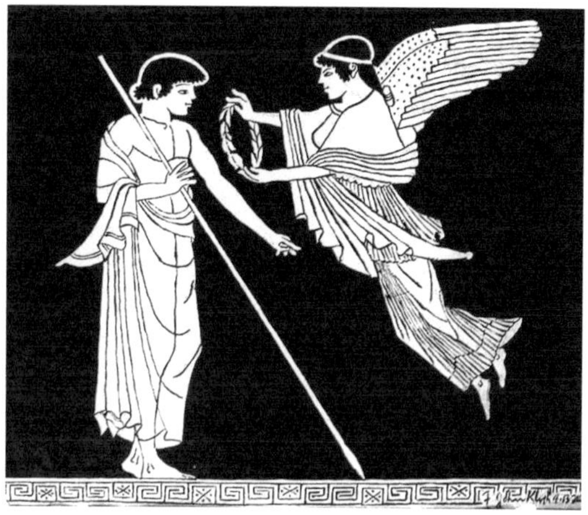

Fig. 2.1 Ancient Greek Athletics: Aretê

Olympic athletes have *aretê*. Since winning the ancient Olympic Games was impossible without the patience and courage to undergo hard training, endure the possibility of defeat and disgrace, and even risk one's life, winning proved the *aretê* of a human being. *Aretê* is that state of self-denial and of personal agony, anguish, and perseverance that was considered to be pleasing to the gods and necessary for accomplishing a superior task. At the coronation ceremony of the winners gathered in front of the Temple of Zeus, the names of the victors, their fathers, and the city were called out loudly. Honor belonged to the individual, to the family, and to the city-state. The Olympics were the best stage for an individual to dedicate themselves to the city-state. Citizens praised the winner's *aretê* with congratulatory poems, songs, and sculptures.

As athletes pursue *aretê*, what should excellent plastic surgeons learn from this concept?

K. Hwang, *Good Physician, Good Plastic Surgeon*, https://doi.org/10.1007/978-981-97 1864-1_2

The biggest threat that hinders one from being an excellent plastic surgeon is the failure to continue to practice. Actual practice with the goal of self-improvement does not simply constitute repeated performance. Progress is not inevitable. Practice involves critical self-analysis of procedures with the goal of performing them perfectly. Therefore, to be excellent plastic surgeons, we also should have *aretê*, the self-discipline of practice [1].

Self-discipline includes the anatomical basis of treatment and the principles of perioperative care, including fluid and electrolyte balance. The ability to choose when to operate and when not to operate is essential, as well as surgical skills. An attitude of honesty and empathy for patients constitutes the moral virtue of a good plastic surgeon [2].

When I come out of the operating theater, I ask myself whether I just carried out the operation exactly as planned. Although I precisely design the procedures and I usually come fairly close, I have never been able to operate in exactly the same way that I conceive of it in my mind [3]. I have empty note papers on which I write or draw to prepare for operations that I expect will involve complicated procedures. Upon arrival to my office, I recall the procedure and fill an empty page with the procedural steps I performed and my regrets regarding the operation. When these operative notes are collected, they can be the basis of case reports, idea and innovation reports, case series, or even original articles [4].

The winners of the Olympic Games will die 1 day. However, those memories of *aretê* are perpetuated from generation to generation and became the soul of the *polis*. Even an excellent plastic surgeon will retire someday. However, the papers published based on the "self-discipline of practice" will serve as a beacon for junior plastic surgeons who will take their place.

2.2 Enigmatic Smiles for Plastic Surgeons

2.2.1 Introduction

Years ago, I visited the Louvre in Paris, where I enjoyed the paintings from the Renaissance period. In the room dedicated to Renaissance paintings, I had the opportunity to see the *Virgin of the Rocks* and the *Mona Lisa*. Several people were looking at the *Virgin of the Rocks*, but there was a very large crowd in front of the *Mona Lisa*.

Because the *Virgin of the Rocks* contains content related to religious doctrines (St. John the Baptist and the young Jesus), which is not the case for the *Mona Lisa*, the former painting was more famous than the latter during Leonardo's lifetime (1452–1519). In contrast, the enigmatic smile of Mona Lisa was revaluated as time went by, with growing appreciation.

On my way home, I thought about the eternal charm of mysterious smiles and resolved to search for historical examples of enigmatic or mysterious smiles.

The aim of this paper is to review famous examples of mysterious or enigmatic smiles in art history that might be interesting for plastic surgeons.

2.2.2 What Is a Smile and Which Muscles Are Responsible for Smiling?

In Webster's Dictionary, a smile is defined as "a change of facial expression involving a brightening of the eyes, an upward curving of the corners of the mouth with no sound and less muscular distortion of the features than in a laugh that may express amusement, pleasure, tender affection, approval, restrained mirth, irony, derision or any of various other emotions."

Rubin wrote that the nasolabial fold is the keystone of the smiling mechanism [5]. He stated that a smile is formed in stages: in the first stage, the levator muscles contract and raise the upper lip to the nasolabial fold, and in the second stage, the levator labii superioris, zygomaticus major, and buccinator muscles raise the lips even more superiorly. He also classified smiles into three categories depending upon the direction of the elevation and depression of the lips and the dominant muscles involved. In commissure smiles, the zygomaticus major muscles pull the upper lip like a Cupid's bow (as in the smile depicted in the

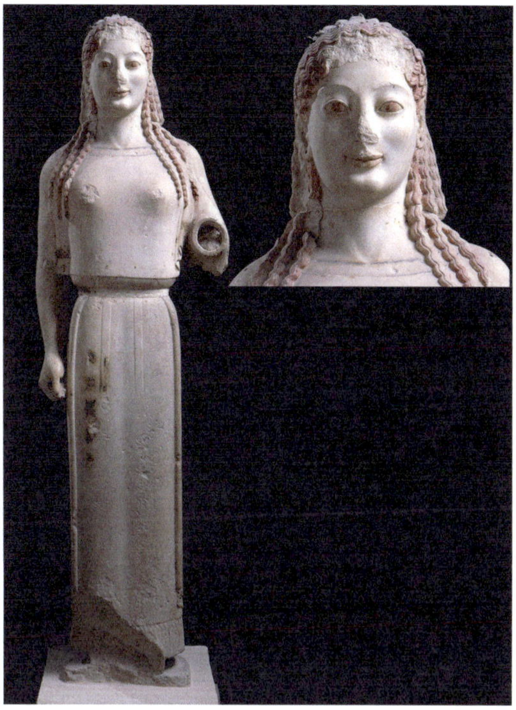

Fig. 2.2 *Peplos Kore (*a statue of a girl, *530 BC)*

Mona Lisa). In canine smiles, the upper lip is elevated uniformly like a diamond, without the corners of the mouth turning upward. In full denture smiles, the lower lip moves inferiorly at the same time as the upper lip moves superiorly.

2.2.3 Famous Enigmatic or Mysterious Smiles in the Arts

Blessing and well-being in smiles from the archaic period (600–480 B.C.) of Ancient Greece

The most famous examples of the archaic smile are the *Kroisos Kouros* (a grave marker for a fallen young warrior named Kroisos) and the *Peplos Kore* (a statue of a girl that was originally colorfully painted) (Fig. 2.2).

It has been theorized that artists felt that the archaic smile represented the blessing of the gods for the actions of the figures portrayed. It is also thought that this smile reflected a state of ideal health and well-being.

Warmth and softness in the smile of the Buddha's face

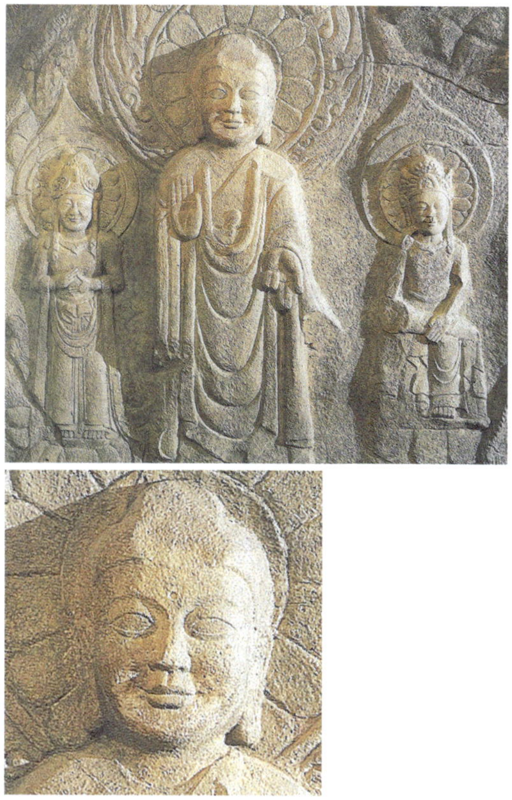

Fig. 2.3 *Rock-Carved Triad Buddha in Seosan* (from the Baekje Kingdom period in Korea; late sixth to early seventh century)

This smile is exemplified by the *Rock-Carved Triad Buddha in Seosan* (from the Baekje Kingdom period in Korea; late sixth to early seventh century) (Fig. 2.3).

Baekje figures express a unique smile that has been described as both enigmatic and subtle. The smile has been also been characterized in many different ways, from "genuinely glowing" to "thin and mild" to "unfathomable and benevolent." Baekje sculpture exhibited distinct characteristics of warmth and softness and used relaxed poses conveying friendliness and an air of pleasantness that is rarely found in other traditions of Buddhist sculpture.

Serene concentration in the Bodhisattva's smile

A gilt-bronze Bodhisattva, in a pensive position (sixth century, 83rd National Treasure of Korea), has a face with a hint of a smile that

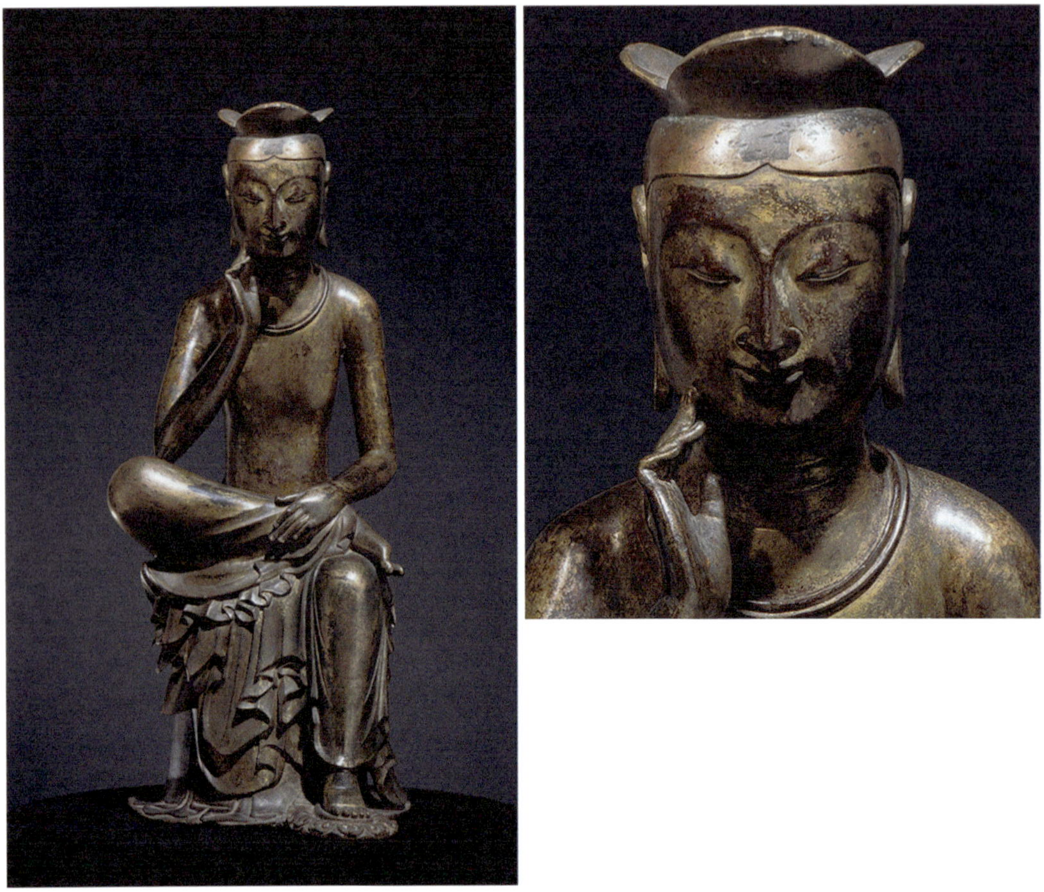

Fig. 2.4 A gilt-bronze Bodhisattva in a pensive position (sixth century, 83rd National Treasure of Korea)

exhibits a sense of serene concentration and gives the viewer the impression of an aura of deep thought (Fig. 2.4).

Hints of happiness and sadness in Gabriel's smile

Reims Cathedral (also known as Notre Dame de Reims) has four statues forming a composition of *Annunciation* and *Visitation*, with two statues each. In *Annunciation*, the angel Gabriel is sent by God to visit the Virgin Mary to give her the news that she will give birth to the Savior. Gabriel's gaze is focused on Mary with a hint of happiness but also sadness (Fig. 2.5). He understands her excitement but also realizes the fate of her unborn son. The Virgin Mary gives Gabriel a slight smile from her youthful face as she receives the news of her child.

Happiness or a non-genuine smile: Mona Lisa's mysterious smile

The painting is thought to be a portrait of the Italian noblewoman Lisa Gherardini, the wife of Francesco del Giocondo, and was painted between 1503 and 1506. Over the years, there have been many debates about the valence of the emotion expressed on her face, but most interpretations agree that the expression depicted in *Mona Lisa* is happiness (Fig. 2.6).

In a recent paper, a neurobiologist wrote that happiness is expressed only on the left side and that her asymmetric smile is a non-genuine smile, which is also thought to occur when an individual lies [6].

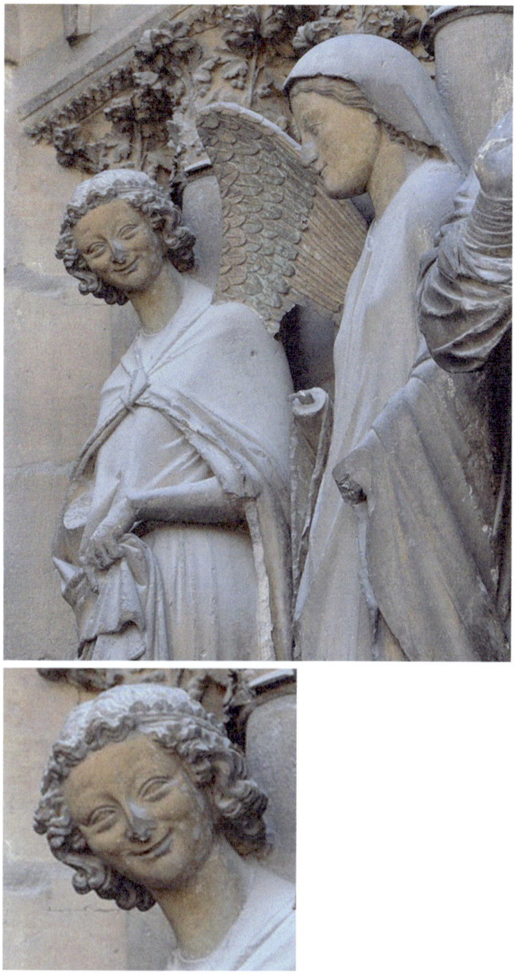

Fig. 2.5 Statue of angel Gabriel (Notre Dame de Reims Cathedral, 1236–1245)

2.2.4 Discussion

Smiles make art history beautiful.

In the archaic period of Greece, smiles represented blessing and well-being. In the sixth century, Buddha's smile conveyed warmth, softness, or serene concentration. Gabriel's smile provided a hint of happiness in response to the Virgin Mary's excitement as well as sadness regarding the fate of her unborn son, who was destined for crucifixion. Mona Lisa's mysterious smile is generally interpreted as showing happiness but has also been interpreted as a non-genuine smile.

The components of the smile should be considered not as rigid boundaries but as artistic guidelines to help the plastic surgeon or orthodontist. It is important for plastic surgeons and orthodontists to make every effort to develop a harmonious balance that will produce the most attractive smile possible for each patient being treated [7].

In our modern competitive society, a charming smile can be a key to open doors and to knock down barriers to success. From the surgeon's point of view, however, there is no universal "ideal" smile.

The most important esthetic goal for surgeons is to obtain a balanced—or preferably, enigmatic—smile, as represented in artistic masterpieces from across the ages.

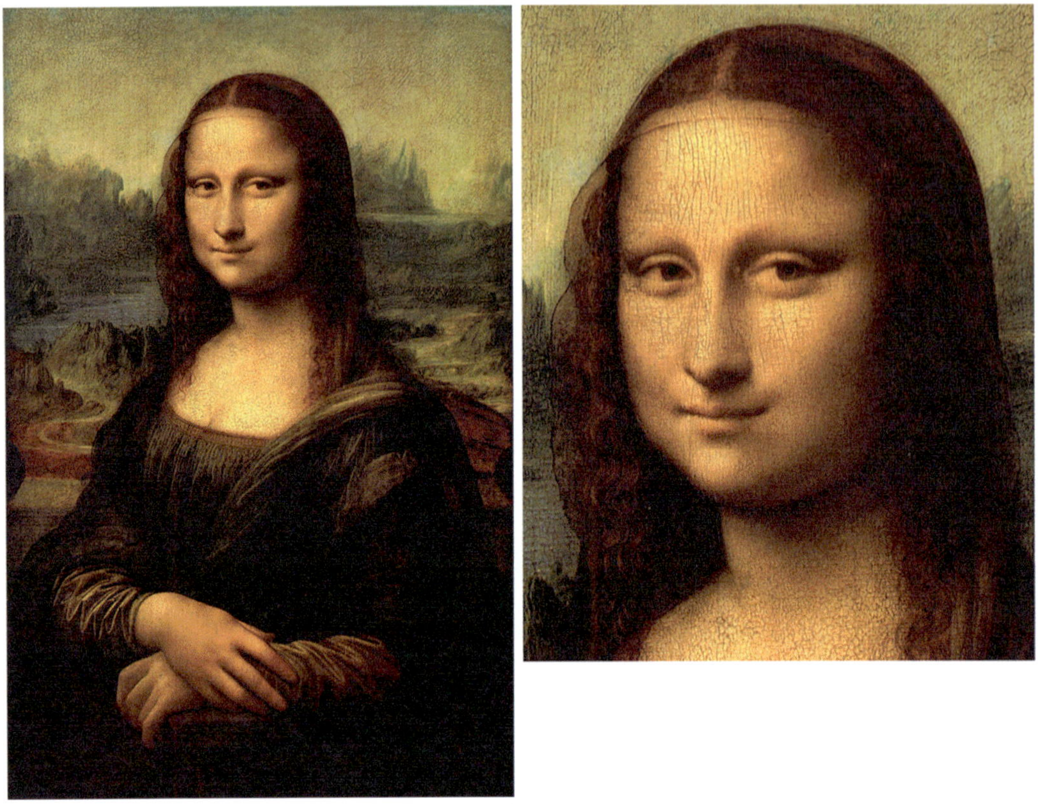

Fig. 2.6 *Mona Lisa* (Louvre Museum, 1503–1506)

2.3 Robbing Peter to Pay Paul

> Your slogan should be: the simplest possible repair with minimum sacrifice of material.—*Thomas Pomfret Kilner (1890–1964)*

Last year, I visited the Hunterian Museum in London and saw Dr. Kilner's relics. Among them, I read the draft for a course of lectures in plastic surgery, arranged by the Postgraduate Education Committee of the Royal College of Surgeons (cleft lip and palate repair, February 23, 1948). While I was reading his lecture draft written 68 years ago, I felt as if I was listening to his lecture in the lecture room downstairs. He emphasized "Your slogan should be: the simplest possible repair with minimum sacrifice of material."

During my stay in London, I also visited two famous churches: St. Paul's Cathedral and Westminster Abbey. Christopher Wren, the architect who designed the Royal Observatory at Greenwich, designed St. Paul's Cathedral, and it is famous because Prince Charles and Princess Diana got married there. The full name of Westminster Abbey is the Collegiate Church of St. Peter at Westminster, and it contains many tombs of famous kings, queens, scientists, and poets. The body of Isaac Newton is placed in this church, as described in *The Da Vinci Code* written by Dan Brown.

The tour guide said that money was taken from the government's allotment for Westminster Abbey, or St. Peter at Westminster, to pay for the construction of St. Paul's after the earlier cathedral on the site was destroyed by a fire in 1666 (Fig. 2.7). She told us that this is the origin of the expression "robbing Peter to pay Paul." This familiar phrase means to take something from one person or thing to pay a debt to another.

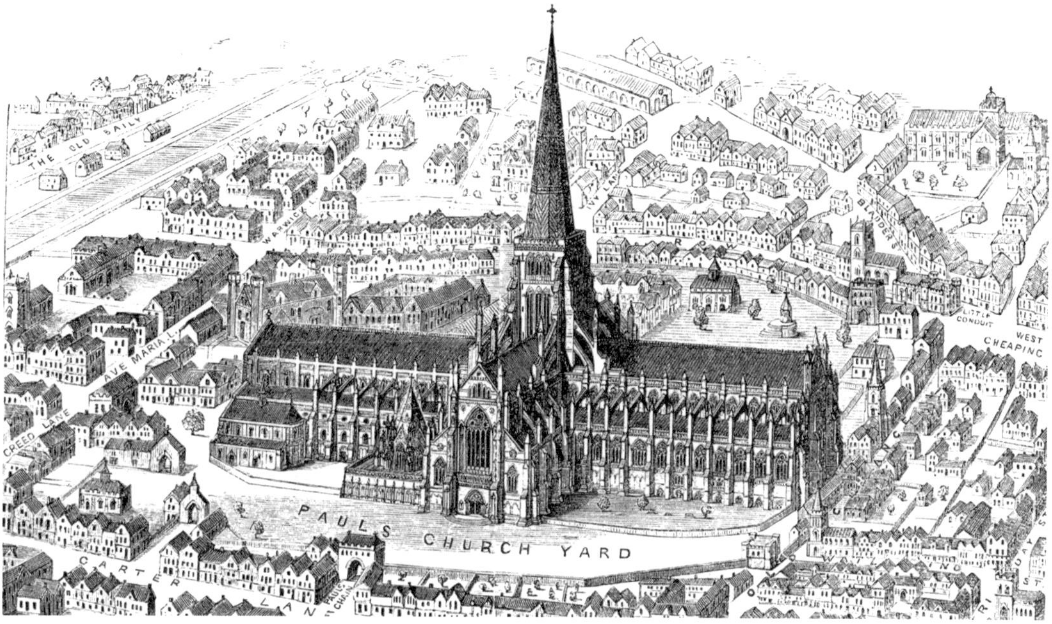

Fig. 2.7 Old St. Paul's Cathedral in London

On my way home, I remembered the "barter principle" I read in the first edition of *Plastic Surgery* when I was a trainee.

"In making a scalping flap or median forehead flap for subtotal reconstruction of the nose, forehead tissue is used for this procedure because of the good color and texture match. A major portion of the flap is replaced in its original site after dividing the pedicle, leaving a portion of the flap to form the reconstructed nose. However, a secondary defect remains on the forehead. This defect is repaired by the most suitable skin available to minimize the secondary deformity. Thereafter full-thickness skin from the supraclavicular area gives a suitable color match. The supraclavicular defect can usually be closed primarily. This is a good barter; by contrast, a split-thickness graft placed upon the forehead represents an unsatisfactory repair of the secondary defect."

Reconstructive ladder and elevator/lift have developed reconstructive plastic surgery. Nowadays, we have free flaps for almost every defect; thereafter, we sometimes overlook simpler means of closing a defect to be inferior to the more sophisticated but complex techniques. However, free flap does not always promise a superior outcome. It is time-consuming, costly, and often involves a number of complementary procedures with considerable donor site morbidity.

In reconstructive plastic surgery, surgeons must remember that good clinical judgment reduces the cost of the barter to a minimum. I do think the slogan "Simplest possible repair with minimum sacrifice of material" is still valid until today. Always remember that "Paul must also be able to pay Peter."

2.4 Metamorphosis From an Ugly Girl to a Beauty

The desire to have a beautiful appearance has been deeply rooted in human beings in all ages and countries. In this era, many women live with an intense interest in their appearance due to the social importance placed on appearance. Some women even suffer from an obsession for a beautiful face and slim body in order to achieve success in employment or marriages, without the discrimination and disadvantages faced by women perceived to be ugly.

Women are often unable to escape from the social emphasis on beauty and the Cinderella complex due to the influence of the mass media and the sociocultural phenomena of discrimination against women based on their appearance and commercialization of women's appearance. The causes of these sociocultural phenomena may be complex, but it is difficult to ignore the influence of children's books and animations of old tales that people encounter in childhood. For many years, the female protagonists in children's fairy tale books and animations have been mostly beautiful-looking princesses, whereas most of the ugly-looking women were witches, cannibals, or evil stepmothers, who symbolized evil or greed, or their daughters.

Is there really no fairy tale in the world where an ugly woman is the main character? In the catalog of international tale types (ATU) based on the Aarne/Thompson system, one (ATU 711. "The Beautiful and the Ugly Twin") has an ugly female protagonist [8]. This tale has been handed down in Europe.

Another tale that is not included in the ATU index has been passed down in Jewish communities living in predominantly Islamic countries, such as Morocco, Yemen, Iraq, and Persia: "The Ugly Wise Girl." In this story. The daughter of a rabbi born with a beast's face finally undergoes a metamorphosis [9].

The summary of the tale is as follows:

Once upon a time in Constantinople lived a girl with a face that resembled a beast. The girl, the only daughter of a rabbi, had a very ugly face, but she was wiser than anyone. Because of her ugliness, her parents locked her up in the attic of the school so that no one else could see her. She received food through a small hole in the door. A young male student from a distant province came to this city to study at the rabbi's school. This young man studied in a room next to where the girl was locked up in the attic. When he was in trouble because he was unable to answer the rabbi's questions, he would find notes with the correct answers written on them. When he realized that the notes were written by the rabbi's daughter in the attic, he was deeply moved by her wisdom and knowledge and finally made a marriage proposal to her. Her parents initially opposed the idea, but later agreed to their marriage. At the wedding ceremony, the groom couldn't see the bride's face, which was covered with a veil. The groom was shocked to see her face on the first night; however, he spent the night with her to keep his marriage vows. When he started on a long journey, she asked for a love token for the child to be born, and a ring and prayer shawl were handed over to the bride. The bride gave birth to a son, but she couldn't raise him, and her parents raised their grandson instead. The son grew up and went to school, where he was teased by his friends for being a fatherless child. After learning the secret of his birth, the son met his mother, who was still staying in the attic. He realized that his mother endured hard times studying the Torah, and the son learned Torah from his knowledgeable and intelligent mother. One day the son asked his mother about the whereabouts of his father and started a journey to his father, carrying the ring and prayer shawl that his father had left behind. After several months of journeys, he arrived in the country where his father lived and entered the synagogue there. When the rabbi saw the prayer shawl embroidered with his son's name, he recognized that this boy was his own bloodline. The son persuaded his father to return to live together with them since his mother was prettiest and wisest person in the world. Hearing his son's words, the rabbi thought that a miracle might have happened, and told him he would return home soon. On the way back to his homeland, the son met an old man, who gave him a mysterious drug. The old man told the son to apply it to his mother's face. Upon returning home, his mother applied it on the face and became as beautiful as the sun and the moon. She prayed to God with thanks for giving a miracle drug through the hand of Prophet Elijah (Fig. 2.8). When the father returned home, he realized that a miracle had indeed happened. This wise son brought peace and happiness to his parents' home.

In this story, the protagonist's transformation was a rite of passage for women entering a soci-

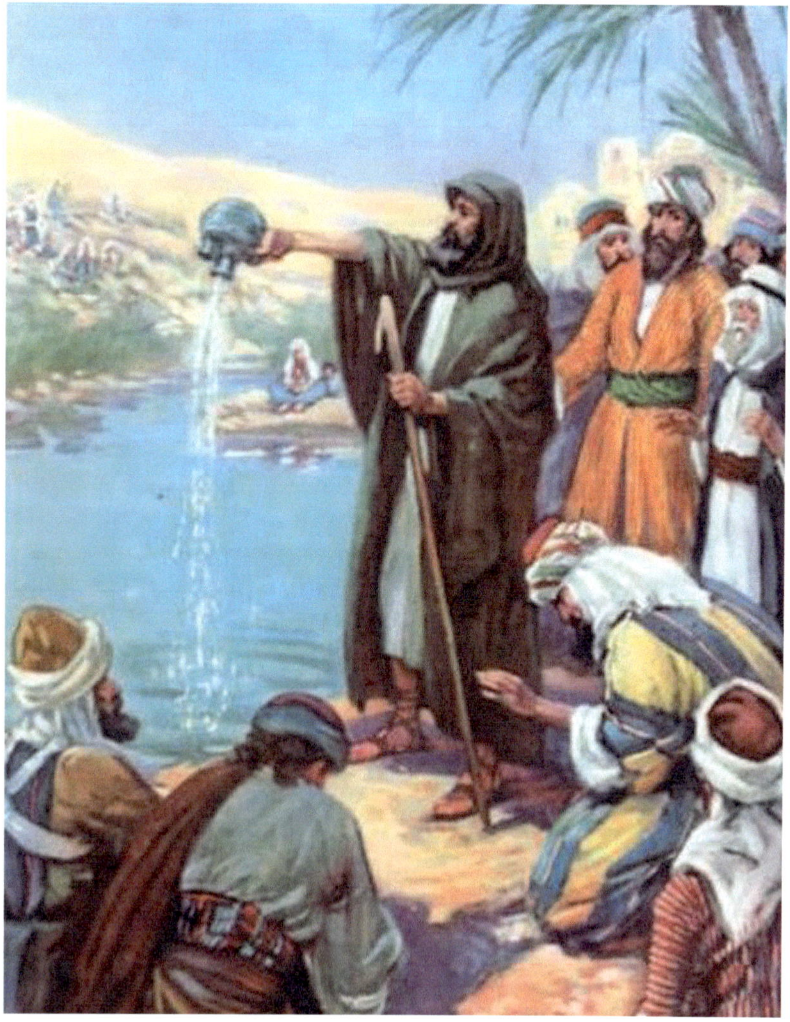

Fig. 2.8 Elijah poured the salt in the water and blessed it. "So the waters were healed unto this day, according to the saying of Elisha which he spake" (2 Kings 2:22)

ety (male-centered, patriarchal society) after enduring trials and pains. The rabbi's daughter was not able to complete a sequence of rites of separation, transition, and incorporation at her birth, and her parents did not assimilate her into their family structure. For this "ugly girl," the marriage ceremony could not function as a rite of incorporation because she was abandoned by her husband on their wedding night and then experienced a transitional period in an enclosed room without integration into society through her husband. After her transformation into a beautiful woman, she was able to complete her rite of passage from separation through transition to incorporation [10]. She overcame her hardships through her wisdom and belief in God. The rabbi's daughter transformed her appearance, thanks to her son, who obtained a bottle of miraculous water from the Prophet Elijah.

In our era, fortunately, women do not have to rely upon God's grace and miraculous water from the Prophet. Instead, plastic surgeons express their imagination by modifying the living bodies of patients like poets or writers of tales expresses themselves through their writings or poems [11]. If women have free will to transform themselves, many miraculous plastic surgical procedures can replace Elijah's water, opening a door to the corresponding rites of passage.

2.5 Designing on Paper and Using a Model

> How many things painters see in shadows and in the foreground that we do not see? Oh, think what you would say if you could see it with Salvator Rosa's eyes.—*Baldinucci*

When I visited St. Peter's Basilica in the Vatican, I saw a sign at the front of the Blessed Sacrament Chapel that read: "Only those who wish to pray may enter." It really was the only quiet place for reflection in the crowded and noisy Basilica. At the front was a beautiful tabernacle designed by Bernini. The 12 apostles and Jesus are perched on top of the cornices of the miniature dome. Two large angels are kneeling on the altar in reverent prayer. In our contemplative mood, gazing at the beautiful spectacle, my wife and I soon became oblivious of the noise of the world.

In the Vatican Museum (Vatican Pinacoteca), I chanced upon a similar angel. The iron armatures of the wings and bundled twigs inside the shoulder exposed by damage. It was the full-sized modello for the kneeling angel of the "Altar of the Blessed Sacrament" (Fig. 2.9).

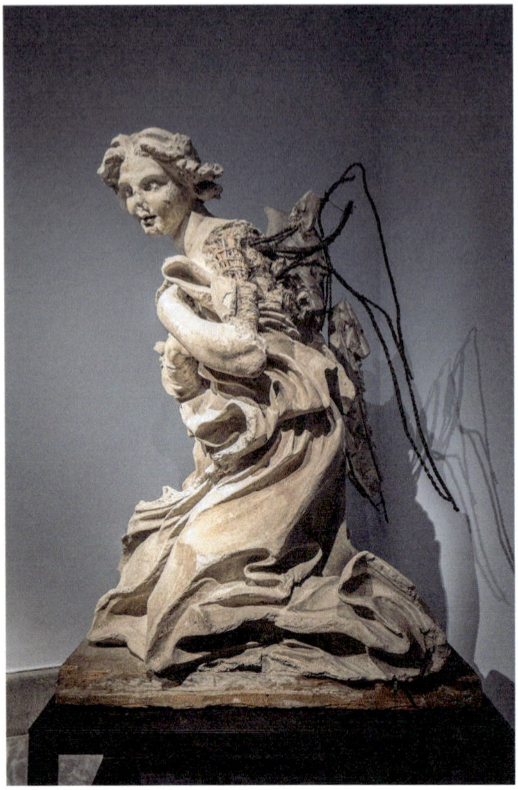

Fig. 2.9 Full-sized modello for the kneeling angel of the "Altar of the Blessed Sacrament" (Vatican Pinacoteca)

After seeing the terracotta models, I acquired a book, *Bernini Sculpting in Clay*, and discovered that Bernini had used drawing and terracotta modeling as preparatory studies for his marble statues. He began with a sketchbook or model stand.

On my way home, I thought about the modello of the kneeling angel and the use of occlusal plane casting and the occlusal wafer for jaw surgery.

Whenever I meet a patient, I would draw a face schema. If a scar is visible, I would draw it precisely on the paper medical record. For a Z-plasty or W-plasty, I usually design a schematic representation of the procedure on the paper drawing of the scar and show it to the patient.

This led me to think about the use of three-dimensional (3D) silicon models for breast reduction. Even if we do not make such 3D models, similar models can be purchased. By designing the procedure on the model and practicing with different methods, we can choose the most proper method for a specific patient.

Bernini's models are appealing because of their vitality and their vivid reflection of the sculptor's touch. The range of his drawings is remarkable in terms of type and quality; Bernini appreciated the versatility offered by various techniques as he grappled with the diverse problems that he encountered in sculptural commissions [12]. Drawings were indispensable to Bernini's design process, linking his thoughts to his clay models and to the final sculptures.

Changes made in surgery are irreversible, like those made in marble or bronze statues. Like Bernini, the famous artist of the Baroque period, we plastic surgeons also need drawings or models for our operations, to make "the field real." Performing numerous imaginary operations prior to real surgery will help plastic surgeons to see their patients with "Salvator Rosa's eyes."

2.6 Critical Appraisal in Plastic Surgery: *Nullius in Verba*

Nullius in verba (Don't take anyone's word for it)

At conferences, many new techniques are introduced to many audience members, often including myself. Sometimes a new technique with dramatic postoperative results may be especially intriguing. The presenter says that all the patients were satisfied and that no complications occurred. In such cases, we are prone to incorporate at least a part of the method into our routines, or even to change our previous operative method. Of course, the famous surgeon, giving the presentation, has already published his methods in a journal article or a book chapter. Some surgeons develop new surgical nomenclature or propose names for a purportedly new anatomical structure because they think that they were the first to innovate the technique or to find the anatomical structure.

Several years later, a modified technique can be introduced by the same surgeon. At this time, the presenter insists that the new modified method obtained better results. He publishes again, this time with modified methods. Usually, he does not mention why he modified the previous method or express regret for the shortcomings of the previous method. He may introduce a new name for a structure similar to one that he previously named.

Since the famous surgeon says that this new method is better or even best, we are put in the position of having to follow this "virtuoso," without knowing whether he will change the method once more. We have to use the new terminology as an indicator of being up to date. If we do not use the new term for a method or anatomical structure, we seem out of date and lose the ability to communicate each other.

With the ever-increasing quantity of medical literature, it is impossible for plastic surgeons to read every article, even in their subspecialties. Thus, the critical appraisal of scientific papers is an important skill for plastic surgeons to master. We must start from a position of skepticism because it is the true starting point of science [13].

It is difficult to distinguish papers written just to meet publication requirements from true gems, and we should have our eyes wide open to distinguish trustworthy papers from theses published for their own sake.

If all the patients are satisfied and no complications occurred, the follow-up period should be checked. If new surgical nomenclature or a name for a purportedly new anatomical structure appears in a paper, we must review previous techniques or go back to the anatomy textbook we used in medical school. Papers that do not cite previous papers on similar topics and insist on their originality should be disregarded. If a paper provokes a letter to the editor and the authors do not respond to this letter, it can be concluded that the authors are attempting to avoid criticism [14, 15].

We should not be "conclusion-of-the-abstract readers." In a systematic review containing a meta-analysis, the data are contained in the few articles that are included in the meta-analysis. Such "evidence-based medicine" is intrinsically dependent on both the direction of the available research and the selection criteria used [15]. Thereafter, when reading a review article, we should consult the guidelines presented in PRISMA (Preferred Statement for Meta-Analytical Studies and Systematic Reviews: http://www.prisma-statement.org) or CONSORT (Consolidated Standard for Reporting Trial 2010 for Randomised Trials: http://www.consort-statement.org).

Nullius in verba (don't take anyone's word for it) was the motto adopted by the Royal Society of London for Improving Natural Knowledge in 1660 (Fig. 2.10). I strongly suggest that this motto should also be applied in the field of plastic surgery.

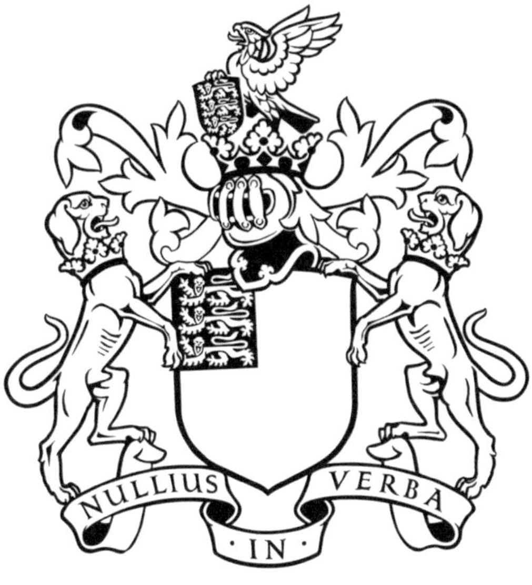

Fig. 2.10 Coat of arms of the Royal Society with the motto Nullius in verba along the bottom

2.7 Clip an Angel's Wings, Make Man's Wings

When I visited Guy's Hospital, London, for my youngest son's medical school commencement, I happened to see the statue of John Keats (1795–1821) (Fig. 2.11). Despite an early interest in literature, Keats was apprenticed to an apothecary and continued his medical training as a surgeon's assistant at Guy's Hospital, obtaining the Licentiate of Apothecaries in 1816. However, he never practiced medicine.

In his poem, "Lamia," I noticed some interesting verses: "Philosophy will clip an Angel's wings."

There was an awful rainbow once in heaven:
We know her woof, her texture; she is given
In the dull catalogue of common things.
Philosophy will clip an Angel's wings,
Conquer all mysteries by rule and line,
Empty the haunted air, and gnomed mine—
Unweave a rainbow, as it erewhile made
The tender-person'd Lamia melt into a shade

According to scholars, Keats [16] claims in "Lamia" that scientific knowledge ruins our sense of beauty. It is thought that sole emphasis on science might stifle the creativity. However, his scientific knowledge surely helped him to create poetry of great beauty, even though he decided to pursue poetry rather than a career in medicine. His medical experience also influenced to some degree his ideas and even his choice of words [17].

Upon arriving home, I thought deeply about whether scientific knowledge spoils plastic surgeons' aesthetic sense and was reminded of a book I have had since my training years: *The Artistry of Reconstructive Surgery: Selected Classic Case Studies* [18]. In the epilogue of this book, the two surgeons posed the question of "Can man have wings?" as a methodological inquiry. Dr. Brent stated that it would be possible through a "thoracobrachial pterygoplasty (making a wing between arm and trunk using tissue expander) powered by split latissimus dorsi muscle transposition flap and bone grafts." In contrast, Dr. Krizek proposed creating muscle-powered wings (tissue expanders and uroepithelial rib grafts made flexible by incorporating interphalangeal joints) and conehead buoyancy.

Although these methods are almost impossible in real-world circumstances, these reflections show the potential growth and evolution that lie in the flexible and creative nature of man's imagination [11]. Commixing the science and creativity lead the plastic surgeons onto innovation.

After reading "Lamia" and the epilogue of *The Artistry of Reconstructive Surgery*, I began to think that scientists and poets are more alike than I thought before.

Just as the medical knowledge of the doctor Keats helped the poet Keats who sang of physical pain and pleasure, our literary sense as surgeons will help our creativity in developing new innovation of techniques through imagination.

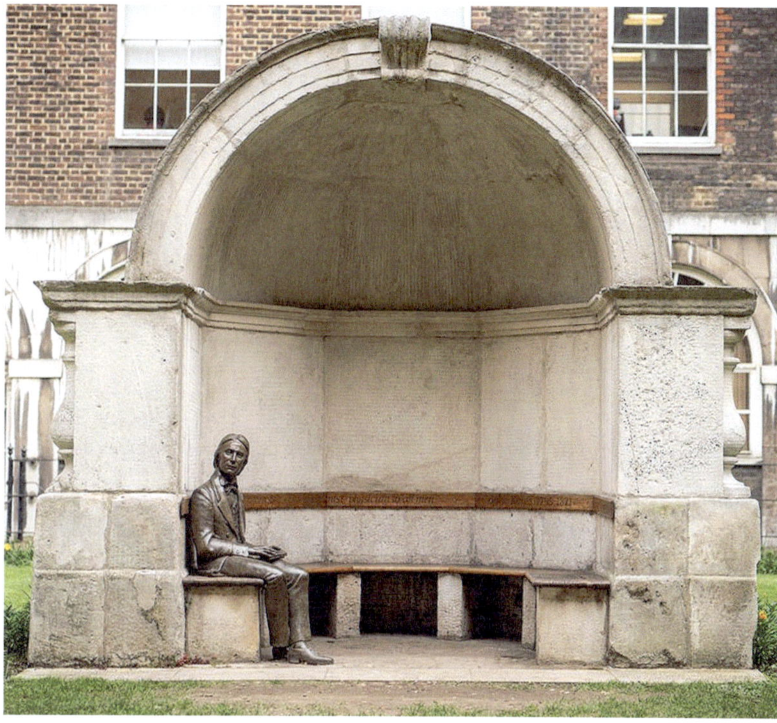

Fig. 2.11 The Keats statue at King's College London, Guy's Campus

2.8 "Brighter Hours Will Come:" The Signet Ring of Florence Nightingale

We hope for the hours that are brighter to come.—Elizabeth Piddocke Roberts

A lady with a lamp I see.—Henry Longfellow

A Gallup poll asked what jobs people considered trustworthy, and the medical doctor was ranked third among the most trusted professions, following nurses and pharmacists. On the contrary, health maintenance organization managers ranked fifth least trusted position [19]. In South Korea, however, assembly passed a bill recently, which allows victims of medical malpractice to begin legal processes without the consent of hospitals and doctors. This bill represents distrust of the patients and relatives to the medical doctors [20].

It is well-known that Florence Nightingale (1820–1910) became a persona of "The Lady with the Lamp," making rounds on wounded soldiers at night during the Crimean War (1853–1856). This powerful and recognizable image first came from Illustrated London News (1855). Henry Longfellow (1807–1880)'s poem "Santa Filomena" written in 1857 ("Lo! in that house of misery, A lady with a lamp I see") fixed forever Florence's image as the lady with the lamp. This image was enhanced by many paintings.

Many of her relics, including her seal press marked with her initials "FN," are displayed in the Florence Nightingale Museum, located near St. Thomas Hospital where she first established a modern nursing school. However, her signet ring has not been described yet.

During my 3 months stay in London, I happen to see Nightingale's seal at Henry Wellcome's Legacy in the Science Museum London (Object number A134207), which she used to impress wax seals on her letters until her death (1910). The figure and the phrase on the signet ring help provide some insight, thus worth describing in detail.

The ring bears an image of a nurse's lamp and the phrase "Brighter Hours Will Come" (Fig. 2.12). This phrase was likely derived from

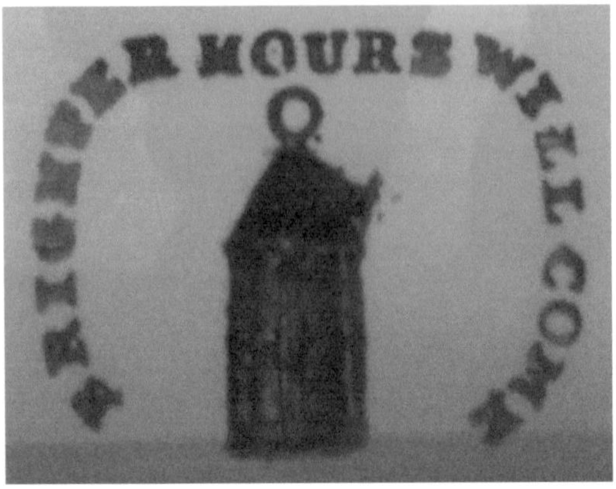

Fig. 2.12 Image of a nurse's lamp and the phrase "Brighter Hours Will Come" in the signet ring of Florence Nightingale

the poem title "Brighter Hours Will Come" in the book "Miscellaneous Poems (1845)" written by Elizabeth Piddocke Roberts [21].

> *When the winter wind howls o'er the desolate plain,*
> *Or agitates madly the billowy main,*
> *With a rush, and a hollow-toned, whistling blast,*
> *As it moans round the sales, or the tall stately mast,*
> *Oh, where is the mariner, exiled from home,*
> *But sighs for the hours that are brighter to come?*
> *And 'this thus with the soul, as it struggles with woe,*
> *While o'er us its billows unceasingly flow;*
> *Through the wildest of sorrow, the bitterest grief,*
> *'Tis in thoughts of the future the mind seeks relief.*
> *Though from happiness now, saddened outcast we roam,*
> *We hope for the hours that are brighter to come.*

As King Solomon had carved on his signet ring the phrase "This too will pass away"—which would always be true in good times or bad—the phase "Brighter hours will come" is thought to be Nightingale's favorite words that gave her hope in difficult times and humility in good times. Then, what was the "brighter hours" for Florence Nightingale? Was it professionalizing nursing roles, or social reforms of improving healthcare? Or was it simply spring the poet was longing for in winter?

As I came out of the museum, I thought about the image of medical doctors depicted in the eyes of the people in these days.

I miss the poets like Henry Longfellow or artists like Sir Luke Fields (1843–1927), who would express the good image of plastic surgeons of this era.

2.9 How to Hold an Osteotome? Michelangelo Grip

> Lorenzo laughed and said, 'But don't you know old people never have all their teeth; there are always some missing.' As soon as Lorenzo had gone away, Michelangelo broke off one of the faun's teeth and dug into the gum so that it looked as if the tooth had fallen out.—Christopher Hibbert

We plastic surgeons, especially craniofacial surgeons, routinely use surgical instruments. It is generally thought that there are no specific rules for how surgeons should hold instruments with their hands. Most surgeons in training learn how to use instruments by observing their teachers. After completion of training, when we have the chance to see other surgeons operate, especially famous surgeons, we carefully observe their hands-on skills and the maneuvers that they use to handle their instruments. If they are sufficiently skillful and their technique seems even better than ours, we can mimic their technique and abandon the technique that we previously used. However, I believe that this rarely occurs because we are stuck in a rut, following the law of inertia.

The osteotome is a surgical instrument that is frequently used in rhinoplasty as well as harvesting bones. When I use an osteotome, I support its bottom with my left thumb and hold it with the remaining four fingers (Fig. 2.13, lower left). When I impact the tip of the osteotome, my eyes are usually focused on the proximal tip of the chisel, which receives the impact of the mallet.

Recently, I visited the Pitti Palace in Florence, where I happened to see a beautiful marble sculpture of a boy making a facial mask of a Satyr (Faun) using a chisel and mallet. This statue captures the legendary artist Michelangelo as an adolescent ("The Young Michelangelo," 1861, by Emilio Zocchi, 105 cm; Fig. 2.13, upper).

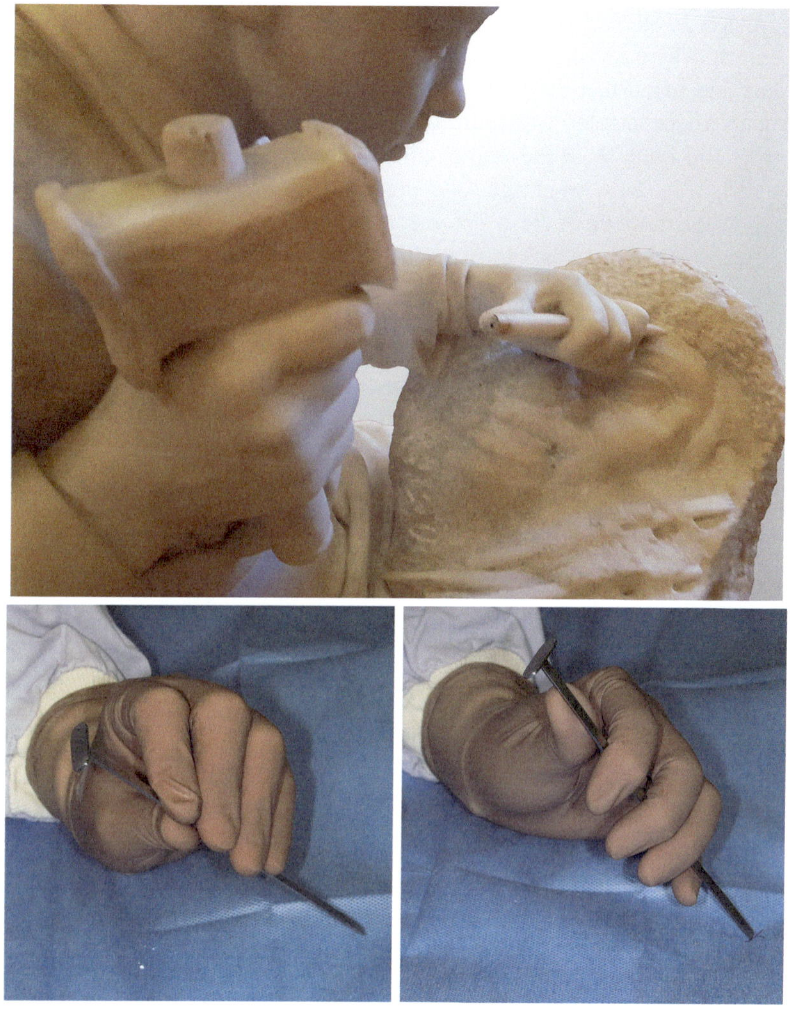

Fig. 2.13 Michelangelo's grip. Upper: part of the "The Young Michelangelo," 1861, by Emilio Zocchi, white marble, Pitti Palace Museum, Florence (Whole statue; 105 cm). Note the left hand holding a chisel. Lower left: supporting the bottom with the thumb and holding it with the remaining four fingers. Lower right: the distal part of the chisel is supported on the extensor surface of the proximal phalanx of the flexed little finger, and the proximal part is pushed by the palmar surface of the distal phalanx of extended thumb. The index finger, middle finger, and ring finger hold the shaft of the chisel

At the age of 15, Michelangelo entered the Garden of the Medici School of San Marco to study sculpture. When Lorenzo de' Medici (known as Lorenzo il Magnifico), the school's founder and patron, came upon Michelangelo replicating an ancient statue of a satyr, Lorenzo was impressed by the youth's talent but commented that the elderly satyr would not have such perfect teeth. In response, Michelangelo spontaneously took up his chisel and broke off a single tooth from his statue. It was at that moment that Lorenzo understood the talent of the young sculptor and invited him to stay in the Palazzo Medici [22, 23].

In "The Young Michelangelo," the boy is so concentrated that he has a glabellar frown. His eyes are focused on the tip of the chisel, which is making contact with the raw marble bone. The distal part of the chisel is supported on the extensor surface of the proximal phalanx of the flexed little finger, and the proximal part is pushed by the palmar surface of the distal phalanx of extended thumb. The index finger, middle finger, and ring finger hold the shaft of the chisel (Fig. 2.13, upper). The contact surface of the mallet is concave. It is thought that this grip can transmit the impact of the mallet to the tip of the chisel effectively, because the chisel is held lightly, with less grasping force of the fingers. Therefore, Michelangelo was able to break off a single tooth in front of his patron immediately.

When I returned to my operating theater, I compared these two methods of holding an osteotome and found that the grip portrayed in "The Young Michelangelo" was more stable than the grip I had used. With the improved stability of this grip (Fig. 2.13, lower right), I could focus my eyes on the distal tip of the osteotome, rather than on the proximal tip, which receives the impact of the mallet.

Although I myself had been stuck in a rut, I changed my method of holding an osteotome, and by doing so, I broke the law of inertia.

References

1. Futrell JW. Aretê. Am J Surg. 1975;130:512–3.
2. Hwang K. A plastic surgeon should be a good physician first. J Craniofac Surg. 2019;30:629.
3. Hwang K. The aging surgeon and the secret of longevity. J Craniofac Surg. 2019;30:12.
4. Hwang K. The poet-physician's note and the plastic surgeon's note. Arch Plast Surg. 2021;48:345–6.
5. Rubin LR, Mishriki Y, Lee G. Anatomy of the nasolabial fold: the keystone of the smiling mechanism. Plast Reconstr Surg. 1989;83:1–8.
6. Marsili L, Ricciardi L, Bologna M. Unraveling the asymmetry of Mona Lisa smile. Cortex. 2019;120:607–10.
7. Manjula WS, Sukumar MR, Kishorekumar S, Gnanashanmugam K, Mahalakshmi K. Smile: a review. J Pharm Bioallied Sci. 2015;7(Suppl 1):S271–5.
8. Uther H. The types of international folktales: a classification and bibliography. Based on the system of Antti Aarne and Stith Thompson, part III. Helsinki: Finnish Academy of Science and Letters; 2011.
9. Frankel E. The ugly wise girl. In: The classic tales: 4000 years of Jewish Lore. Northvale: Jason Aronson Inc; 1993. p. 588–94.
10. Kim HH. The rites of passage of the ugly girls transformed into beauties: a comparative study of the ugly-girl Tales from Korean and Jewish traditions. Comp Korean Stud. 2014;22:117–54.
11. Hwang K. Metamorphosis in the imagination of poets, artists, and plastic surgeons. J Craniofac Surg. 2020;31:3.
12. Wardropper I, Polizzotti M. Sketching on paper and in clay: Bernini's use of preparatory drawings and models. In: Bernini: Sculpting in clay. 1st ed. New York: MetPublications; 2012.
13. Lehman RS. Nullius in verba: don't take anyone's word for it. JAMA Intern Med. 2013;173:1049–50.
14. Hwang K. Appropriate roles for the subscriber, publisher, author, and reviewer in the archives of plastic surgery. Arch Plast Surg. 2013;40:663–5.
15. Hwang K, Hwang SH. Selecting trustworthy papers. J Craniofac Surg. 2017;28:591.
16. Ruston S. John Keats, Poet-physician [British Library web site]; 2014. https://www.bl.uk/romantics-and-victorians/articles/john-keats-poet-physician#. Accessed 17 Feb 2021.
17. Smith H. John Keats: poet, patient, physician. Rev Infect Dis. 1984;6:390–404.
18. Brent B, Brent BP. The artistry of reconstructive surgery: selected classic case studies. St Louis: Mosby; 1987. p. 947–70.
19. Jeressi L. What are the most trusted and least trusted professions? http://943thepoint.com/what-are-the-most-trusted-and-least-trusted-professions/?trackback=tsmclip. Accessed 2 Apr 2013.
20. Korea Herald. Assembly passes undisputed bill in final session. 2016. http://www.koreaherald.com/view.php?ud=20160519000882. Accessed 30 June 2016.
21. Roberts EP. Miscellaneous poems. London: Darton and Clarke; 1845. p. 16.
22. Vasari G. Lives of the painters, sculptors, and architects (Le Vita De' Piu Eccellenti Architetti, Pittori, et scultori). Florence: Appresso I Giunti; 1568.
23. Hibbert C. The rise and fall of the house of Medici. London: Penguin; 1974.

3 Anatomy and Plastic Surgery

3.1 Stiff Twin Compasses: Anatomy and Plastic Surgery

> As stiff twin compasses are two;
> Thy soul, the fix'd foot, makes no show
> To move, but doth, if th' other do.—*John Donne*

Years ago, I visited Guy's campus of King's College London to meet Professor Harold Ellis, the author of "Clinical Anatomy." As I explored the campus, I happened to come across Guy's chapel, where I saw the tomb of Thomas Guy (1644–1724), who was a British bookseller, speculator, and the de facto founder of Guy's Hospital.

Among the several tombs in the chapel, a lead-lined stone sarcophagus caught my eye: Astley Paston Cooper (1768–1841). His name reminded me of his famous quote. In his days, without anesthetics, surgeons had to work quickly, precisely, and with indifference to the pain they inflicted. Therefore, he said that "A good surgeon must have an eagle's eye, a lady's hand, and a lion's heart." However, even in the nineteenth century, a sound knowledge of human anatomy was more important than the above three virtues [1].

Over the centuries, most surgeons, such as Dr. Cooper, were "surgeon-anatomists," who self-pursued knowledge and understanding of anatomy as the foundation of successful surgical results.

However, recent advances in medical education have ironically led to the separation of anatomy and surgery. In some medical schools, including my college, cadaver dissection time has been reduced and replaced with prosections, plastic models, and computer-based multimedia learning [2].

In my department, year 3 students in the 4-year medical program complete clerkships. Some of them still remember the structures of the head and face, but most forget them as soon as they take the corresponding examination in their first year.

As cadaveric training may be best suited for surgical residents, we had weekly cadaver dissection seminars for 5 weeks every year when I was the program director of my department. Residents dissected and exposed structures for days and then demonstrated the structures in front of the surgeons and anatomists of the department.

In workshops of American Society of Maxillofacial Surgeons and Arbeitsgemeinschaft für Osteosynthesefragen craniomaxillofacial division (AOCMF) courses, they use a saw-bone, but participants cannot directly experience the cadaver dissection. If anatomy is included on board certification examinations, especially in the form of an objective structured clinical evaluation, as well as on the written examination, the training staff will prepare their trainees by teaching them the anatomic details of the surgical procedures that they study.

There are many opportunities for anatomists and surgeons to work together to improve

K. Hwang, *Good Physician, Good Plastic Surgeon*, https://doi.org/10.1007/978-981-97-1864-1_3

educational instruction about anatomical regions known to be difficult, to refine procedural training, and to develop new techniques and procedures.

During surgical procedures, some surgeons are prone to think that they are the first to find a "new structure" that has never been described before. In these occasions, anatomists and histologists play a vital role in helping surgeons, if our forerunners have already defined and named a structure or if vigorous discussions have already been conducted in forums such as "Nomina Anatomica." Surgeons and anatomists could thereby share a mutually beneficial relationship and greatly enhance each other's academic productivity.

The next day, I visited the National Portrait Gallery and saw the portrait of John Donne (1572–1631) (Fig. 3.1), the author of the famous poem "*A Valediction: Forbidding Mourning.*"

If they be two, they are two so
As stiff twin compasses are two;
Thy soul, the fix'd foot, makes no show
To move, but doth, if th' other do.
And though it in the centre sit,
Yet, when the other far doth roam,
It leans, and hearkens after it,
And grows erect, as that comes home.

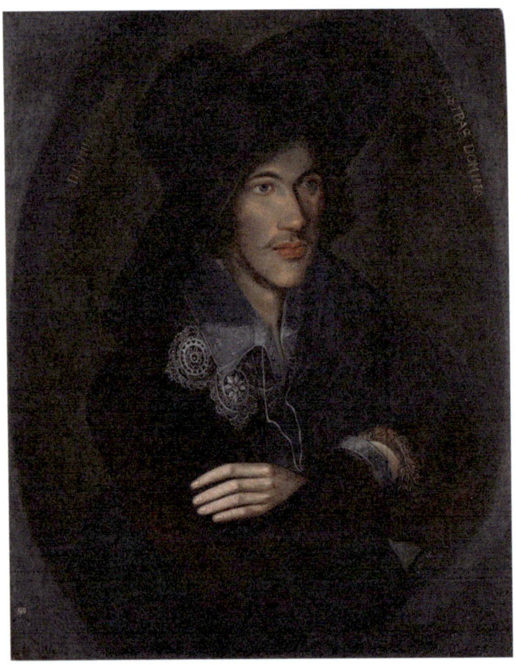

Fig. 3.1 A portrait of John Donne as a young man, c. 1595, reproduced with permission from the National Portrait Gallery, London

I believe that anatomy and surgery are 2 feet of stiff twin compasses, just as John Donne wrote. Anatomy is the center foot, which is fixed but leans toward the other moving foot. Surgery, in contrast, is the moving foot, which comes home.

3.2 An Oculist and a Musician in Leipzig

I was present at a feast of St. Lucia, so famous for curing defects of sight (

Fig. 3.2).—*John Taylor*

I recently visited Leipzig to collaborate with a physicist who is involved in a European Research Council project. In that city, I visited the St. Thomas Church (Thomaskirche), where Johann

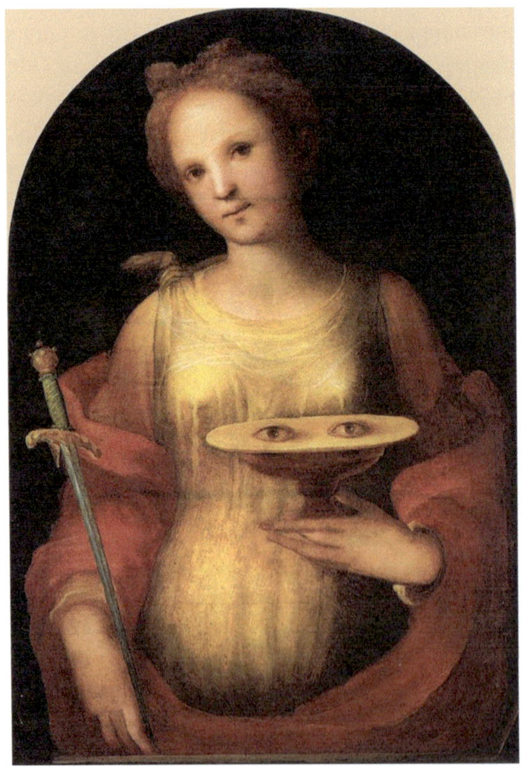

Fig. 3.2 Saint Lucy (Domenico Beccafurni, 1521, Pinacoteca Nazionale, Siena)

Sebastian Bach worked as a music director from 1723 until his death in 1750.

My colleague said that Bach had cataracts in his late years and underwent cataract surgery performed by an oculist named John Taylor (1703–1772). Because of two surgical errors of couching (a needle was poked into the eye and the cataract-clouded lens was pushed into the rear of the eye, out of the field of vision), Bach developed a painful postoperative infection and was treated with laxatives and the favorite cure of his day: bleeding. He was blind when he dictated his final work and died a few months later.

It is not widely known that Taylor performed many aesthetic procedures, including repairs of blepharoptosis, which became common a century later in the age of Dieffenbach. He also removed a cicatrix from the lower eyelid of a burn patient [3]. Since there were no local anesthetics at the time, the pain was excruciating, and the patient shouted repeatedly "You hurt me!" Taylor replied, "Remember, Lady, Beauty! [4, 5]." When he finished, the women's friends were astonished and the postoperative result looked like a miracle. Despite his skill, Taylor was considered a "quack" by the Edinburgh Royal College of Physicians, which excoriated him in print [3].

Thus, when do we suspect quackery, and what is the difference between orthodox plastic surgery and quackery?

When Taylor arrived into town, he was heralded by placards and handbills, and his coach was decorated with paintings of eyeballs and the motto: *Qui dat videre dat vivere* (He who gives sight, gives life) [6]. In modern days, on the outside of buses and inside the subway, we can easily find advertisements for plastic surgery clinics and their preoperative and postoperative pictures.

According to Coats, Taylor's knowledge was good; he was a shrewd observer and not without original ideas, but his actual practice was deeply tainted with the "dishonest arts" of the quack. The characteristics of charlatans are bombast, effrontery, dishonesty, and ignorance. Taylor showed all these elements except ignorance, and this is his chief condemnation [7, 8]. Thus, Coats concluded that that a knowledgeable but dishonest doctor should be condemned.

The difference between medicine and quackery is that medicine should be based on high-quality evidence, and surgery on anatomical basis, not on opinion [9]. We surgeons need to be much more honest about what we do not know.

3.3 A Plastic Surgeon Striving for Anatomical Knowledge

Wer immer strebend sich bemüht, Den können wir erlösen (He who ever strives, he can be redeemed).—*Goethe* (1749–1832)

Recently, I visited Leipzig to collaborate with a physicist who works at the Max Planck Institute. While in Leipzig, I visited Leipzig University, the home of many renowned researchers, such as August Möbius (famous for the Möbius strip) and Werner Heisenberg (known as his uncertainty principle). There, I saw the statue of Goethe (*Goethedenkmal*), which reminded me of the name of a pub (Auerbachs Keller) located in Leipzig.

My accompanying Korean researcher led me to the tavern and said that Goethe (1749–1832) was a regular at Auerbachs Keller as a university student from 1765 to 1768, so he later made the tavern a household name in *Faust*.

In *Faust*, Mephistopheles leads Dr. Faust to this pub as the first destination on their travels to show him the pleasures of the tavern (Fig. 3.3). The first edition of *Faust* contains a figure illustrating the tavern, where four men were drinking. Goethe describes the tavern here as the "devil's ride on a wine barrel:" "Doctor Faustus at this tide, Out of Auerbach's cellar did ride, Upon a wine-cask up sped he, As many a mother's son did see."

In a classic German legend, Dr. Faust was highly successful but dissatisfied with his life and made a pact with Mephistopheles, exchanging his soul for unlimited knowledge and worldly pleasures. The term "Faustian" implies an ambitious person who surrenders moral integrity to achieve power and success for a delimited term.

Nowadays, many areas of plastic surgery have bloomed, especially aesthetic plastic surgery. On

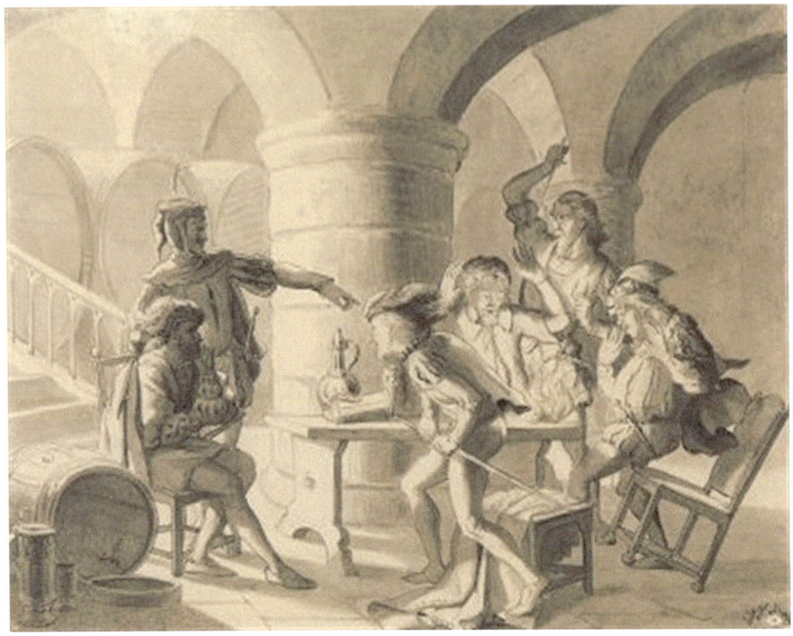

Fig. 3.3 Dr. Faust and Mephistopheles in Auerbachs Keller

the sides of buses, inside the subway, and on the Internet, we can easily find advertisements for plastic surgery clinics and their pre- and postoperative pictures. Some surgeons make presentations at a conference primarily to have pictures taken for their homepage. Some surgeons write papers just for the sake of being able to advertise that they have written articles. In certain clinics, the surgeon who owns the clinic employs a "ghost surgeon" who operates on patients instead of the surgeon who interviews the patients. I am afraid that some successful surgeons are likely to be "Faustian."

As a plastic surgeon and an anatomist, the soft tissue anatomy of the face is my lifetime project. I visited Leipzig to meet with a physicist who is working on a high resolution 7-T magnetic resonance imaging system. During my stay at his institute, he took magnetic resonance imaging scans of my face four times with different facial coils and at different resolutions, and he shared the images with me. I hope that this development will be a major milestone in imaging, but we have a long way to go.

In that tavern, with a Korean researcher who is working there, we acknowledged the work of Gotthold Lessing (1729–1781), the poet who first made Faust saved rather than damned. At the end of the work, a celestial voice was to cry: "Don't gloat. You have not triumphed over Man and Knowledge. God has not given Man the noblest of impulses only to make him eternally miserable."

As a plastic surgeon striving for anatomical knowledge, I encourage myself with the phrase, "Wer immer strebend sich bemüht, Den können wir erlösen (He who ever strives, he can be redeemed)."

3.4 Corrugator: Muscle of Empathy and Determination

> Never give in. Never give in. Never, never, never, never—in nothing, great or small, large or petty—never give in, except to convictions of honour and good sense.—Sir Winston Churchill

According to *Gray's Anatomy*, the corrugator supercilii muscle arises from the medial end of the superciliary arch and inserts into the deep surface of the skin, above the middle of the orbital arch. The corrugator draws the eyebrow downward and medially, producing the vertical wrinkles known as glabellar frowns.

These wrinkles are regarded as an expression of suffering and might produce the picture of premature aging even in a young person [10]. Thereafter, many treatments to reduce or abolish the action of corrugator have been developed and are being performed as if this muscle is "the muscle of suffering."

Then, will we be all happy without glabellar frown wrinkles if we have nonfunctioning corrugator?

We should not forget that the corrugator also contracts to prevent high sun glare, pulling the eyebrows toward the bridge of the nose, making a roof over the area above the middle corner of the eye [11].

de Wied et al. compared the electromyography (EMG) activity of the corrugator and zygomaticus in patients with disruptive behavior disorder (DBD) and normal controls. The corrugator muscle response pattern was less pronounced for patients with DBD than for the normal controls. Since lower empathy scores were obtained for patients with DBD than for normal controls, the authors concluded that facial mimicry responses to angry facial expressions were subnormal in patients with DBD, and this may be sign of a deficient early component in the process of emotional empathy [12]. Varcin et al. measured the EMG activity of the corrugator supercilii and zygomaticus major muscle in patients with schizophrenia and controls with viewed images of happy and angry facial expressions. In contrast to controls, individuals with schizophrenia showed atypical facial mimicry reactions that were not associated with any clinical features of the disorder. The authors concluded that the low EMG of corrugator and zygomaticus major is the evidence for a low-level disruption of empathizing deficits in schizophrenia [13]. Through these papers we can see that the corrugator plays a role in empathic responding and regard it as the "muscle of empathy."

This April, I met an English dermatologist at a conference and he showed me the picture of Sir Winston Churchill with his deep glabellar frowns (Fig. 3.4), which shows his image of "determination" [14]. I agreed with his opinion because Churchill perpetually demonstrated enthusiasm, determination, and optimism—if not at all times in private, then at least always in public [15].

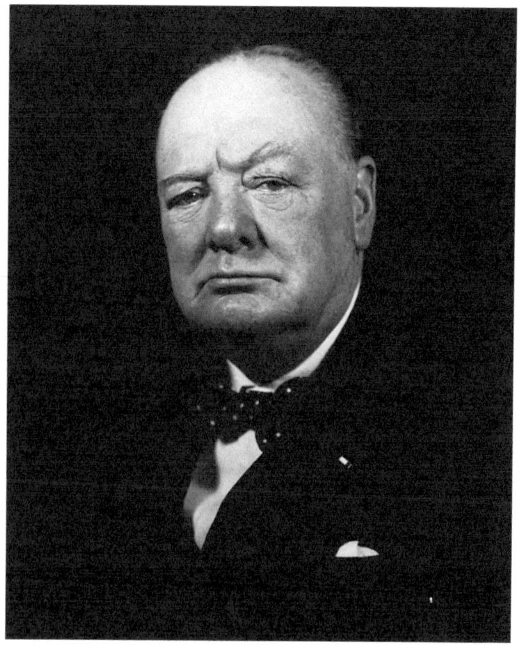

Fig. 3.4 Sir Winston Churchill (1874–1965)

The corrugator should not be despised as a "muscle of suffering." It should be respected as a "muscle of empathy and determination."

3.5 An Anatomist's Contribution to Blepharoptosis Surgery: 100th Anniversary of the Whitnall Ligament

Most plastic surgeons or ophthalmologists who deal with blepharoptosis are expected to have heard about the Whitnall ligament. In *Gray's Anatomy, 39th Edition* [16], Fig. 41.5, which shows sagittal and horizontal sections of orbital fascia, is reproduced from Whitnall [17].

Despite his famous name, his publications or his careers are not widely known to many plastic surgeons. I have carried out a survey about the publications and careers of Dr. Whitnall among Korean plastic surgeons. Most of the respondents knew about the Whitnall ligament; however, their knowledge of Dr. Whitnall himself was rather superficial.

This article is not a bibliography of Dr. Whitnall. It aimed to elucidate who he was, what he wrote, and how he contributed to blepharoptosis surgery.

Anatomy of the Human Orbit and Accessory Organs of Vision was first published in 1922, and its second edition in 1932 (Fig. 3.5) [17]. I first encountered this famous book in 1991 just after my completion of plastic surgery residency. I borrowed the book from the British Council Library in Seoul, South Korea, and cited it in some of my articles, including one published 1998 in the *British Journal of Plastic Surgery*. According to a

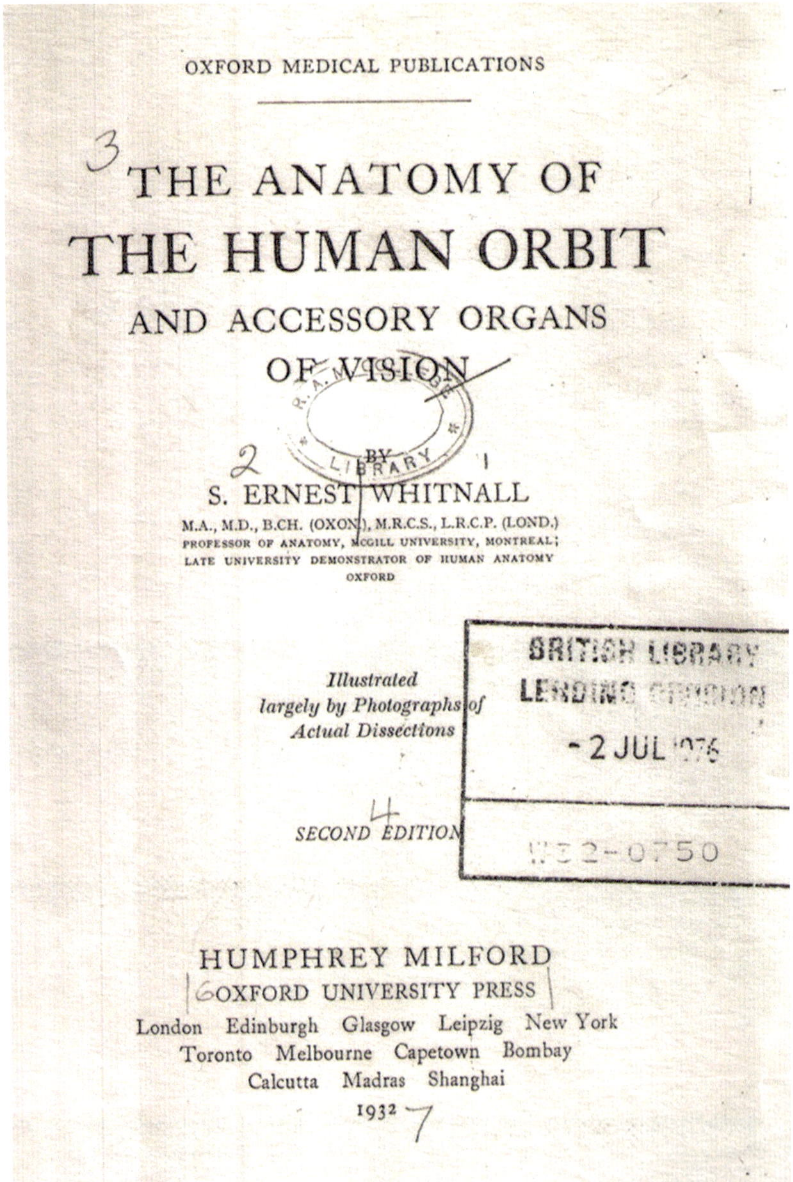

OXFORD MEDICAL PUBLICATIONS

THE ANATOMY OF
THE HUMAN ORBIT
AND ACCESSORY ORGANS
OF VISION

BY
S. ERNEST WHITNALL
M.A., M.D., B.CH. (OXON.), M.R.C.S., L.R.C.P. (LOND.)
PROFESSOR OF ANATOMY, MCGILL UNIVERSITY, MONTREAL;
LATE UNIVERSITY DEMONSTRATOR OF HUMAN ANATOMY
OXFORD

Illustrated largely by Photographs of Actual Dissections

SECOND EDITION

HUMPHREY MILFORD
OXFORD UNIVERSITY PRESS
London Edinburgh Glasgow Leipzig New York
Toronto Melbourne Capetown Bombay
Calcutta Madras Shanghai
1932

Fig. 3.5 Anatomy of the Human Orbit and Accessory Organs of Vision by Whitnall in 1932

Google search, the book has been cited 281 times, which is more frequent than *Wolff's Anatomy of the Eye and Orbit* [18], which is cited 211 times.

Although the structure so-called Whitnall ligament is described in his book, it is first described in his article titled, "On a ligament acting as a check to the action of the levator palpebrae superioris muscle [19]," in 1911, exactly 100 years ago.

In this article, he described, "The superficial layer of the fascial sheath of the levator palpebrae superioris is very thin over the posterior half of the muscle, but traced forwards is seen to become gradually thicker, until just before the levator expands to form the palpebral aponeurosis, the overlying sheath of connective tissue becomes condensed to form a ligament which stretches transversely across the muscle and extends laterally to the walls of the orbit on either side, to which it has the following attachments: on the inner side the main connection is with the pulley of the superior oblique muscle, but behind this some fibres can be traced directly to the bone, whilst in front of the pulley a well-marked slip of fascia passes forward to bridge across the supraorbital notch, being inserted into the bone at either side of it. Externally, the ligament is fixed to the capsule of the lacrymal gland, and also directly to the bone. The ligament lies free above the aponeurosis for the most part, but laterally a few strands of tissue connect the two."

He first described the ligament that stretches transversely across the muscle, which was later renamed as "superior transverse ligament of Whitnall" by other surgeons [20–23].

In a memoriam in 1950 in the *Journal of Anatomy* [24], the details of his life was revealed. Samuel Ernest Whitnall was born on 1876, at Eccles in Lancashire, United Kingdom. He obtained his doctorate MD and BCh degrees at Magdalen College, Oxford, in 1905, and he worked there from 1908 to 1919 as a demonstrator of anatomy. In 1919, he was called to the McGill University as professor of anatomy and spent the next 15 years in Canada, where, in 1921, the *Anatomy of the Orbit* was published. It was in 1935 that Whitnall returned to England to occupy the chair of anatomy position at Bristol University, a post that he held until his retirement in 1941. On February 19, 1950, at the age of 74, he died.

I have tried to find some relics belonging to him, such as books or instruments he used while working at Oxford University, McGill University, and Bristol University but without success.

Recently, I obtained a booklet published in 1933 titled, *The Study of Anatomy: Written for the Medical Student* [25] by Dr., Whitnall (Fig. 3.6). It was written as a student's guide-a vade mecum. It was a most attractive and extremely sane piece of writing, and *JAMA*'s book notice wrote, "The students who read it will be influenced through it to be happier and sounder doctors, wiser friends and better gentlemen [26]." After reading this, I was convinced that he was a good teacher as well as a famous anatomy professor.

The condensation of the levator sheath Dr. Whitnall described is now widely known as the "superior transverse ligament of Whitnall," which is an unassailable landmark in blepharoptosis surgery. Dr. Whitnall should be remembered as a pioneering anatomist and a fine teacher. He left an indelible mark on clinical anatomy with his masterpiece, *Anatomy of the Human Orbit*, which is still being cited in many articles.

There is an Oriental saying, "Tigers leave fine hides when they die, and people leave their name on their departure." Dr. Whitnall has surely left his good name, which will be remembered for generations to come.

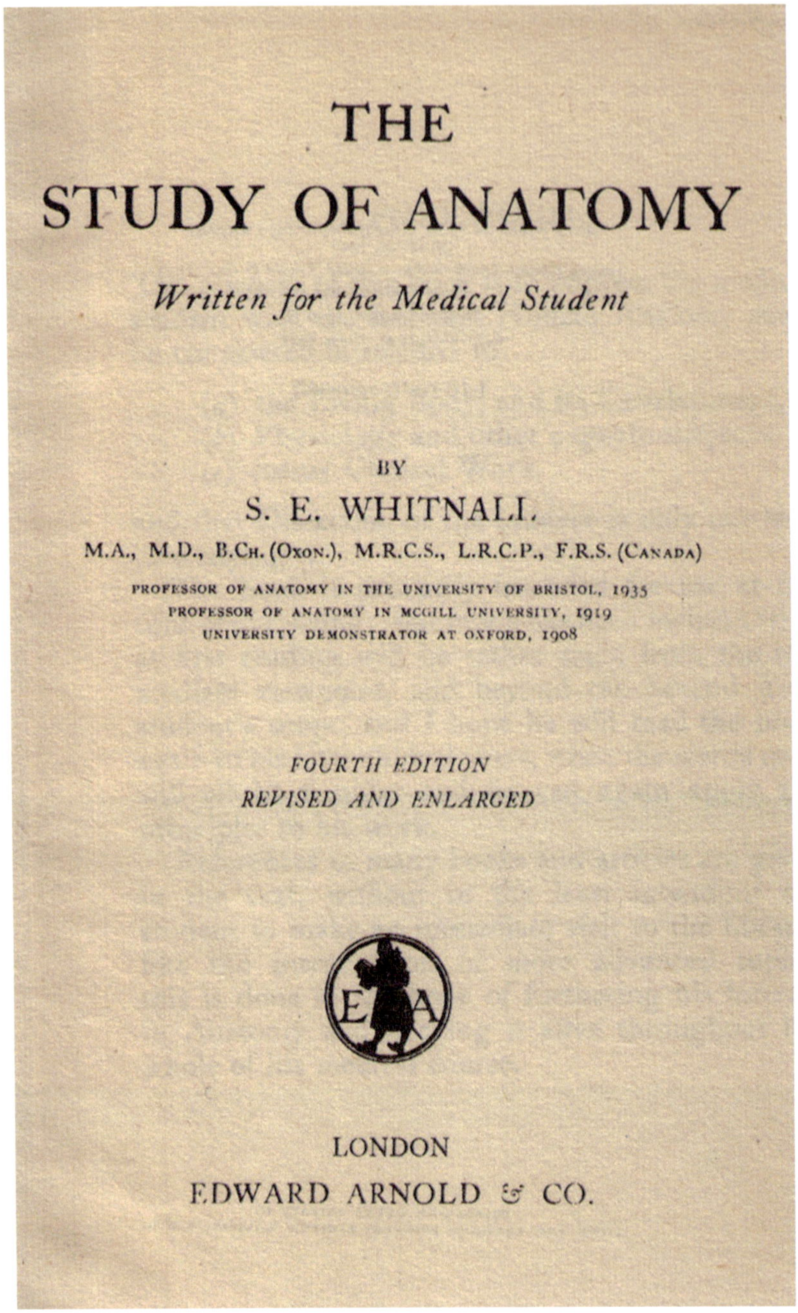

THE

STUDY OF ANATOMY

Written for the Medical Student

BY

S. E. WHITNALL

M.A., M.D., B.CH. (OXON.), M.R.C.S., L.R.C.P., F.R.S. (CANADA)

PROFESSOR OF ANATOMY IN THE UNIVERSITY OF BRISTOL, 1935
PROFESSOR OF ANATOMY IN MCGILL UNIVERSITY, 1919
UNIVERSITY DEMONSTRATOR AT OXFORD, 1908

FOURTH EDITION
REVISED AND ENLARGED

LONDON
EDWARD ARNOLD & CO.

Fig. 3.6 The Study of Anatomy: Written for the Medical Student by Whitnall in 1933

3.6 Form Follows Function, Function Follows Form

> Whether it be the sweeping eagle in his flight, or the open apple blossom, the toiling work-horse, the blithe swan, the branching oak, the winding stream at its base, the drifting clouds, over all the coursing sun, form ever follows function, and this is the law.—Louis Sullivan

"Form follows function," a famous maxim coined by architect Louis Sullivan (1856–1924), articulates the principle that the shape of a building or object should directly relate to its intended function or purpose. This principle has been a guiding light of twentieth-century modernist architecture and industrial design.

He wrote "Where function does not change, form does not change" and stated that "It is the pervading law of all things organic and inorganic, of all things physical and metaphysical, of all things human and all things superhuman, of all true manifestations of the head, of the heart, of the soul, that the life is recognizable in its expression, that form ever follows function. This is the law [27]."

This credo has been applied in different fields, including product design, software engineering, and automobile design.

In biology, this principle means that the form and shape of a body structure is related to the function of that structure. The systems of the body do not have structures that are planned in advance; instead, over the course of evolution, structures change to allow novel ways of functioning, and organisms with those structural innovations survive to produce the next generation [28].

As a surgical anatomist, I believe that human structures have been structured according to the functions their associated with use, and that form is altered by the required function (form follows function), as in Lamarckian evolution.

As a plastic surgeon, I think otherwise. I know that changing the form can improve the function (function follows form). For example, blepharoplasty improves peripheral vision in aging eyelids, jaw surgery results in precise occlusion in malocclusion patients, and palatoplasty is necessary for speech in children with cleft palate.

Recently, I enjoyed the movie "Ando Tadao," a documentary about a self-taught Japanese architect characterized by "critical regionalism." Ando Tadao (1941–) said: "Dwelling in a house is not only a functional issue, but also a spiritual one. In a spiritual place, people find peace in their heart (*kokoro*), as in their homeland."

In the Church of the Light in Ibaraki, Osaka, light enters from behind the altar from a cross cut in the concrete wall that extends vertically from the floor to ceiling and horizontally from wall to wall, aligning perfectly with the joints in the concrete (Fig. 3.7). In the Water Temple in Honpukuji, a statue of the Buddha is hidden behind two concrete walls, and only the roof, a pond, can be seen. However, it was built such that a ray of light hits the statue at the hour of sunset. Ando's buildings are certainly exceptional to the credo "form follows function," as their form is designed to induce a new function.

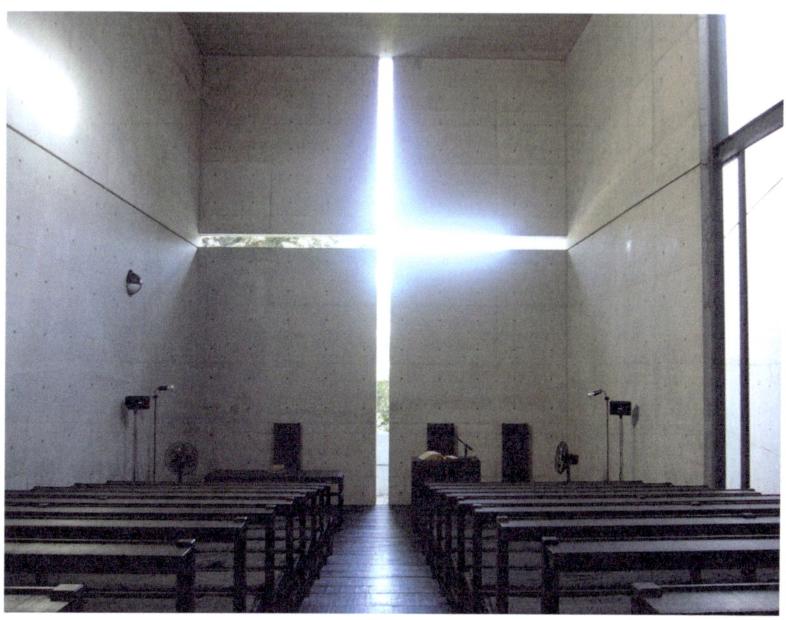

Fig. 3.7 Church of the Light in Ibaraki, Osaka

Plastic surgeons are continuing to develop new methods to improve their techniques for changing the form of the human body. The human body, like a dwelling place, is not only a functional issue but also a spiritual one. We should consider patients' spirit, as well as their body, and remember that function follows form.

3.7 Surgeon-Friendly Anatomy

> Doctors without anatomy are similar to moles: they work in the dark and their daily tasks are mole hills [29].—*Friedrich Tiedemann* (1781–1861)

Ever since submitting my first anatomy paper to the *Journal of Craniofacial Surgery* just over 20 years ago [30], I have been confident that my anatomy papers would be useful to my plastic surgeon colleagues. The reason for my pride was because I started every study to fulfill the curiosity arisen from my own surgical experiences. In almost every paper, I wrote the following phrase: "The aim of this study is to elucidate the precise anatomical detail of (a structure) relating to (an operation)."

However, my belief of "user-friendly papers" may not have been so correct. Recently, I have received a letter from an American board-certified plastic surgeon. He sent me a picture of his sub-superficial muscular aponeurotic system (SMAS) dissection and asked me the name of a strand cephalad to the zygomatic major muscle as it goes under the orbicularis oculi muscle. He also asked me if it is a sensory nerve. As I could not identify the nerve within the photograph, I sent him a paper from my previous work, which I thought would answer his question. Cheek and lower eyelid en bloc from the bone was harvested and dissected from the periosteum to find the branches of facial nerve in the study [31]. Several days later, there was a discussion regarding the anatomical structure with him, face to face. He said that he could not find the answer to his question as the paper was "not user friendly." Since he found the branch in sub-SMAS dissection, the topographical anatomy, though clearly showing the most distal branches deep to the muscles, could not quench his thirst for the surgical anatomy.

After the discussion, I searched for the "surgeon-friendly anatomy" and answered myself that surgeon-friendly anatomy should have several surgical perspectives.

The structures should be localized in topography relating to the anatomic landmarks. A landmark is anything that helps us know where we are. If we're sailing from Plymouth to New York, the Statue of Liberty will be the landmark that lets us know we're in the right port. Similarly, an anatomic landmark is a morphologic feature of the anatomy that is readily recognizable and may be used as a reference point for other body features [32]. The structures should be demonstrated in layer-by-layer dissections along the surgical plane as "the field real." Additionally, the depth of the structure should be displayed using histology or tomography.

Since facial appearance, including several intraoral and extraoral parameters, varies in different ethnic origins [33–35], transracial anatomy should also be in consideration to enhance the safety of the patients in different races.

Finally, I hope my further anatomy papers move "from strength to strength" (a medieval homiletic phrase) with the constructive feedback given from the plastic surgeon colleagues.

References

1. Bell A. The anatomy of Astley. Lancet. 2007;369:1510.
2. Phitayakorn R, Lachman N. Getting back together after a break-up: relationship advice for anatomists and surgeons. Clin Anat. 2015;28:931–4.
3. Gilman SL. Making the body beautiful: a cultural history of aesthetic surgery a cultural history of aesthetic surgery. Princeton: Princeton University Press; 2000.
4. Jameson E. The natural history of quackery. London: Michael Joseph; 1961.
5. Porter R. Health for sale: quackery in England, 1660–1850. Manchester: Manchester University Press; 1989.
6. Albert D. Men of vision: lives of notable figures in ophthalmology. San Diego: Harcourt College Pub; 1993.
7. Coats G. The chevalier Taylor. London: Adlard; 1915.

8. Jackson DM. Bach, Handel, and the chevalier Taylor. Med Hist. 1968;12:385–93.
9. McCartney M. The difference between medicine and quackery is that medicine is based on evidence, not opinion. http://www.telegraph.co.uk/news/health/11037159/The-difference-between-medicine-and-quackery-is-that-medicine-is-based-on-evidence-not-opinion.html. Assessed 18 Jan 2018.
10. Bartolin C, Lalo J. The corrugator supercilii muscle. A review. Morphologie. 2008;92:145–53.
11. Eye, human. Encyclopedia Britannica 2006 Ultimate Reference Suite DVD. 2009. Accessed 24 Apr 2016.
12. de Wied M, van Boxtel A, Zaalberg R, et al. Facial EMG responses to dynamic emotional facial expressions in boys with disruptive behavior disorders. J Psychiatr Res. 2006;40:112–21.
13. Varcin KJ, Bailey PE, Henry JD. Empathic deficits in schizophrenia: the potential role of rapid facial mimicry. J Int Neuropsychol Soc. 2010;16:621–9.
14. Payne CR. Multi mini botulinum. In: Presented at masters world aesthetic congress, London: 2016.
15. The Churchill Centre. Churchill: leader and statesman. http://www.winstonchurchill.org/the-life-of-churchill/life/414-churchill-leader-and-statesman. Accessed 24 Apr 2016.
16. Standring S. Gray's anatomy: the anatomical basis of clinical practice. 39th ed. Edinburgh: Churchill Livingstone; 2005.
17. Whitnall SE. Anatomy of the human orbit and accessory organs of vision. 2nd ed. London: Oxford University Press; 1932.
18. Bron AJ, Tripathi RC, Tripathi BJ. Wolff's anatomy of the eye and orbit. 8th ed. London: A Hodder Arnold Publication; 1997.
19. Whitnall SE. On a ligament acting as a check to the action of the levator palpebrae superioris muscle. J Anat Physiol. 1911;45:131–9.
20. Anderson RL, Dixon RS. The role of Whitnall ligament in ptosis surgery. Arch Ophthalmol. 1979;95:705–7.
21. Lukas JR, Priglinger S, Denk M, et al. Two fibromuscular transverse ligaments related to the levator palpebrae superioris: Whitnall's ligament and an intermuscular transverse ligament. Anat Rec. 1996;246:415–22.
22. Ettl A, Priglinger S, Kramer J, et al. Functional anatomy of the levator palpebrae superioris muscle and its connective tissue system. Br J Ophthalmol. 1996;80:702–8.
23. Codère F, Tucker NA, Renaldi B. The anatomy of Whitnall ligament. Ophthalmology. 1995;102:2016–9.
24. In Memoriam: Samuel Ernest Whitnall, M.A., M.D., B.Ch. (Oxon), M.R.C.S., L.R.C.P. (Lond.). J Anat. 1950;84:395–396.
25. Whitnall SE. The study of anatomy: written for the medical student. 2nd ed. London: Edward Arnold; 1933.
26. Whitnall SE. The study of anatomy written for the medical student. JAMA. 1934;102:2139.
27. Sullivan LH. The tall office building artistically considered. Lippincott's Magazine; 1896. p. 403–9.
28. Fowler S, Roush R, Wise J. Concept of biology. 1st ed. OpenStax College: Houston; 2013.
29. University of Heidelberg Digital Library. Friedrich Tiedemann. http://www.ub.uni-heidelberg.de/Englisch/helios/digi/anatomie/tiedemann.html. Assessed 7 Feb 2016.
30. Hwang K, Kim JH, Baik SH. Thickness map of parietal bone in Korean adults. J Craniofac Surg. 1997;8:208–12.
31. Hwang K, Lee DK, Lee EJ, et al. Innervation of the lower eyelid in relation to blepharoplasty and midface lift: clinical observation and cadaveric study. Ann Plast Surg. 2001;47:1–5.
32. Medical Dictionary for the Dental Professions. Anatomic landmark. http://medical-dictionary.thefreedictionary.com/anatomic+landmark. Accessed 5 Jan 2016.
33. Owens EG, Goodacre CJ, Loh PL, et al. A multicenter interracial study of facial appearance. Part 1: a comparison of extraoral parameters. Int J Prosthodont. 2002;15:273–82.
34. Owens EG, Goodacre CJ, Loh PL, et al. A multicenter interracial study of facial appearance. Part 2: a comparison of intraoral parameters. Int J Prosthodont. 2002;15:283–8.
35. Packiriswamy V, Kumar P, Rao M. Identification of facial shape by applying golden ratio to the facial measurements: an interracial study in Malaysian population. N Am J Med Sci. 2012;4:624–9.

4 What Is "Beauty" Which Plastic Surgeon Pursue?

4.1 Queen Nefertiti's Eye and the Beauty of Incompleteness

When I stayed in Germany for a month, I visited the Neues Museum located in Berlin. There, I saw the bust of Queen Nefertiti (1370–1330 BC), the royal wife of the Egyptian Pharaoh Amenhotep IV and mother of the boy king Tutankhamun (Fig. 4.1). Since the profile of the bust appears on the title page of a scientific journal and the technique of botulinum toxin injection is used to create a similar appearance to her elongated, thin neck, I enjoyed looking at it carefully.

The bust was life-sized (47 cm) and her face was almost intact and symmetrical. It was made from a limestone core and covered with painted stucco layers. She had a long neck, elegantly arched brows, and eyelids outlined in black. Her inner canthi descended abruptly and abutted the upper lid, forming epicanthal folds. She had high cheekbones, a slender nose, and an enigmatic smile around her red lips and slender neck. However, I could not see the pupil on her left eye, as the background of the eye socket was just unadorned limestone.

This bust was found in 1912 at Amarna in the studio of the sculptor Tuthmosis, a royal artist who made statues or paintings of the king and a few nobles. Her missing left eye has been an archaeological mystery, with no satisfactory consensus regarding possible explanations.

An ophthalmologist speculated that she might have suffered from an ophthalmic infection and a dermatologist suspected uveitis from Behçet disease [1]. However, these theories were abandoned when new figures were found showing the queen, some at an older age, with both eyes in perfectly good condition. Another opinion is that the artist's work was interrupted and he left the studio, never to return [2]. Yet another theory is that the bust was a model (*modello*) for official portraits and was used by the master sculptor for teaching his pupils how to carve the internal structure of the eye, and thus, the left iris was not added [3].

This mysterious eye reminded me a famous Chinese idiom; "Adding eyes to a painted dragon (畵龍點睛)." The expression comes from a Chinese legend. According to the legend, a great painter named Zhang Sengyou (張僧繇, 502–549) of the Southern and Northern Dynasties painted four dragons on the wall of a temple, where he spent his leisure time. People were dumfounded when they saw that he had not painted the eyes, and asked him why (Fig. 4.2). He told them that if he had painted the eyes, the dragons would fly into the skies.

K. Hwang, *Good Physician, Good Plastic Surgeon*, https://doi.org/10.1007/978-981-97-1864-1_4

People did not believe him and urged him to add the eyes. As soon as he painted the eyes of the two dragons, dark clouds covered the sky, followed by thunder and lightning. The dragons then freed themselves from the wall and flew to the sky.

I think Tuthmosis thoroughly understood "the beauty of incompleteness" and therefore did not complete the "final touch." Like the old legend of the Chinese painter, if the great sculptor had completed Nefertiti's left eye, she might have blinked her eyes and animated all of her facial muscles, like Galatea in Ovid's *Metamorphoses*.

Artists and plastic surgeons have the common trait of pursuing completeness but never reaching it. Artists express their imagination by making sculptures or paintings. Plastic surgeons express their imagination on patients' living bodies. Both of these tasks are a difficult way to pursue completeness, and one must take a moment to stop just before reaching "completeness."

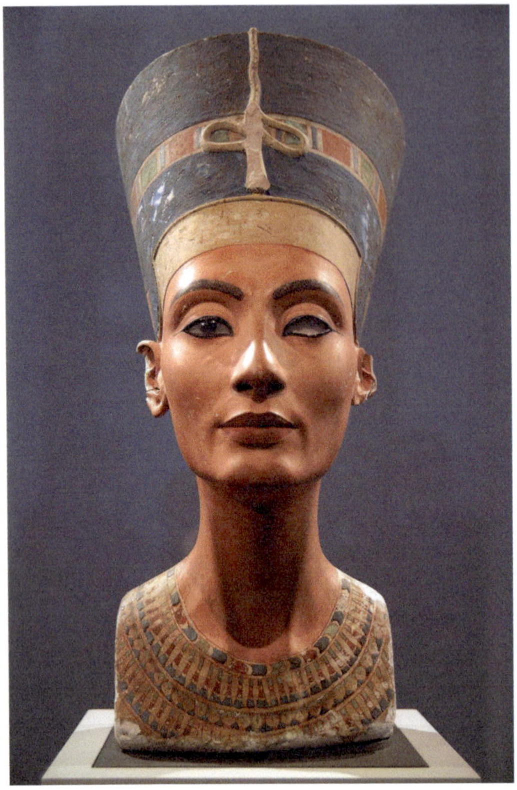

Fig. 4.1 Bust of Queen Nefertiti (1370–1330 BC), Neues Museum, Berlin

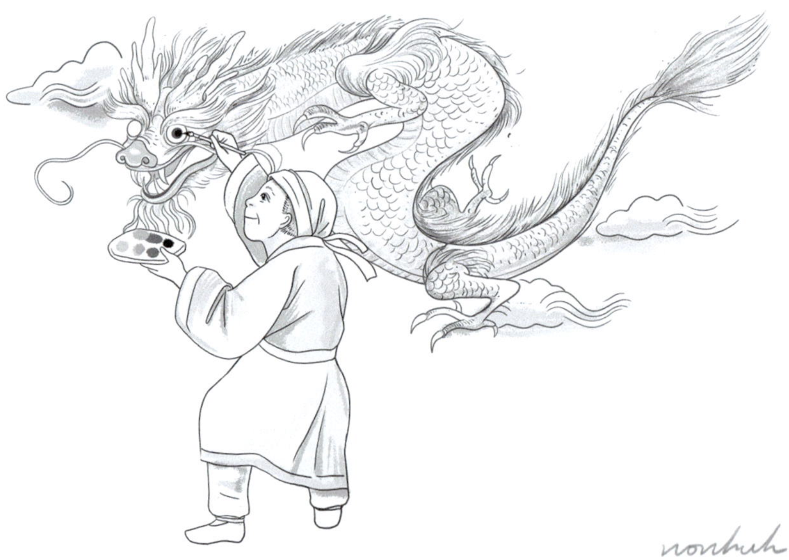

Fig. 4.2 Adding eyes to a painted dragon (畵龍點睛). [Illustration was drawn by Hye Won Hu, M.F.A. (1986–)]

4.2 The Faces that Launched a Thousand Ships and Gathered Thousands of Horses and Soldiers

Was this the face that launch'd a thousand ships/ And burnt the topless towers of Ilium?— Christopher Marlowe (1564–1593)

Who was the most beautiful woman in world history? Most people would agree that she was Helen of Troy from Greek mythology. Although she was believed to be the daughter of the god Zeus and the human Leda, fragments of her putative biography can be found from classical authors, especially Homer *(Iliad and Odyssey)*.

She is generally described as "the face that launched a thousand ships" because the Trojan war was mounted on her behalf. She was also called Helen of Sparta, as she was the wife of King Menelaus of Mycenaean Sparta. Paris, the Prince of Troy, abducted her. Accordingly, Menelaus led a war against Troy, which resulted in the destruction of Troy and the rescue of Helen. It is widely believed that the Trojan war actually happened, but it is not certain whether Helen of Troy really existed.

Christopher Marlowe (1564–1593), an English playwright of the Elizabethan era, first used the term "the face that launched a thousand ships" in his "The Tragical History of the Life and Death of Doctor Faustus" (1588–1592): "Was this the face that launch'd a thousand ships/ And burnt the topless towers of Ilium?" This verse is still used to describe the unsurpassed beauty of Helen of Troy, as well as the beauty of any woman [4].

Because of Helen's long-lasting fame, as portrayed in many movies and dramas, we plastic surgeons are curious about the appearance of her face.

The *Iliad* and the *Odyssey* refer to Helen as "white-armed" (λευκλευος; *leuklenos)*, "long-dressed" (ταυπεπλος; *tanýpe- plos)*, and "lovely-haired" (καλλκομος; *kallíkomos)*, which are not particularly descriptive. In a surviving fragment (Fragment 23) of a lyric poem by Sappho (630–570 BC), she is described as "jαυθή" (xanthḗ). This word is usually translated as "blonde-haired." She is also described as "κυαυώπιζ" (kyanôpis), which means "having gleaming blue eyes" in other lyric poems. A description gives the appearance of Helen and her brothers Castor and Pollux: "As for Castor and Pollux, he learned from the Trojans what they were like and how they looked: they were twins, blond haired, large eyed, fair complexioned, and well-built with trim bodies. Helen resembled Castor and Pollux. She was beautiful, ingenuous, and charming. Her legs were the best; her mouth the cutest. There was a beauty-mark between her eyebrows [4]."

In ancient China, a similar legendary beauty really existed and thousands of horses and soldiers gathered on her behalf. Bao Si (褒姒, 792–779 BC) as the concubine of the King You of Zhou (周幽王, 795–771 BC) (Fig. 4.3). She was considered to be one of the most beautiful

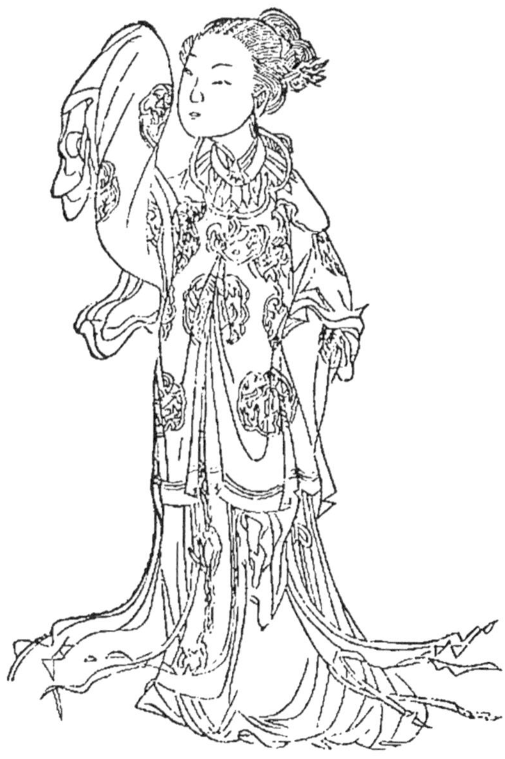

Fig. 4.3 An eighteenth-century depiction of Bao Si (褒姒, 792–779 BC), in "Yan XY (顏希源). Baimei xinyong tuzhuan (百美新詠圖傳, Illustrated biographies of one hundred beauties with new verses). Nanjing, China: Jiyexuan (集腋軒), 1792. 顏希源.百美新.南京:集腋軒, 1792"

Chinese women ever. She was stunningly gorgeous woman and had an icy beauty. No matter how many precious Teasing the seiginors with beacon fire (烽火戲諸侯). Shanghai, China: Shanghai people's fine arts publishing house, 2008" clothes and jewellery the king gave her, or how many fancy palaces were built for her, or how many jesters were hired to make her laugh, she never smiled. Even after the king gave her the queen's crown, she still was a "lady of ice" with a "poker face." Since she was still melancholy, the King offered a thousand ounces of gold to anyone who could make her laugh. Someone at his cabinet suggested lighting the warning beacons usually used to summon armies from the surrounding vassal states in times of danger. The feudal lords with their armies and horses duly arrived at the court only to find that Bao Si laughed at them (Fig. 4.4). In order to make her laugh, the King continued to abuse the system of warning beacons, thereby losing the trust of the feudal lords. The former queen's father was angry about the deposition of his daughter and grandson and attacked the King in conjunction with nomads. The King called for the nobles with the beacons but none came, as they no longer trusted him. Tragically, the King was killed and Bao Si committed suicide.

Feng Menglong (馮夢龍, 1574–1646), a Chinese historian, described the appearance of Bao Si in his "Dong zhou lieguozhi" (東周列國志) [5].

"She had bright eyes and clean eyebrows, red lips and white teeth."

Her hair was abundant like a bleak cloud and her fingers seemed to have been cut with jade. Her appearance was just like flowers or the moon [5].

Through the above descriptions, it is thought that legendary beauties have been imagined in many different ways throughout history. Because the descriptions of the facial beauty of them are metaphysical in old literatures without concreate records nor specific pictures, people of each era have remade legendary beauties to match their own standards of perfect beauty. Today, we are also free to imagine Helen or Bao Si just as every other generation has been free to imagine them before us. Bao Si depicted in twenty-first century drawing is quite different from that depicted in eighteenth century drawing (Figs. 4.3 and 4.4).

However, it is striking that when describing these beauties, historians and poets focused on the eyes, eyebrows, hair, lips, and teeth, which compose the elements of the face. Modern plastic surgeons can manipulate and improve the appearance of these components by plastic surgery.

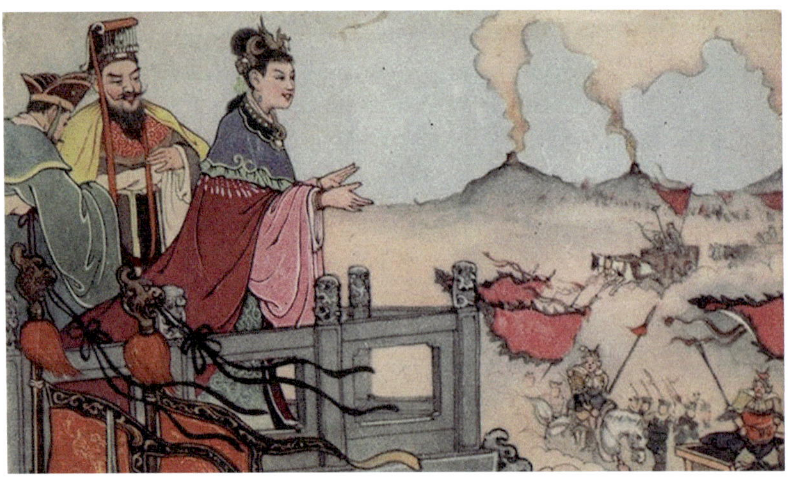

Fig. 4.4 A twenty-first-century depiction (2018) of Bao Si. In "Wang Jing (王井)

4.3 Metamorphosis from an Ugly Girl to a Beauty

The desire to have a beautiful appearance has been deeply rooted in human beings in all ages and countries. In this era, many women live with an intense interest in their appearance due to the social importance placed on appearance. Some women even suffer from an obsession for a beautiful face and slim body in order to achieve success in employment or marriages, without the discrimination and disadvantages faced by women perceived to be ugly.

Women are often unable to escape from the social emphasis on beauty and the Cinderella complex due to the influence of the mass media and the sociocultural phenomena of discrimination against women based on their appearance and commercialization of women's appearance. The causes of these sociocultural phenomena may be complex, but it is difficult to ignore the influence of children's books and animations of old tales that people encounter in childhood. For many years, the female protagonists in children's fairy tale books and animations have been mostly beautiful-looking princesses, whereas most of the ugly-looking women were witches, cannibals, or evil stepmothers, who symbolized evil or greed, or their daughters.

Is there really no fairy tale in the world where an ugly woman is the main character? In the catalog of international tale types Aarne–Thompson–Uther Index (ATU) based on the Aarne/Thompson system, one (ATU 711. "The Beautiful and the Ugly Twin") has an ugly female protagonist [6]. This tale has been handed down in Europe.

Another tale that is not included in the ATU index has been passed down in Jewish communities living in predominantly Islamic countries, such as Morocco, Yemen, Iraq, and Persia: "The Ugly Wise Girl." In this story. The daughter of a rabbi born with a beast's face finally undergoes a metamorphosis [7].

The summary of the tale is as follows:

Once upon a time in Constantinople, there lived a girl with a face that resembled a beast. The girl, the only daughter of a rabbi, had a very ugly face, but she was wiser than anyone. Because of her ugliness, her parents locked her up in the attic of the school so that no one else could see her. She received food through a small hole in the door. A young male student from a distant province came to this city to study at the rabbi's school. This young man studied in a room next to where the girl was locked up in the attic. When he was in trouble because he was unable to answer the rabbi's questions, he would find notes with the correct answers written on them. When he realized that the notes were written by the rabbi's daughter in the attic, he was deeply moved by her wisdom and knowledge and finally made a marriage proposal to her. Her parents initially opposed the idea but later agreed to their marriage. At the wedding ceremony, the groom couldn't see the bride's face, which was covered with a veil. The groom was shocked to see her face on the first night; however, he spent the night with her to keep his marriage vows. When he started on a long journey, she asked for a love token for the child to be born, and a ring and prayer shawl were handed over to the bride. The bride gave birth to a son, but she couldn't raise him, and her parents raised their grandson instead. The son grew up and went to school, where he was teased by his friends for being a fatherless child. After learning the secret of his birth, the son met his mother, who was still staying in the attic. He realized that his mother endured hard times studying the Torah, and the son learned Torah from his knowledgeable and intelligent mother. One day the son asked his mother about the whereabouts of his father and started a journey to his father, carrying the ring and prayer shawl that his father had left behind. After several months of journeys, he arrived in the country where his father lived and entered the synagogue there. When the rabbi saw the prayer shawl embroidered with his son's name, he recognized that this boy was his own bloodline. The son persuaded his father to return to live together with them since his mother was prettiest and wisest person in the world. Hearing his son's words, the rabbi thought that a miracle might have happened, and told him he would return home soon. On the way back to his homeland, the son met an old man, who gave him a mysterious drug. The old man told the son to apply it to his mother's face. Upon returning home, his mother applied it on the face and became as beautiful as the sun and the moon. She prayed to God with thanks for giving her a miracle drug through the hand of Prophet Elijah (Fig. 4.5). When the father returned home, he realized that a miracle had indeed happened. This wise son brought peace and happiness to his parents' home.

In this story, the protagonist's transformation was a rite of passage for women entering a society (male-centered, patriarchal society) after enduring trials and pains. The rabbi's daughter was not able to complete a sequence of rites of separation, transition, and incorporation at her birth, and her parents did not assimilate her into their family structure. For this "ugly girl," the marriage ceremony could not function as a rite of incorporation because she was abandoned by her husband on their wedding night and then experienced a transitional period in an enclosed room without integration into society through her husband. After her transformation into a beautiful woman, she was able to complete her rite of passage from separation through transition to incorporation [8]. She overcame her hardships through her wisdom and belief in God. The rabbi's daughter transformed her appearance, thanks to her son, who obtained a bottle of miraculous water from the Prophet Elijah.

In our era, fortunately, women do not have to rely upon God's grace and miraculous water from

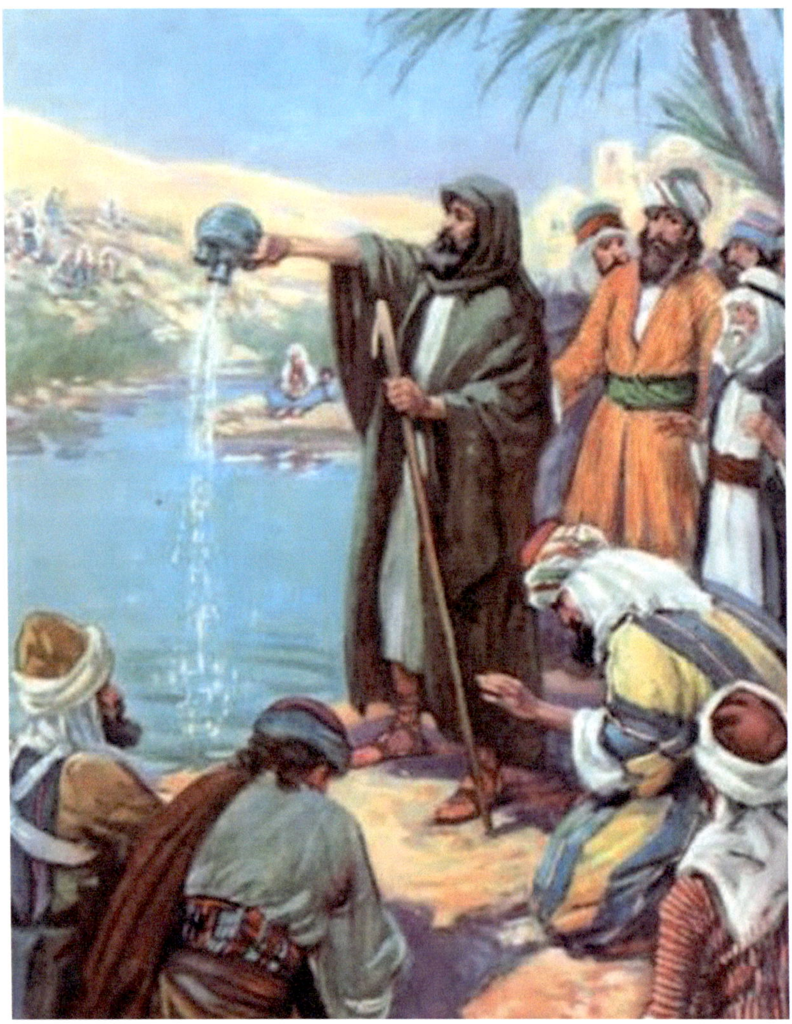

Fig. 4.5 Elijah poured the salt in the water and blessed it. "So the waters were healed unto this day, according to the saying of Elisha which he spake" (2 Kings 2:22)

the Prophet. Instead, plastic surgeons express their imagination by modifying the living bodies of patients like poets or writers of tales expresses themselves through their writings or poems [9]. If women have free will to transform themselves, many miraculous plastic surgical procedures can replace Elijah's water, opening a door to the corresponding rites of passage.

4.4 The Young Lady Who Made the Old Man Forget His Age

Have you ever met a woman who is so beautiful that you completely forget your age and take a risk to please her? If you have and felt your heart beating, you are young regardless of your age.

Attractive women have been found to have advantages over unattractive women. For instance, attractive ladies in distress received more offers of aid than unattractive ladies in distress, and physical attractiveness played a part in inducing aiding behavior [10, 11].

I introduce an example of a young lady who made an old man completely forget his age and aid her about 1500 years ago in Korea.

On a narrow coastal road along the East Sea of a peninsula, a new provincial governor and his party were traveling to a new post. They had left the capital the day before or very early that morning and were now making leisurely progress to the north. They stopped for lunch at the foot of the cliff. The governor was on horseback, and his beautiful young wife, Lady Suro, rode along—perhaps in a carriage. They paused to admire the splendid scenery. It might have been Lady Suro's first journey out of the capital city. She was struck by the scenery before her, the sparkling East Sea and the rocky cliffs. What she saw high up on the cliff, near the very top, was a beautiful flower in full bloom, perhaps a red azalea. It almost took her breath away. "Oh, I wish I could have that flower! I would give anything, if someone would only get it for me!" she said loudly. The attendants, in the meantime, muttered among themselves loudly enough for Lady Suro to hear: "That cliff is clearly a thousand feet high, and there are neither trails nor any tracks leading to where the flower is. It is impossible for anybody to get it."

At this point, an old man appeared leading a cow. Upon hearing the request made by the governor's beautiful young wife, he approached and offered to clamber up the rocky cliff and pick the flower for her (Fig. 4.6):

If you would let me leave
The cattle tethered to the brown rocks,
And feel no shame for me,
I would pluck and dedicate the flower [12]*!*

Why did he say he would climb to pluck the flower only if she would "feel no shame for (him)"? Was it because he felt self-conscious about his age, his weathered skin cracked and scaled with dirt, and his face blackened and wrinkled from too much exposure to the sun?

The "Flower Dedication Song," composed of four lines, has been passed down to us across the silence of more than a thousand years, and yet it shows us a living, breathing picture. In this brief ancient poem, through the painstakingly restored words, we can listen in on the living voices of the beautiful Lady Suro and an unnamed man who, though old in years, is still young at heart. There is almost a mythic quality to the homage he pays her, a kind of exemplary homage that has always been paid to beautiful, young women by ordinary, aged men.

The story of Lady Suro of Silla (in the reign of King Seongdeok, 702–737) was recorded in the *Surobuin* section of the *Samgungnyusa* (Memorabilia of the Three Kingdoms) written by Iryon (1206–1289), a Buddhist monk. The *Samgungnyusa* was assembled as a supplement to Kim Pu-sik's *Samguk Sagi.* The *Samgungnyusa* draws together a wide assortment of myths, legends, genealogies, histories, Buddhist tales, observations by the compiler, and other materials [13].

Researchers in the field of Korean literature concluded that the statement "the beauty of Suro cannot be compared with any other things in the world" implies that the beauty of Suro is much more sensual and voluptuous in terms of physical meaning [14, 15].

Reading this poem, I remember the scene in *A Portrait of the Artist as a Young Man* where

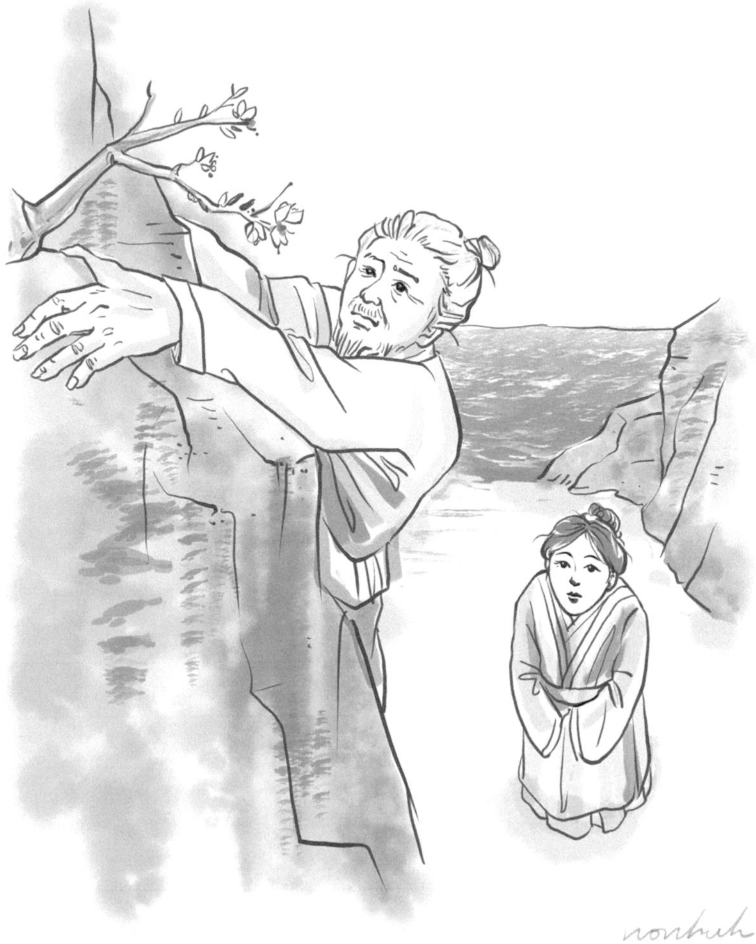

Fig. 4.6 An old man is climbing up the rocky cliff and picking the flower for governor's beautiful young wife. [Illustration by Hye Won Hu, MA (1986)]

Stephen Dedalus found perfect beauty in a girl. "Her long slender bare legs were delicate as a crane's and pure save where an emerald trail of seaweed had fashioned itself as a sign upon the flesh. Her thighs, fuller and soft hued as ivory, were bared almost to the hips, where the white fringes of her drawers were like feathering of soft white down. Her slate blue skirts were kilted boldly about her waist and dovetailed behind her. Her bosom was as a bird's, soft and slight, slight and soft as the breast of some dark plumaged dove. But her long fair hair was girlish: and girlish, and touched with the wonder of mortal beauty, her face [16]."

As a plastic surgeon, one of my ultimate goals would be to make a beautiful and young lady, for whom an old man would completely forget his age and be willing to take a risk to please her. For this purpose, one requires an understanding of a surgical anatomy, as well as skillful surgical technique. Of course, a keen eye and imagination are also mandatory.

4.5 The Characteristics of Ancient Chinese Beauty Represented in "Ode to the Goddess of the Luo River"

Long eyebrows delicately arched/Red lips that shed their light abroad/White teeth gleaming within/Bright eyes skilled at glances/A dimple to round off the base of the cheek.—Cao Zhi (曹植, 192–232)

Years ago, I was invited to be a speaker at a conference on blepharoptosis surgery held in Shenyang, China. In that city, I had the chance to visit the Liaoning Provincial Museum.

Among the many collections, a painting scroll intrigued me. It was not wide (27 cm), but it was quite long (5.7 m). The title of this painting was "Nymph of the Luo River" (Fig. 4.7). It was one of the three remaining duplicates made by painters of the Song Dynasty (960–1279) because the original one created by GuiKaizhi (顧愷之, 348–409) in the Eastern Jin Dynasty had been lost.

A prose-poem (fu, 賦) with the same name (or "Ode to the Goddess of the Luo River") inspired this painting. The poem was written during the Three Kingdoms Period (220–280) by the literary genius Cao Zhi (曹植, 192–232). This famous poem uses the dream world to portray a romantic encounter and sorrowful departure between the writer and the Luo River nymph.

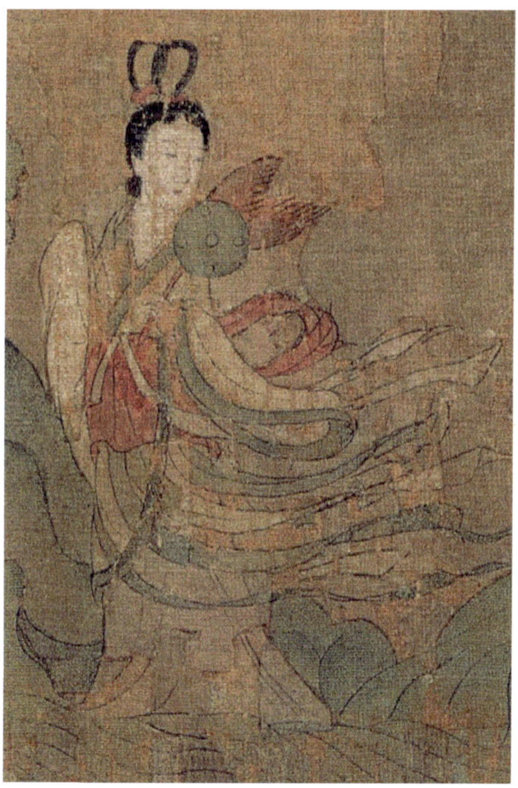

Fig. 4.7 "Nymph of the Luo River" in Beijing Palace Museum

Upon returning home, I searched for the history of the poet Cao Zhi and the background of creation of the poem, which is considered to be one of the best poems ever written describing female beauty.

In the "Romance of Three Kingdoms (三國志演義)," two beautiful women appear: Diaochan (貂蟬, –192) and Zhen Ji (甄姬). Zhen Ji became queen (文昭甄皇后, 183–221) but was eventually executed by the jealous Emperor Cao Pi (曹丕), the elder brother of Cao Zhi. When Zhen Ji was killed, Cao Zhi, who adored his sister-in-law, fell into sorrow and wrote the poem using the "Legend of Mi Fei (宓妃)."

From the entire prose-poem, as a plastic surgeon, I particularly noted the verses that portray the woman's beauty, reflecting the characteristics of beauty in ancient Chinese culture.

"Her body soars lightly like a startled swan, Gracefully, like a dragon in flight (其形也 翩若驚鴻 婉若遊龍). The tall and short of her are justly proportioned, With shoulders shaped as if by carving, Waist narrow as though bound with white cords; (脩短合度 肩若削成 腰如約素). At her slim throat and curving neck (延頸秀項 皓質呈露). Cloud-bank coiffure rising steeply, Long eyebrows delicately arched (雲髻峩峩 脩眉聯娟). Red lips that shed their light abroad, White teeth gleaming within (丹脣外朗 皓齒內鮮). Bright eyes skilled at glances, A dimple to round off the base of the cheek (明眸善睞 靨輔承權) [17–19]."

Reading this poem written about 1900 years ago, I realized that the characteristics of beauty had not changed much through the years.

As plastic surgeons, we can make a "narrow waist" by liposuction or abdominoplasty. We can pursue a "slim throat and curving neck" through neck lifting. The goal of brow lift is to achieve "delicately arched long eyebrows." Jaw surgery would be the basis of "red lips and white teeth within." Blepharoplasty is the most popular procedure for "bright eyes." Plastic surgeons also make cheek dimples. If the poet Cao Zhi could see modern women who have received plastic surgery, he would certainly be surprised by the "nymphs of the Luo River" that we plastic surgeons have made.

The beautiful beloved woman was ephemeral, since she died at the age of 34. However, by being depicted in the famous poem and paintings, she became a source of timeless beauty.

4.6 How Did the Beauties of the Joseon Dynasty (1392–1910) of Korea Look?

Things change, and the eyes through which we see things also change. As plastic surgeons, we know the old axiom, "beauty is in the eye of the beholder." Therefore, if we want to know about changes in beauty—or beautiful people—over time, we have to trace the "eyes of the beholders" of each era. To investigate the appearance of "beauties" in the era before the invention of cameras, we have to rely upon literature or paintings as historical records from that period.

In Korea, there has been a "rule of three" regarding the characteristics of beauties: the three "bigs," the three "smalls," the thee "blacks," the three "whites," and the three "reds." The three "bigs" are the breasts, buttocks, and thighs; the three "smalls" are the hands, feet, and mouth; the three "blacks" are hair, eyebrows, and pupils; the three "whites" are the skin, teeth, and hands; and the three "reds" are the lips, cheeks, and nails (Fig. 4.8).

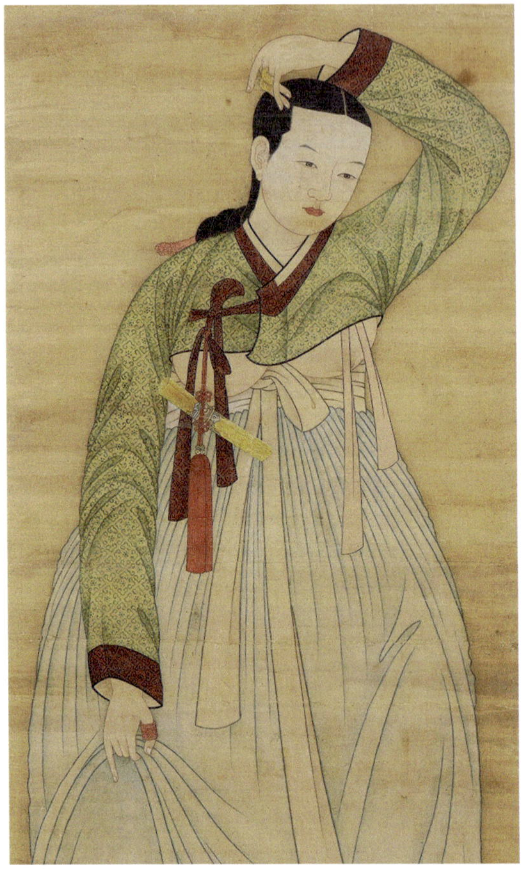

Fig. 4.8 The three "reds" of beautiful women: lips, cheeks, and nails

The first novel of the Joseon dynasty was written by Kim, Si-seup (1435–1493), and many novels were then written by other authors until the end of the Joseon dynasty in 1910. Each novel had a protagonist—a man, a woman, or both—and the heroines of novels were usually beautiful women.

Regarding the appearance of the Joseon beauties, Kim [20] analyzed 50 novels from the Joseon dynasty and found that beautiful protagonists had common aspects of their appearance, which could be summarized in 11 items:

- Hair: well-groomed (cloud-like hair, orchid-like hair presses both ears)
- Eyebrows: thin, black, and rounded
- Eyes: clear as starlight and wet (an amorous glance)
- Lips: luscious and red like a cherry (like a parrot biting a single yarn)
- Cheeks: moderately round and reddish
- Skin: white (in particular, the skin below the ears should be white, as it is the window through which one sees the woman's hidden flesh)
- Body shape: slender and soft (a thin waist like a willow tree, stocking feet like cucumber seeds)
- Teeth: white and even
- Voice: sweet and small (like rolling jade beads on a silver tray)
- Breasts: small and luscious
- Height: not tall

Relatively few paintings of young women were created in the Joseon dynasty. In an analysis of 24 paintings of Joseon beauties, Lee and Ku wrote that beauties had the following facial compositions: a round-forehead, thin crescent-shaped eyebrows (a sign of wisdom and sensitivity), single long thin eyelids (longevity), a round curved nose (as a symbol of being a wise mother or good wife), small concave lips (a sign of gentleness and intelligence), and a round face (as an indicator of insight and good memory) [21].

Comparing the shape of eyebrows in the Joseon dynasty to those in present Korea, different preferences are noted. Although the preferred eyebrow shape of the Joseon dynasty was thin and rounded, the preference of present Koreans is for eyebrows to be relatively thick with a specific shape: a prior study found that the "Anastasia type" (brow starts on a perpendicular line drawn from the middle of the nostril, arches on a line drawn from the center of the nose through the center of the pupil, and ends on a line drawn from the edge of the corresponding nasal ala through the outer edge of the eye) was the most preferred. The middle brow height was most preferred (the distance from the lateral canthus to the lateral end of the eyebrow is two thirds of the eye width). A thick brow was most frequently preferred as healthy looking by women (52.2%), whereas the thinnest type (40.8%) was most often considered to be sexy looking.

Regarding lip shape, similar preferences are found between the Joseon dynasty and present Korea. Present-day Koreans also replied that thick lips were attractive. The most attractive VUL (upper vermillion thickness-to-upper lip height ratio) was VUL-1/2 (thickness of the upper vermillion is 1/2 of upper lip height, 60.3%).

It is interesting that writers of the Joseon dynasty preferred small and luscious breasts over large ones. It is thought that traditional Korean dresses compress the breasts and that small-breasted women had advantages in terms of fitting those dresses well. On the contrary, in Western poems and paintings, large breasts are preferred.

Because beauty is characterized by individual and subjective pleasure, plastic surgeons must synthesize classical ideas of beauty with patients' desires, cultural nuances, and ethnic considerations, all while maintaining a natural appearance and results. Anyone can tell that a face is distorted or ugly. However, we plastic surgeons need special eyes to know why it is distorted and skillful hands that can alter it to become beautiful. We have to fix any deficiencies before we leave the operating theater. To fix faces properly, we must have special eyes and skillful hands.

4.7 Chinese Ghosts, Chinese Beauties

I recently enjoyed a movie entitled "Painted Skin." This story is one of the widely known Liaozhai stories (聊齋誌異, *Strange Stories from a Chinese Studio*) that has a well-developed narrative (Fig. 4.9). It focuses on a hideous monster disguised as a beautiful ghost.

As a plastic surgeon, I found it interesting that the heroine of the ghost story is a "beautiful

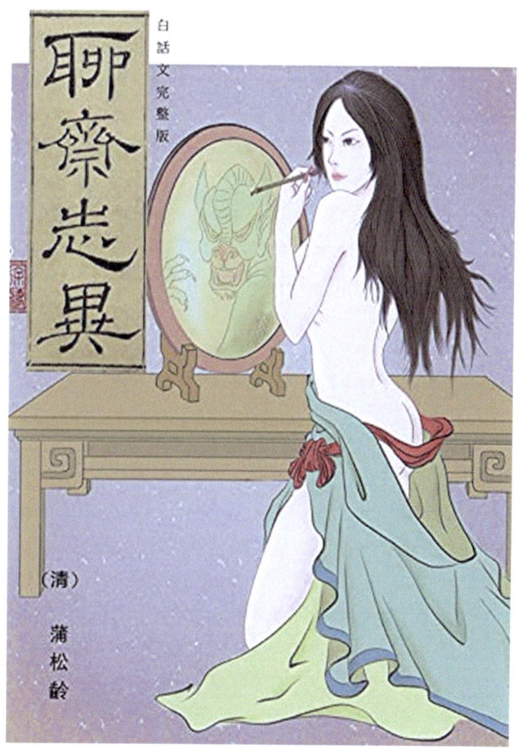

Fig. 4.9 Title page of Strange Stories from a Chinese Studio written by Pu Songling

ghost" in this ancient tale. This prompted me to read the book and search for papers about the Liaozhai tales [22].

The Liaozhai stories, which are viewed as belonging to the genre of Chinese romance fantasy, are a collection of classical Chinese stories compiled by the Qing dynasty writer Pu Songling (蒲松齡, 1640–1715), comprising close to 500 "marvel tales."

The typical Liaozhai ghost, in the Chinese popular imagination, is female, beautiful, and sexual. Although they are not necessarily always beautiful, the ghosts are predominantly female. A considerable number of Liaozhai anecdotes portray the ghost characters as grotesque and dangerous [23, 24].

According to Wang Fenling (汪玢玲), of ~500 Liaozhai tales, ghosts and spirits appear in 258. She placed the fox stories (82) into a separate typology and divided the remaining 176 Liaozhai ghost stories into eight categories: ghost–human love stories (28); governance of the underworld (24); demons and malicious ghosts (18); benign ghosts and reciprocity (10); transcendents, immortals, and spirits (38); karmic retribution (29); obsession and object spirits (6); and souls (23) [25].

Chen classified 41 ghost–human interaction stories into four groups: the affection type (16), the compassion type (11), the revenge type (7), and the eradication type (7). According to his analysis, the shape of the female figure is a beautiful figure pursued by contemporary men. In addition, a commonality of female ghosts is that they have sexual relations with the male protagonist, breaking the taboo of childhood and expressing desires that cannot be revealed in real society [26].

In the tales, I found several verses that describe the external appearance of female ghosts: "He then seized a chop-stick and threw it into the moon, whereupon a lovely girl stepped forth from its beams. At first she was only a foot high, but on reaching the ground lengthened to the ordinary size of women. She had a slender waist and a beautiful neck, and went most gracefully through the Red Garment figure." "She was between thirteen and fourteen years old, and had beautiful eyes with a very intelligent expression in them, and a most graceful figure besides." "This Mr. K'ung acceded to, and accordingly saw Miss Chiao-no come out with a lovely girl—her black eyebrows beautifully arched, and her tiny feet encased in phœnix-shaped shoes—as like one another as they well could be." "Looking closely at her, he observed that she had a beautiful complexion, and feet as small as bamboo shoots, being altogether much prettier now that he came to see her by daylight."

I previously analyzed another Chinese work, *Portrait and Biography of 100 Beauties* (1792). Forty-six women had specific descriptions of their appearance, most often of their face (33.5%), followed by their body (16.5%), manners (7.3%), fragrance (4.3%), and clothes (2.4%). The most frequent descriptions of specific attributes were found for the hair (7.4%), eyebrows (6.7%), eyes (5.5%), skin (5.5%), and body shape (4.9%) [27].

Comparing the "ghost disguised of a beautiful woman" to the "historical 100 beauties," I found some commonalities: they are graceful, have good manners, and are slender and intelligent. Chinese ghosts, which are basically hideous monsters disguised as beautiful women, have the external appearance of a "beautiful figure" pursued by contemporary people.

Nonetheless, as plastic surgeons, we "make" beautiful faces rather than "disguise" the real appearance.

4.8 Appearance of the Japanese Beauty Described in the *Yuki-Onna* (雪女, Snow Woman) Story

When I visited Niigata University, I noticed a peculiar picture of a Japanese woman in a home I was invited to visit. A plastic surgeon at that university explained about the picture and the legend of the *Yuki-onna* (snow woman). The story intrigued me because the protagonist of the legend never becomes old-looking, *even after* having 10 children.

The story of the snow woman has been passed down through the generations in several provinces of Japan, especially in ones that have heavy snows in winter. In 1904, the Greek-Japanese writer Lafcadio Hearn (Koizumi Yakumo, 1850–1904) merged similar stories from several regions and published his version (Fig. 4.10) [28]. The plot summary of the story is as follows:

[A long time ago, there lived 2 woodcutters, Minokichi and Mosaku. Minokichi was young and Mosaku was very old. One winter day, they could not come back home because of a snowstorm. They found a hut in the mountain and decided to sleep there. On this particular evening, Minokichi woke up and found a beautiful lady with white clothes. She breathed on old Mosaku and he was frozen to death. The white woman bent down over Minokichi, lower and lower, until her face almost touched him; and he saw that she was very beautiful—though her eyes made him afraid. She approached to breathe on him, but stared at him for a while and said, "You are a pretty boy, Minokichi; and I will not hurt you now. You must not tell anyone about this incident. If you tell anyone about me, I will kill you." One evening, in the winter of the following year, as he was on his way home, Minokichi overtook a girl who happened to be traveling by the same road. She was a tall, slim girl, very good-looking; and she answered Minokichi's greeting in a voice as pleasant to the ear as the voice of a song-bird. Minokichi soon felt charmed by this strange girl; and the more that he looked at her, the handsomer she appeared to be. Her name was O-yuki (*yuki* means snow), and he married her and they lived happily for years. She was a good wife. Most peasant-women age early; but O-Yuki, even after becoming the mother of 10 children, looked as young and fresh as on the day when she had first come to the village. One night, after the children were asleep, Minokichi said to O-yuki: "Whenever I see you, I am reminded of a mysterious incident that happened to me. When I was a lad of eighteen. I then saw somebody as beautiful and white as you are now—indeed, she was very like you. I do not know if it was a dream or if she was a *Yuki-onna*..." After finishing his story, O-yuki

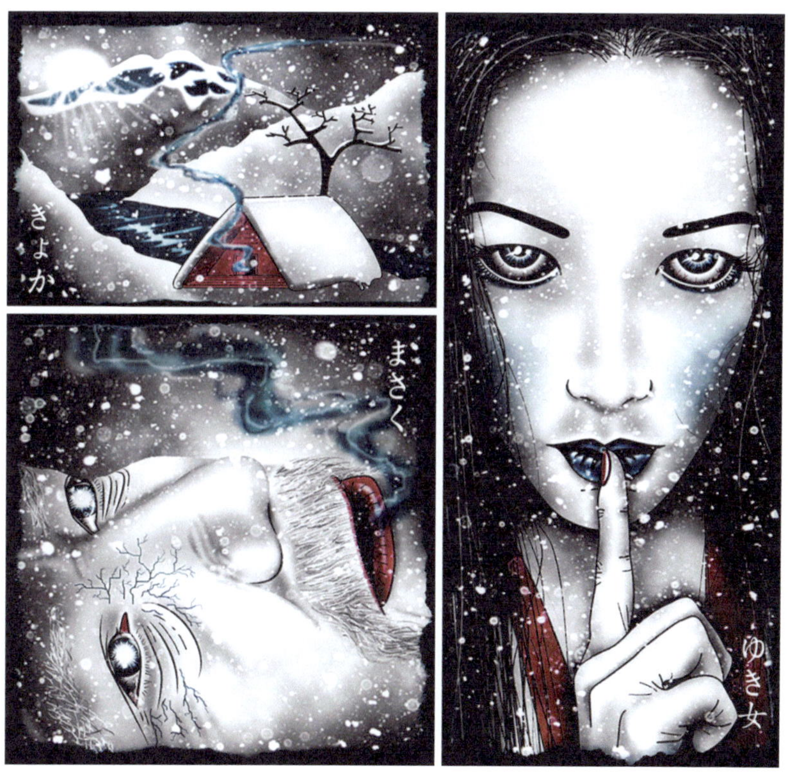

Fig. 4.10 Title page of "Yuki-onna" written by Lafcadio Hearn

suddenly stood up and said "That woman you met was me! I told you that I would kill you if you ever told anyone about that incident. However, I can't kill you because of our children. And now you had better take very, very good care of them; for if ever they have reason to complain of you, I will treat you as you deserve!." Then she melted and disappeared. No one saw her again.]

In this story, the ghost *Yuki-onna* and O-yuki have the same appearance. A ghost becomes human and returns to a ghost again. The ghost was beautiful despite her eyes, which made the male protagonist "afraid." Like the ghost, the transformed human girl was "tall and slim," with a "song-bird voice." The peculiar phenomenon was that she looked as young and fresh as the first day she arrived at the village, even after having 10 children.

Based on this story, I infer that the preferred Japanese woman (regardless of whether she is a femme fatale or not) should have "white skin" (representing the pure whiteness of virginity), a "tall and slim" stature, a sweet voice, an ageless appearance, and a maternal instinct for her children. The snow woman turned into a scary mother who threatened her unreliable husband when she had to leave her children with him; however, she saved his life, since he was the only one who could take care of their children [29, 30]. Among these characteristics, the most important one is that of timeless beauty. Because this tale contains interesting images of the femme fatale, beautiful woman, and maternal affection, many cultural productions, such as movies or animations, have adapted the plot of *Yuki-onna* [31].

At our dinner, the surgeon's wife wore a kimono. She had white face paint with make-up, as many Japanese wives do. Traditionally, many Japanese husbands did not see their wives' bare face (i.e., a face that does not have any make-up on) until death. Their wives pursued white skin and timeless beauty for their male protagonists in a play called "life."

We plastic surgeons can help our patients obtain a slim body, pristine skin, and wrinkleless face in order to achieve "ageless beauty," like that of O-Yuki.

4.9 Eye of the Beholder

A thing of beauty is a joy forever.—*John Keats*, 1795–1821

Because a plastic surgeon and a patient with bandages appeared on a poster advertising the show, I recently enjoyed an episode of an old TV drama, "The Twilight Zone" ("Eye of the Beholder", 1959; director: Douglas Heyes, starring Donna Douglas, and 2003; director: David Ellis, starring Molly Sims) (Fig. 4.11).

In this episode, Janet Tyler, a woman with facial deformities in a totalitarian society that emphasizes conformity even in in physical appearance, is undergoing her 12th surgery in an attempt to make her appear normal. It is the last chance she can legally receive to alter her looks, and if the operation succeeds, she will fit in with those around her for the first time in her life. If it fails, she will be transported to a "segregated" colony of those who look like her, rather than as "normal" people do. Tyler is first shown with her head bandaged completely, so that her face cannot be seen. She is described as being "not normal" by the nurses and doctor, whose own faces are always either in shadows or off-camera. Her bandages are due to come off any day now and she is terribly worried as to the outcome.

When the bandages were removed, I noticed that she had a beautiful face. However, the reaction of the doctor and nurses was complete disappointment, to the point that the shocked surgeon dropped his scissors. Janet tried to run, but they restrained her and turned on the lights. At this point, the doctor, nurses, and other people in the hospital, whose faces had not been shown clearly before, are now revealed to be grotesquely deformed, looking like monsters (1959 version) or burn victims (2002 version). Mr. Smith, from the congregate separatist group for the "freaks", tells Tyler the old axiom, "beauty is in the eye of the beholder" as they walk off.

After watching the drama, I investigated the concept of beauty from an aesthetic standpoint and in the setting of plastic surgery.

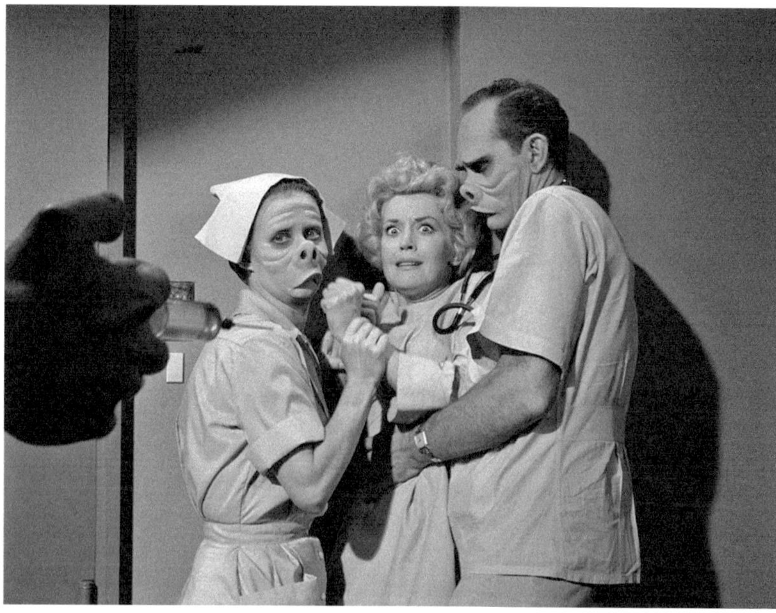

Fig. 4.11 Doctor and nurse restraining Janet and turning on the light. In "The Twilight Zone" ("Eye of the Beholder," 1959; director: Douglas Heyes, starring Donna Douglas)

According to Tatarkiewicz, theories of beauty have conceptualized beauty in three different ways [32].

1. A broad sense of beauty: The Greek concept of beauty was broader than the modern concept, encompassing not only beautiful things, shapes, colors, and sounds but also beautiful thoughts and customs. With the passage of time, the Greeks began to use *beauty* in the narrower sense, so that the word forced *symmetry* and *harmony* into the background. In the fifth century BC, the sophists of Athens had narrowed the original conception of beauty in Greek culture to define it as "that which is pleasant to sight or hearing."
2. A purely aesthetic sense of beauty: This notion of beauty extends only to that which evokes aesthetic experience but embraces everything in this category, including mental products no less than colors and sounds.
3. An aesthetic sense of beauty, restricted to things apprehended by the sight: In this sense of the word, only shape and color could be beautiful. The Stoics partially adopted this concept of beauty.

The Great Theory was developed by the Pythagoreans, but only in a narrower version. This theory was based on observation of the harmony of sounds, but the idea of beauty quickly appeared in an analogous form in the visual arts. The words *harmonia* and *symmetria* were closely connected with the theory's application to the domains of hearing and sight, respectively.

The only detailed exposition is found in Vitruvius' *Ten Books on Architecture*. According to Vitruvius, beauty is achieved in a building when all its parts have the appropriate proportions of height to breadth and breadth to length and, in general, fulfill all the demands of symmetry. He thought that the same was true in sculpture and painting and believed that nature "has created the human body in such a way that the skull from the chin to the upper brow and hairline makes up one tenth of the entire length of the body." His view enabled him to present the just proportions of both buildings and human bodies. The Stoics thought that "the beauty of the body resides in the proportion of the limbs in relation to one another and to the whole." They also took an analogous view of the beauty of the soul, as consisting in a proportion of the parts.

Thus, the proportion theory of beauty was both universal and lasted long. The Pythagoreans and Plato in the fifth century BC, Aristotle in the fourth century BC, the Stoics in the third century BC, Vitruvius in the first century BC, and even artists and thinkers during the Renaissance era accepted it. The decline of the theory came in the eighteenth century when beauty began to be approached differently and the theory of taste appeared. In light of this trend, old beauty standards, as determined by anthropometric, photogrammetric, and cephalometric data, do not correspond to the current public perceptions of facial beauty.

Leo Tolstoy (1828–1910) wrote that "people will come to understand the meaning of art only when they cease to consider that the aim of that activity is beauty, that is, pleasure." Influenced by Tolstoy, Ludwig Wittgenstein (1889–1951) presented the core idea of modern aesthetics that "the end of art is the beautiful." He also wrote that "[...] the beautiful is what makes happy" (Notebook 21.10.16). In *Lectures on Aesthetics* (1938), he wrote, "It is remarkable that in real life, when aesthetic judgments are made, aesthetic adjectives such as 'beautiful', 'fine', etc., play hardly any role at all" (Lecture, I, 8) [33].

In the modern world, social media and fashion trends exert a central influence on common ideals of beauty and on the field of plastic surgery. Compared with the technologically innovative progress, discussion regarding the central question "What is beauty?" is sometimes missing [34].

Recently, Di Stefano raised two biases that affect the idea of beauty often embodied in aesthetic surgery. The first one is that the living body is the sum of different parts; the second one claims that beauty results from the sum of beautiful elements [35]. I believe that most plastic surgeons, including Dr. Stefano, know that our standards and ideals are based on neoclassical models of beauty from Greek and Roman art and architecture; however, we encounter a wide range of variation in patients' desires and perceptions of beauty.

Because beauty is characterized by an individual and subjective pleasure, plastic surgeons must synthesize classical ideas of beauty with patients' desires, cultural nuances, and ethnic considerations, all while maintaining a natural appearance and result. Bueller suggested four goals for patients seeking to enhance their appearance: (1) classical definitions of beauty as they relate to symmetry, proportion, and youth; (2) achieving a natural and unoperated look for the patient; (3) current cultural trends and ideals; and (4) patients' personal preferences and desires [36].

Anyone can tell a face is distorted or ugly. However, we plastic surgeons need special eyes to know why it is distorted and skillful hands that can alter it to become beautiful. Before finishing each operation, we should remember the quote of Albrecht Dürer (1471–1528), "In putting a finished work before the public, most of the time what will be noticed is what is wrong. If so, fix it accordingly." We have to fix the incomplete part before we leave the operating theater. To fix it properly, we must have special eyes and skillful hands.

4.10 Purpose of Zygoma Reduction: Not Just for a Smaller Cheek Bone

Beauty is in the eye of the beholder.—*Margaret Wolfe Hungerford*

Reduction malarplasty is currently one of the most popular surgical procedures for facial contouring in Asians (Fig. 4.12). However, this operation can cause serious complications [37].

This operation was first introduced over 30 years ago. Onizuka, in 1983, first published a description of this procedure, and this paper has been cited many times (90 hits in Google Scholar, 56 in Web of Science) [38].

In the beginning of this historic paper, he cited Agban's paper [39] and stated "Caucasians have a dolicocephaly and Orientals have a mesocephaly. Width of the face is wider and the malar curve is more prominent in Orientals than in Caucasians [38]."

Onizuka devised this procedure to satisfy patients who complain of having the deformity of a prominent zygoma, as can be seen in the *Noh* (skill or talent) mask known as *Yase onna* (thin woman) (Fig. 4.13, left). He wrote that a person with a prominent zygoma shows an aged and

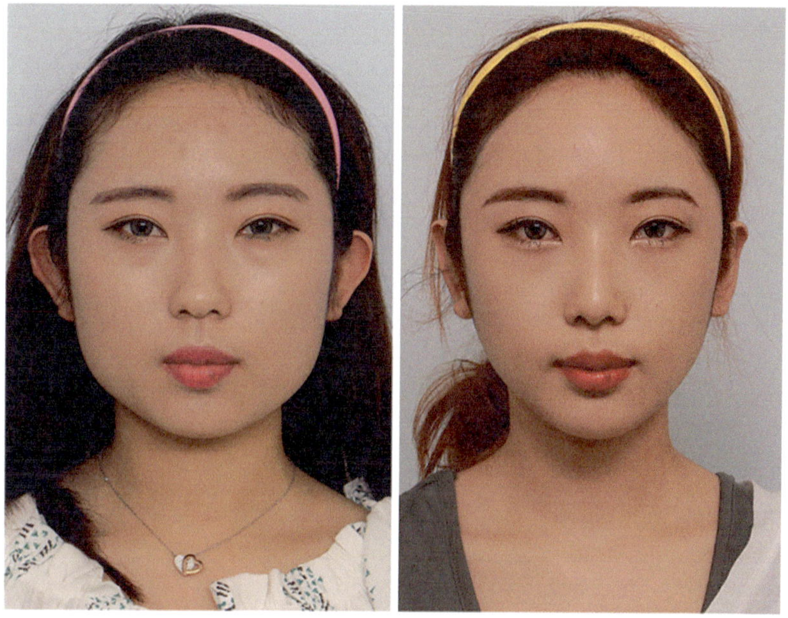

Fig. 4.12 A pre- (left) and postoperative 12 months (right) photo of a 29-year-old patient who had malar reduction, mandible angle ostectomy, bilateral otoplasty for prominent ear, and dorsal nasal implant insertion

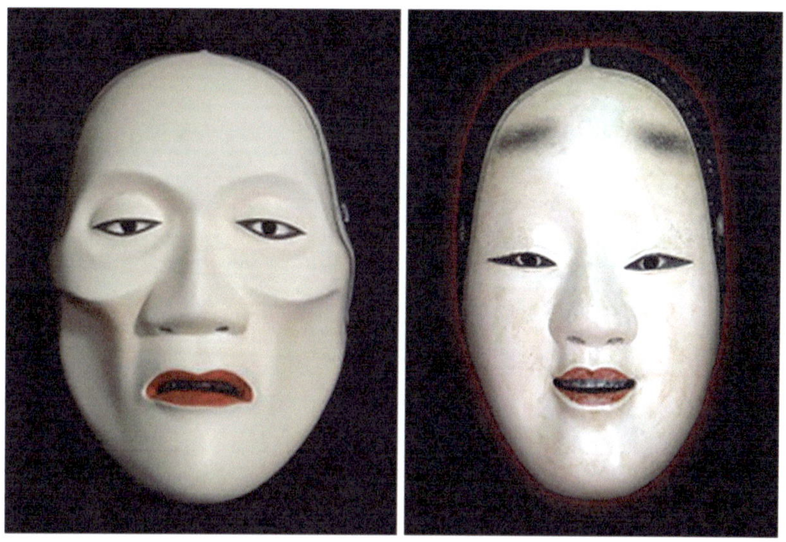

Fig. 4.13 Noh masks. Left: Yase onna (thin woman). Right: Kohime (beautiful lady)

melancholic face, as demonstrated in *Yase onna*. If this prominence is removed, the facial contour becomes soft, cheerful, and young as seen in *Kohime* (beautiful lady) (Fig. 4.13, right) [38].

I have a divergence of opinion regarding Onizuka's remarks that Asians desire malar reduction because Orientals exhibit mesocephaly.

The two masks in the paper do not represent the difference between Caucasians and Asians but merely compare an old thin woman and a young healthy woman. Not all Asians are mesocephalic, and not all Caucasians are dolicocephalic.

Why, then, is reduction malarplasty not frequently performed in Caucasians? The reasons include the following: Western surgeons are concerned about the drooping lateral cheek with age; liposculpture has been the focus of facial recontouring, not facial width reduction [40]; the Caucasian patient does not look unfavorably on a prominent cheek bone the way an Asian patient does; and there is high liability for medical malpractice in Western countries.

Lastly, "mesocephalic" means having a head that is not particularly short or long from front to back relative to its width from left to right; it does not mean having a prominent zygoma.

What, then, is the purpose of zygoma reduction? Because the zygoma become prominent with aging, the aim of reduction malarplasty is to camouflage the strong and masculine appearance caused by the prominent zygoma.

Since the aging of the face involves deflation and descent [41], I think that zygoma reduction should not just aim for a smaller cheek bone. For the purpose of avoiding cheek drooping after reduction malarplasty, the coronal approach, which repositions the malar complex superiorly, might be a better choice than the intraoral approach [42].

With aging, facial fat descends and facial shape changes. The youthful face is full of well-supported fat [43]. It is characterized by full, rounded cheeks, which are high up on the face, with little to no bony areas obviously seen [44].

Asian facial reshaping, cosmetic procedures are not designed to achieve a Western appearance but rather to achieve an attractive Asian, aesthetic appearance. That is suggestive of a youthful, healthy, physically active, and gentle appearance. If marked individuality and elegance can be added, better results will be obtained.

References

1. Ascaso FJ, Lizana J, Singh AD, Dua HS. One eyed beauty: queen Nefertiti's bust. Br J Ophthalmol. 2011;95:161.
2. Ertman EL. Nefertiti's eyes: did the queen's distinctive feature become a symbol of Egyptian royalty? https://archive.archaeology.org/0803/etc/nefertiti.html. Accessed 5 Aug 2020.
3. Lorenzi R. Scholar: Nefertiti was an aging beauty. http://dsc.discovery.com/news/2006/09/05/nefertiti_arc.html. Accessed 5 Aug 2020.
4. McDaniel S. What did Helen of Troy Look Like? https://talesoftimesforgotten.com/2019/08/24/what-did-helen-of-troy-look-like/. Accessed 5 Aug 2021.
5. Feng M. To make Bao Si laugh, king you lighted the warning beacons and feudal lords arrived. In: Feng M, editor. Dong Zhou Lieguozhi. China: People's Literature Publishing House; 1979. p. 9–15.
6. Uther H. The types of international folktales: a classification and bibliography based on the system of Antti Aarne and Stith Thompson, part III. Helsinki: Finnish Academy of Science and Letters; 2011.
7. Frankel FE. The ugly wise girl. The classic Tales: 4000 years of Jewish Lore. Northvale: Jason Aronson Inc.; 1993. p. 588–94.
8. Kim HH. The rites of passage of the ugly girls transformed into beauties: a comparative study of the ugly-girl tales from Korean and Jewish traditions. Comp Korean Stud. 2014;22:117–54.
9. Hwang K. Metamorphosis in the imagination of poets, artists, and plastic surgeons. J Craniofac Surg. 2020;31:3.
10. Athanasiou R, Greene P. Physical attractiveness and helping behavior. Proceedings of the Annual Convention of the American Psychological Association; 1973. p. 289–90.
11. Hwang K. Why do we quest for youth? J Craniofac Surg. 2021;32:e848–9.
12. World History Encyclopedia. 15 Complete Hyangga songs from Ancient Korea. 2016. https://www.worldhistory.org/article/970/15-complete-hyangga-songs-from-ancient-korea/. Accessed 15 Mar 2022.
13. Ha TH. Samguk Yusa: legends and history of the three kingdoms of ancient Korea. Seoul: Yonsei University Press; 1972.
14. Kim JR. The meaning of 'beauty' in lady Suro's legend of Samkuk-Yusa. Fem Korean Lit. 2014;33:193–224.
15. Lee SN. What is the beauty of Suro like? The communication of narrative meaning in Surobuin story and Heonhwaga. Stud Korean Lit. 2009;37:5–39.
16. Joyce J. The portrait of an artist as a young man. 2003. https://www.gutenberg.org/files/4217/4217-h/4217-h.htm#link2HCH0001. Accessed 5 Feb 2021.
17. Watson B. The Columbia book of Chinese poetry: from early times to the thirteenth century. New York: Columbia University Press; 1984. p. 116–21.
18. Owen S. An anthology of Chinese literature: beginnings to 1911. New York: W. W. Norton & Company; 1997. p. 194–7.
19. Minford J, Lau JSM. Classical Chinese literature: an anthology of translations. In: Antiquity to the Tang Dynasty, vol. 1. Hong Kong: The Chinese University of Hong Kong Press; 2002. p. 314–8.
20. Kim JT. An outlook on the traditional beauty of Korean. J Women Probl Res Inst. 1979;8:5–17.
21. Lee HO, Ku YS. Aesthetic characteristics of face in the late Joseon-dynasty's beauty paintings. Fash Text Res J. 2012;14:918–27.
22. Pu S. The project Gutenberg EBook of strange stories from a Chinese studio (*translated by* Giles HA). London: Thomas De La Rue & Co; 1880.
23. Luo H. The ghost of Liaozhai: Pu Songling's Ghostlore and its history of reception [a thesis submitted in conformity with the requirements for the degree of doctor of philosophy]. Toronto: University of Toronto; 2009.

24. Dodd SL. Monsters and monstrosity in Liaozhai zhiyi (submitted in accordance with the requirements for the degree of PhD). Leeds: The University of Leeds; 2013.
25. Wang F. Discussion of ghosts and foxes: Liaozhai Zhiyi and folk culture Guihu Fengqing. Hirbin. 2003;187:219–20.
26. Chen CJ. Ghost fence in Korean and Chinese literature-focusing on works before 18th century. Dongnam J Korean Lang Lit. 2019;47:227–52.
27. Hwang K, Wu X. What did the historical Chinese beauties look like? An analysis of portrait and biography of 100 beauties (1792). J Craniofac Surg. 2022;33:1782. https://doi.org/10.1097/SCS.0000000000008416.
28. Hearn L. Kwaidan-stories and studies of strange things. https://cpb-us-e1.wpmucdn.com/share.nanjing-school.com/dist/a/38/files/2013/02/Yuki-Onna-Snow-Lady-by-Lafcadio-Hearn-2c9tbki.pdf. Assessed 18 Mar 2022.
29. Shin JS. A study on the relation between acceptance of literature and social values: a comparison of Lafcadio Hearn's [雪女YUKIONNA] and Matsutani Miyoko's [snow woman (雪女)]. JAST. 2015;65:247–66.
30. Park HY. The creation and duality of structure of female Yokai in the Japanese Yokai culture: with a special attention to female Yokai Yukionna, Ubume, Yabanba. JMAK. 2013;42:285–99.
31. Park HY. In the east Asian grotesque culture Yokai tradition and the flow: Japanese Yokai, in a cultural history of Yukionna. JMAK. 2013;40:143–62.
32. Tatarkiewicz W. The great theory of beauty and its decline. J Aesthet Art Crit. 1972;31:165–80.
33. Tomasi G. Wittgenstein on "beautiful" and "the beautiful". Aisthesis Pratiche linguaggi e saperi dell'estetico. 2003;6:115–37.
34. Harth W. Was ist Schönheit?: manifest einer ästhetischen Charaktermedizin (What is beauty? Manifest for an aesthetic character medicine). Hautarzt. 2017;68:950–8.
35. Di Stefano N. The idea of beauty and its biases: critical notes on the aesthetics of plastic surgery. Plast Reconstr Surg Glob Open. 2017;5:e1523.
36. Bueller H. Ideal facial relationships and goals. Facial Plast Surg. 2018;34:458–65.
37. Hwang K. Lateral rectus muscle injury, orbital fracture, mouth locking, and facial palsy resulting from reduction malarplasty. J Craniofac Surg. 2011;22:151–4.
38. Onizuka T, Watanabe K, Takasu K, et al. Reduction malar plasty. Aesth Plast Surg. 1983;7:121–5.
39. Agban GM. Augmentation and corrective malarplasty. Ann Plast Surg. 1979;2:306–15.
40. Shirakabe Y, Suzuki Y, Lam SM. A new paradigm for the aging Asian face. Aesthet Plast Surg. 2003;27:397–402.
41. Goldberg RA. The three periorbital hollows: a paradigm for periorbital rejuvenation. Plast Reconstr Surg. 2005;116:1796–804.
42. Baek RM, Lee SW. Face lift with reposition malarplasty. Plast Reconstr Surg. 2009;123:701–8.
43. Stuzin JM, Neligan PC. Facelift: the extended SMAS technique in facial rejuvenation. Plastic surgery, vol. II, vol. 239. Philadelphia: Elsevier Saunders; 2013.
44. Sin LT. Instant youth: non-surgical and minimally painful liquid face lifts. 2012. http://cosmedmd.blogspot.kr/2012/09/instant-youth-non-surgical-and.html. Accessed 14 Aug 2017.

5 Aging from the Perspective of a Plastic Surgeon

5.1 Form in the Country for Old Men

Years ago, I enjoyed a movie entitled "No Country for Old Men" (2007, directed by Ethan Coen and Joel Coen). This film was based on Cormac McCarthy's novel (2005) of the same name. After enjoying this thriller, I figured out that the "old man" refers to the old Sheriff Ed Tom Bell (played by Tommy Lee Jones), who encounters horror and violence as a lawman. However, he is no longer cut out to deal with them.

Later, I learned that this film title was derived from the first verse of the poem "Sailing to Byzantium," which William Butler Yeats wrote at the age of 61.

He wrote about aging:

That is no country for old men. The young
In one another's arms, birds in the trees,
An aged man is but a paltry thing,
A tattered coat upon a stick, unless
He desires to sail to Byzantium, which is a "land for old men," and articulates the appearance that he desires.
Once out of nature I shall never take
My bodily form from any natural thing,
But such a form as Grecian goldsmiths make
Of hammered gold and gold enameling

As Yeats wrote, Byzantium is symbolic of a place that resolves the eternal struggle between the limitations of the physical world and the aspirations of the immortal spirit. Yeats' solution for the agony of old age was to leave the country of the young and travel to Byzantium, where the sages in the city's famous gold mosaics could become the "singing-masters" of his soul. Using bright stones, gold mosaics, wall paintings, carved ivory, and metals, Byzantine artists beautified everything in their surroundings, and their most lasting legacy is the icons that continue to decorate Christian churches.

I had no idea about the "form of hammered gold and gold enameling" until I visited Constantinople (Istanbul), where I enjoyed many icons. Icons, which are images of holy persons, have been an important part of the Byzantine Christian Church from the third century onward. The most common icons are of religious figures: Christ, the Virgin Mary, saints, or angels.

Most icons show holy figures with youthful appearances. However, some saints who had not been executed and did not die at a young age, and instead lived until old age, appear as old men in their icons. These include are St. Nicholas, St. Basil, St Nektarios, St. Pachomius the Great, St. Gherasim, St. Clement, St. Patrick, St. Paisios, St. Gregory, St. Luke, St. John, and St. Anthony. They all show dignity with hammered gold and gold enameling and wisdom embedded in their wrinkles (Fig. 5.1) [1].

In one of the icons of the "old saints," there is a medallion with Saint John the Evangelist portrayed in enamel worked in cloisonné. In this icon, we can see clear forehead wrinkles and

K. Hwang, *Good Physician, Good Plastic Surgeon*, https://doi.org/10.1007/978-981-97-1864-1_5

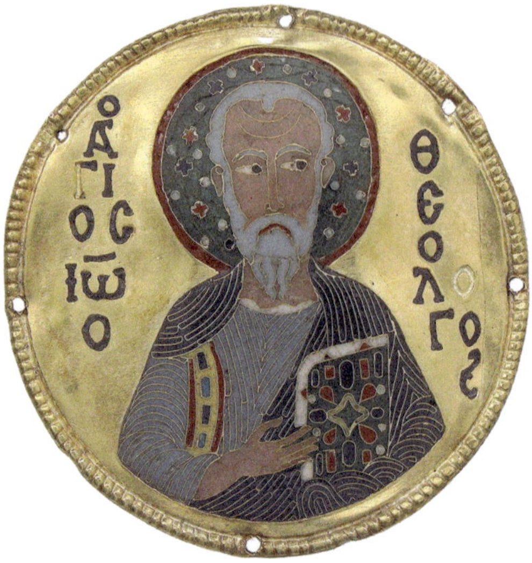

Fig. 5.1 Medallion with Saint John the Evangelist from an Icon Frame. Medium: gold, silver, and enamel worked in cloisonné. (Available at: https://www.metmuseum.org/art/collection/search/464549. Accessed 30 Sept 2021)

marionette lines. Through this icon, we can envision how this wise evangelist, who wrote a Gospel, two letters, and the Apocalypse, looks like his bitter and honorable experiences have melted and filled every furrow of his skin, making him wise and glorious in the "land for old men," Byzantium.

Polyester sheet plastination has been used for over a decade [2]. Sheet plastination is a technology for tissue preservation that provides materials for the study of sectional anatomical structures. This method of creating transparent sectional specimens has the advantage of displaying fibers of connective tissue and myofascial structures in situ [3]. Of the various techniques that have been developed, P45 plastination provides a natural color [4]. Using P45 plastination, skin wrinkles, as well as the underlying superficial fascia of the face and neck, can be visualized in a natural golden hue. Recent studies have used P45 plastination to determine the extent of the superficial fascia of the cheek [5] and the relationships between the nasolabial fold and superficial fascia [6].

Like the golden enameled wrinkles of the saints, golden sheet plastination provides information on the anatomical details of the major wrinkles of the face.

As Byzantine theologian-artists reflected upon the characteristics of the old saints through the form of gold and enameling in the icons that represent the virtues of saints of that period, plastic surgeons can identify the nature of wrinkles through detailed cross-sectional anatomy using histology or sheet plastination. On this basis, plastic surgeons can develop rhytidectomy techniques for the "old men" who have sailed to the "land for old men".

5.2 From Old to Young: Rejuvenation in the Waste Land

As life expectancy increases, senescence is also prolonged. Older adults might hope to live long or even think of asking God for eternal life, as has been portrayed in scenes in popular culture.

There is a well-known mythological example of a woman who was granted eternal life. Years ago, I saw the portrait of the Cumaean Sibyl on the Sistine Chapel ceiling drawn by Michelangelo (Fig. 5.2). She was capable of foretelling the future. She had been granted immortality by Apollo but forgot to ask for perpetual youth. Thereafter, she shrank into withered old age, and her authority declined.

"The Waste Land" (1922), written by Thomas Sterns Eliot, starts with the inscription, "I have seen with my own eyes the Sibyl hanging in a jar, and when the boys asked her, 'What do you want?' She answered, 'I want to die [7].'" Eliot wrote this poem about the crisis of modern culture and the breakup of civilization just after World War I (1914–1918) [8].

The shortest of the five sections (IV. Death by Water, only 10 verses, of the total 433 verses) rebuts ideas of renewal and regeneration.

Phlebas the Phoenician, a fortnight dead,
Forgot the cry of gulls, and the deep sea swell
And the profit and loss.
A current under sea
Picked his bones in whispers. As he rose and fell
He passed the stages of his age and youth

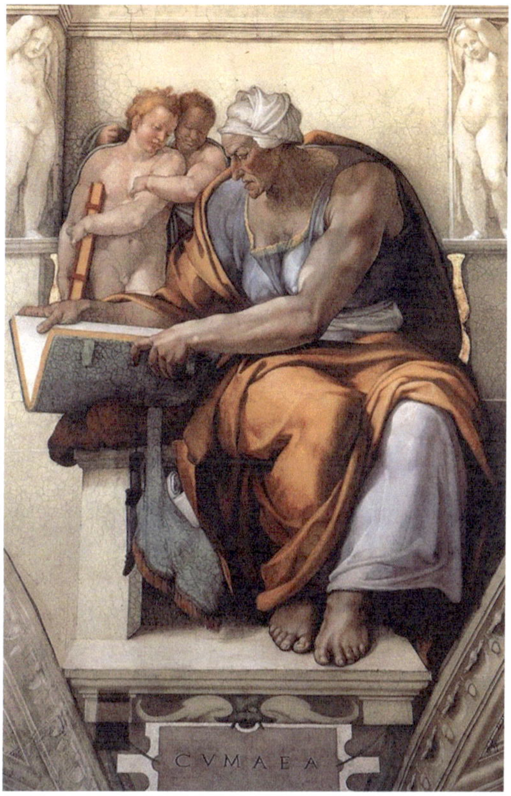

Fig. 5.2 Cumaean Sibyl by Michelangelo (1475–1564) on the Sistine Chapel Ceiling, Rome, Vatican. From public domain through https://commons.wikimedia.org/wiki/File:%27Cumaean_Sibyl_Sistine_Chapel_ceiling%27_by_Michelangelo_JBU35.jpg#filelinks. (This image by Jörg Bittner Unna is licensed under the Creative Commons Attribution 3.0 Unported license)

Entering the whirlpool.
Gentile or Jew
O you who turn the wheel and look to windward,
Consider Phlebas, who was once handsome and tall as you.

Literary critics say that this section represents *samsara*: the cycle of birth, death, and rebirth. Water symbolizes baptism, rebirth, relief, and regeneration. When Phlebas drowns, he seems to forget all his worries and cares from his mortal life. Sins are washed away in the moment of death, and the soul is clean and pure. This theme is related to regeneration and rejuvenation when the soul is cleansed of impurities, like a second chance [9]. The name "Phlebas" originates from *phleps* (the genitive is *phlebos*), the Greek word for "vein."

Eliot (1888–1965) lived in the same era as Harold Gillies (1882–1960), when the techniques of plastic surgery had not been established. Gillies' experiences with head and facial injuries during World War I formed the basis of craniofacial surgery. The surgical experiences that plastic surgeons accumulated by treating injured faces led to the development of aesthetic surgery [10]. Plastic surgeons can now bypass the stages of age and rejuvenate the appearance of older adults by performing rhytidectomy. We can use the whirlpool of their own blood flow to make them as handsome as young people.

In "The Burial of the Dead," the author writes that human eyes look like pearls. "Here, said she/ Is your card, the drowned Phoenician Sailor/ Those are pearls that were his eyes. Look!" Although our patients are becoming older, we might be able to give them a perpetually young appearance if only they maintain a firm will to remain young, like the "pearl eyes."

5.3 Humankind's Endless Quest for Youth

In the morning, my hair was black like silk bundles. In the evening, it became white like snow.—
Li Bai

Humans have tried to maintain a youthful appearance using beauty treatments long before the development of aesthetic plastic surgery. Descriptions of yearning for youth can be found even in ancient literature.

The first emperor of the Qin dynasty in China (Qin Shi Huang, 259–210 BC) commanded scholars to search for a potion that would give him eternal life. He was thought to have consumed cinnabar (or mercury sulfide) hoping it would prolong his life; however, mercury is poisonous, and he passed away at the age of 39.

During my stay in Leipzig for coworking at the Max Planck Institute, I visited the Gemäldegalerie in Berlin, which is only an hour from Leipzig by the InterCity Express train. In that gallery, I happened to see an interesting painting created by Lucas Cranach (1472–1553), who is famous for the "Portrait of Martin Luther."

In this painting (Der Jungbrunnen), more than 30 women are shown around a rectangular bath, with a fountain in its center. On the left half of the painting, older women are taking their clothes off and entering the bath. On the right half, rejuvenated women indulge in music and dance (Fig. 5.3). This painting was based on the belief that certain baths might heal and rejuvenate. The fountain of youth was first described by Herodotus (484–425 BC).

It is believed that the discovery of Florida was due to the curiosity of the famous Spanish explorer Ponce de Leon (1460–1521) about the fountain of youth. Ponce de Leon heard a legend about a fountain that makes people young again. This story piqued his curiosity and he embarked on a journey to find this mystical place. Although he was not able to discover the fountain of youth, he did discover Florida. Florida has continued to capitalize on this legend, and nowadays, hundreds of tourists drink each day from the stone well at St. Augustine's Fountain of Youth Archaeological Park.

Through these examples, ranging from the Chinese emperor's search for the potion of eternal life to the wanderings of Ponce de Leon, we can realize that humankind's quest for youth has been endless. A wrinkled face is the harshest expression of the reality of aging.

Numerous panaceas could not aid furrowed profiles until the modern era. The only pragmatic alternative to the inevitability of aging is plastic surgery.

It is generally accepted that the first operation for eyelid correction was performed by Charles Miller in 1906. Facelift procedures continued to be developed through the twentieth century by many innovative plastic surgeons, including Tord Skoog (1915–1977). His revolutionary idea of the "superficial fascia" (1974) was succeeded by the "superficial musculo-aponeurotic system" (1976) [11–13].

After Skoog, many famous plastic surgeons introduced their own methods of facelift surgery, which sometimes cause confusion for readers. It is time to compare the advantages and disadvantages of these numerous methods. A thorough comparison of these methods will open even the beginner's eye and might lead to the narrow path to the fountain of youth.

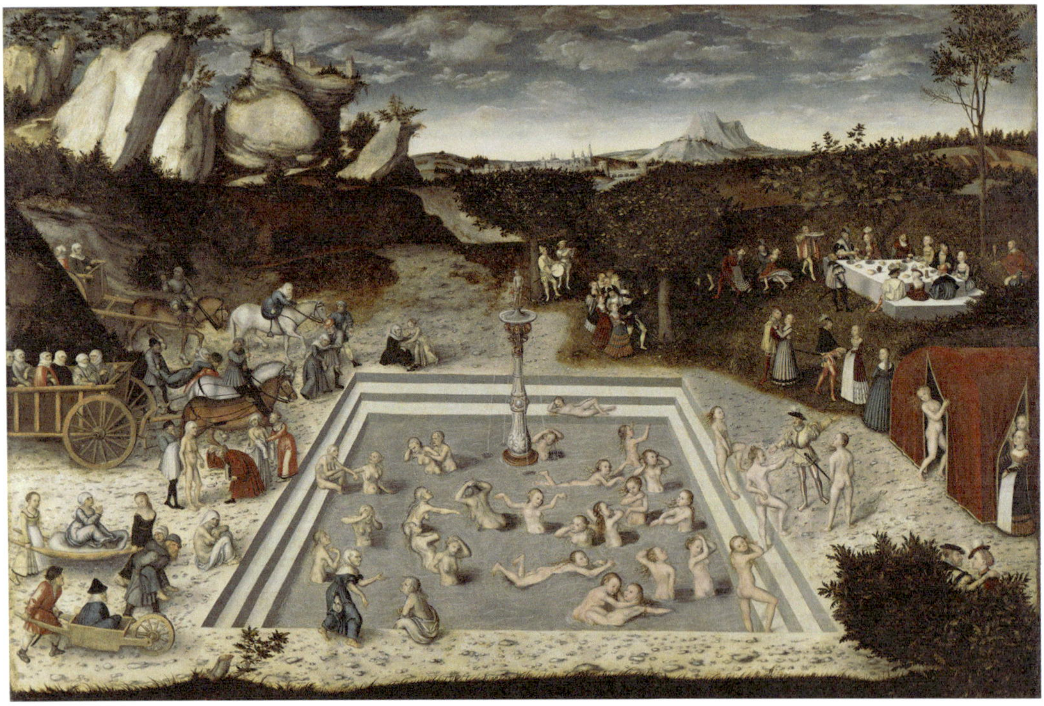

Fig. 5.3 Der Jungbrunnen (The Fountain of Youth), 1546. Lucas Cranach (1472–1553), Gemäldegalerie, Berlin

5.4 Song of Lamenting Old Age

The rosy face fades away and silver threads return.—*From 'Spinning work song' of Korea*

When enjoying fine arts, I like to observe the wrinkles of the face, especially in portraits of old people. I usually see forehead wrinkles, glabellar frown lines, crow's feet, deepened nasolabial grooves, marionette lines, and the turkey gobbler deformity. If the painting contains a skull or a human skeleton, I can estimate the anatomical knowledge of the artist by comparing it with the atlas in my mind.

Recently, a retired general surgeon who lives in Connecticut sent me a photograph of a piece of fine art displayed at the Wadsworth Atheneum Museum of Art near his home. It intrigued me since it contains an old man as well as a skeleton (Fig. 5.4). In this painting, an old man recoils in horror before a skeleton that represents death. The skeleton is coming for the old woodcutter with his arms apart. The poor man is trying to stop the skeleton with his left hand while holding the tied woodcuts with his right hand.

The story is derived from one of Aesop's fables: An old man, "bent double with age and toil," is gathering sticks for a fire. Exhausted, he cries out: "I cannot bear this life any longer! Ah, I wish Death would only come and take me!" On cue, the skeleton appears, bearing a menacing spear. "What wouldst thou, Mortal? I heard thee call me." The old woodcutter pulls back from the ledge. "Please, sir," he says, "would you kindly help me to lift this bundle of sticks onto my shoulder?" According to Aesop, the message is "Be careful what you wish for. You may be sorry."

This painting reminded me of a traditional three-line Korean poem (*sijo*, 時調) written by

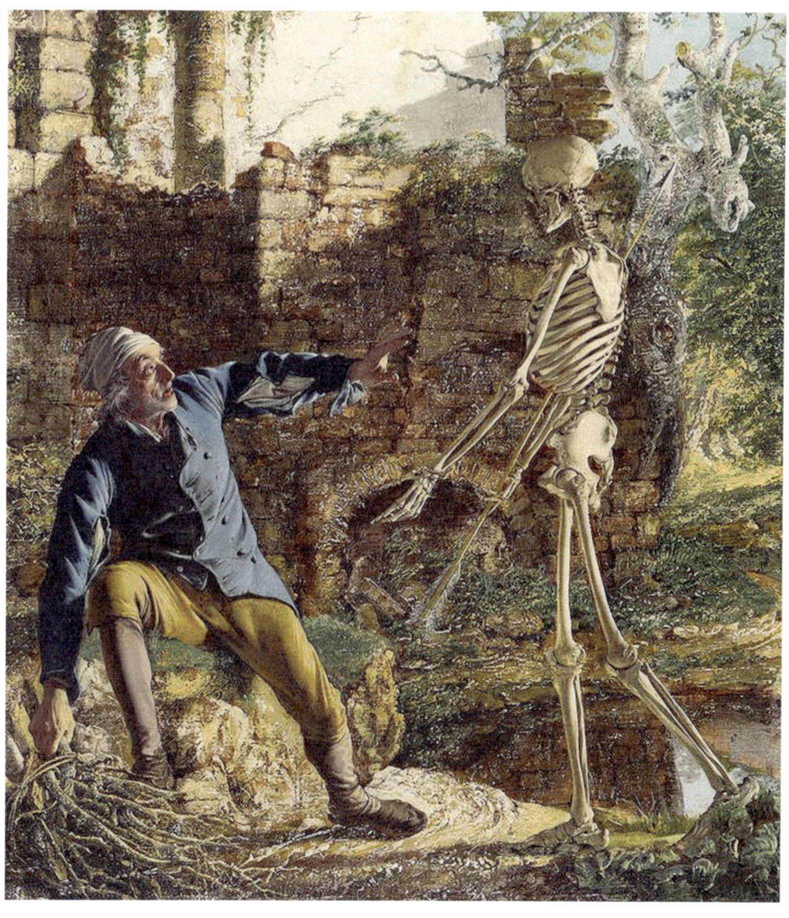

Fig. 5.4 "Old Man and Death" (1774) painted by Joseph Wright (1734–1797)

Woo Tark (禹倬, 1262–1342, late Goryeo dynasty), which I learned in my schooldays.

Holding a stick in one hand, and a thorn in another hand,
I'm trying to block aging with the thorn, and to stop silver hairs with the stick.
Read my intention: silver hairs have already arrived through a shortcut.

In this "Song of Lamenting Old Age, 嘆老歌)," the writer shows his intention to prevent or at least delay the aging process through his will, like the old man reaching out his left hand to stay away from the skeleton in the painting of Joseph Wright (1734–1797).

This poem has been modified to create the "Song of White Hair (白髮歌)," which is sung to accompany spinning work.

This version states:

Holding an ax in the right hand, and a thorn in the left hand,
I'm hitting silver hairs, hooking a rosy face, and tying it up with blue threads.
However, the rosy face fades away and silver threads return.
Crumpled skin below the ears, black hair becomes white.

Numerous panaceas could not aid furrowed profiles until the modern era. The only pragmatic alternative to the inevitability of aging is plastic surgery [14, 15].

Only plastic surgeons can "hook the fading rosy face" and tie it up with "threads."

5.5 Why Do Elderly Men Desire Youth Instead of Aging? An Analysis of Kangnoseonsaeng-Jeon (却老先生傳) by Lee Ok (李鈺)

In the morning, my hair was black like silk bundles. In the evening, it became white like snow (朝如青絲暮成雪).—Li Bai (李白, 701–762 AD, a Chinese poet)

With the snapping of smartphone cameras, photographs are everywhere these days. In our visual society, everybody's insecurities are stamped in time in the annals of the internet. Therefore, troublesome physical features prompt both men and women to undergo plastic surgery.

Recently, I read a book written in Korea 200 years ago (during the Joseon period). The writer, Lee Ok (李鈺, 1760–1815), wrote *Kangnoseonsaeng-Jeon* (却老先生傳, Chronicle of Mr. Tweezer) at the age of 50. This book personifies a tweezer as a narrator and is structured as a set of questions and answers that express psychological anxiety about aging. The author was sensitively aware of aging and described the aging process of the body in detail. The descriptions of changes in hair color and locations are especially impressive [16]. The author would like to delay aging—if not the aging process itself, then at least aging of one's external appearance—by plucking out gray hairs (Fig. 5.5).

In this book, the following reasons for plucking out gray hairs are given: (1) in order to serve in a governmental post, men must avoid looking old; (2) if one's parents are still alive, their son should not look older than his parents; (3) if a man marries a young wife, the husband's old appearance must be avoided; or (4) society treats elderly men poorly.

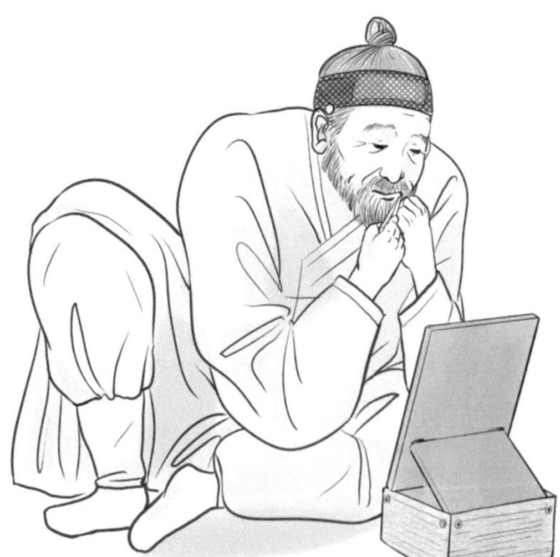

Fig. 5.5 An old writer is tweezing gray hairs. [Illustration by Hye Won Hu, MFA, Division of Biomedical Art, Incheon Catholic University Graduate School (Incheon, Korea)]

From this book, we realize that 200 years ago in Korea, aristocrats (兩班) desired to look young for reasons related to their jobs, social treatment, and marital relationships, just as is the case now. The only difference relates to filial duty, as a good son was expected to avoid looking older than his parents.

It is notable that the author wrote, "It is not sad to die, but it is sad to grow old. People hate aging because they are getting closer to death," which expresses a remarkably modern sentiment but was written 200 years ago.

In our times, elderly men dye their gray hair rather than plucking it out. Cosmetic surgery for men is becoming increasingly common throughout the world. If the author lived in Seoul today, he might have written the "Chronicle of Mr. #15 Blade" instead of the "Chronicle of Mr. Tweezer".

5.6 You Finished the Goose, with the Bones

> And the muscular strength, which it gave to my jaw, Has lasted the rest of my life.—Lewis Carroll (1832–1898)

When I stayed in London for 3 months in 2016, I visited the British Library to borrow a book written by Dr. Grabb. In the lobby, I happened to see a special exhibition entitled "Happy 150th Birthday Alice!" to celebrate the passage of 150 years of the publication of *Alice's Adventures in Wonderland*. I was lucky to see Lewis Carroll's original article with hand-drawn illustrations.

Among them, one illustration particularly intrigued me. While removing the cover from a platter, a youth is surprised and asks his old father something (Fig. 5.6). The legend for this drawing is as follows:

> *"You are old," said the youth, "and your jaws are too weak*
> *For anything tougher than suet;*
> *Yet you finished the goose, with the bones and the beak —*
> *Pray, how did you manage to do it?"*
> *"In my youth," said his father, "I took to the law,*
> *And argued each case with my wife;*
> *And the muscular strength, which it gave to my jaw,*
> *Has lasted the rest of my life.*

This poem, "You Are Old, Father William" is found in Chap. 5, "Advice from a Caterpillar," in the 1865 book *Alice's Adventures in Wonderland*.

Based on this poem, I understood that the aged man was proud of his jaw power (biting force).

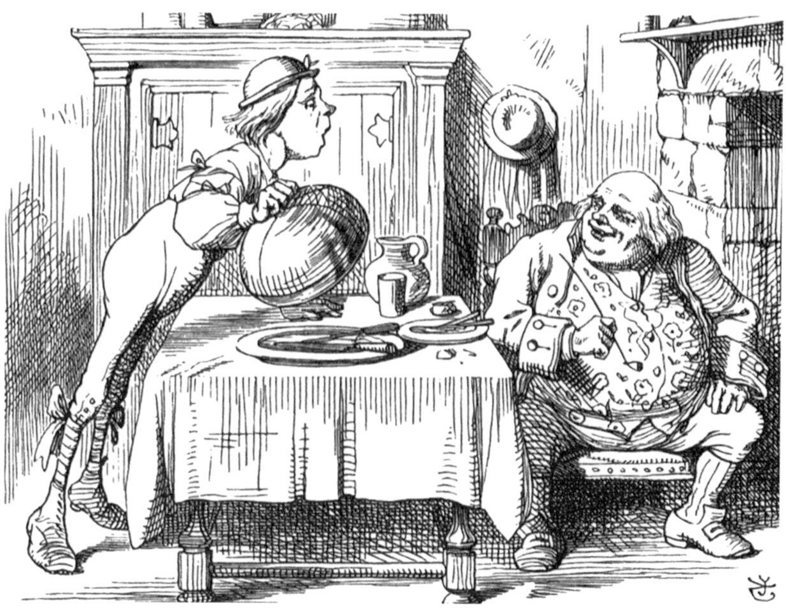

Fig. 5.6 Illustration of "Yet you finished the goose, with the bones and the beak." (Available at: http://bytesdaily.blogspot.com/2010/10/quote-lewis-carroll.html. Accessed 21 Oct 2021)

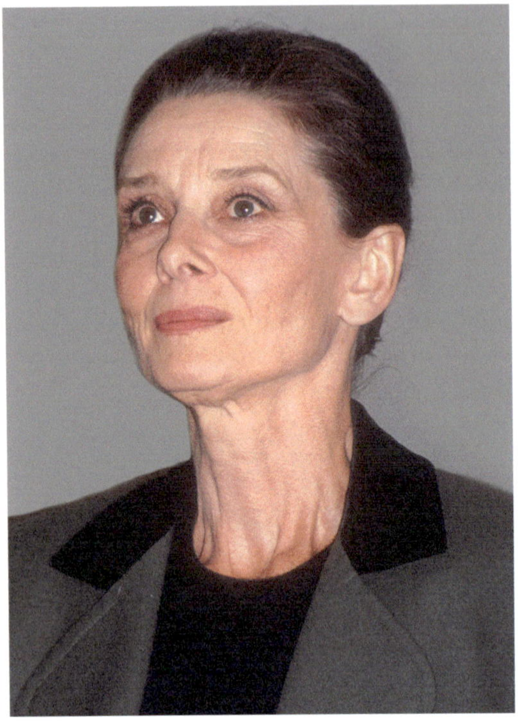

Fig. 5.7 Audrey Hepburn in her old age in 1991. [Photograph was taken by John Barrett and reproduced with permission from Alamy Limited (https://alamy.com)]

When I think of *Alice's Adventures in Wonderland*, my favorite movie star (Audrey Hepburn) comes to mind because she reminds me of the Queen of Hearts due to her regal demeanor. I do not believe that anyone would think that her mandibular angle and masseter muscle made her less charming even in old age (Fig. 5.7). In Asia, however, mandible angle ostectomy to achieve a slim chin has been popular for decades, and masseteric hypertrophy is now corrected using botulinum A toxin injections.

In my training days, a senior resident in my department wrote a dissertation for his master's degree and published it [17]. He made angle ostectomies in rabbit jaws and observed the masseter muscle histologically. He concluded that masseter muscle atrophy after ostectomy of the mandibular angle is not due to connective-tissue changes but instead occurs as a result of individual muscle fiber atrophy accompanied by functional adaptation of sarcomeres and changes in muscle fiber types.

Another author measured the occlusal force of masseteric muscles after intramuscular injections of botulinum toxin A and proved that it reduces the occlusal force [18]. This treatment was found to be effective for temporomandibular joint disorder. However, the biting force must be reduced when treating masseteric hypertrophy for esthetic purposes.

As Alice recites in the poem above, elderly people need healthy teeth and four masticatory muscles (temporalis, masseter, medial, and lateral pterygoid). With regard to procedures to create a slim chin, beauty is in the eye of the beholder. For good biting power in old age, I do think that the temporalis and masseter muscles are very important for the ability to finish a goose with its bones.

5.7 *The Picture of Dorian Gray*: A Plastic Surgeon's View

> We women, as someone says, love with our ears, just as you men love with your eyes, if you ever love at all.—Oscar Wilde (1854–1900)

Years ago, I participated in an annual meeting of the Anatomical Society held in Dublin. After the conference, all the participants were invited to the "literary walk," a tour program in the literary city. We visited a pub (The Duke) where James Joyce was a regular, and Trinity College, where Oscar Wilde studied. At the end of the tour, which lasted until late at night, a tour guide gave us a quiz: Which sport did Oscar Wilde love best? I did not know the answer. An anatomist raised her hand and won a T-shirt as a prize by giving the correct answer: polo. Although I remembered short stories written by Wilde, such as "The Happy Prince" and "The Selfish Giant," I learned during the tour that his father, William Wilde (1815–1876), began the era of modern mastoidectomy with his introduction of the eponymous retroauricular incision and that Oscar Wilde suffered from chronic otorrhea and died from meningitis caused by otitis.

On arrival home, I read the only full-length novel written by him and enjoyed the movie of the same name: *The Picture of Dorian Gray*. This is the story of a very handsome young man (Dorian Gray), who admires and envies his portrait and wishes that the portrait would grow old, instead of him (Fig. 5.8). To resist the physical

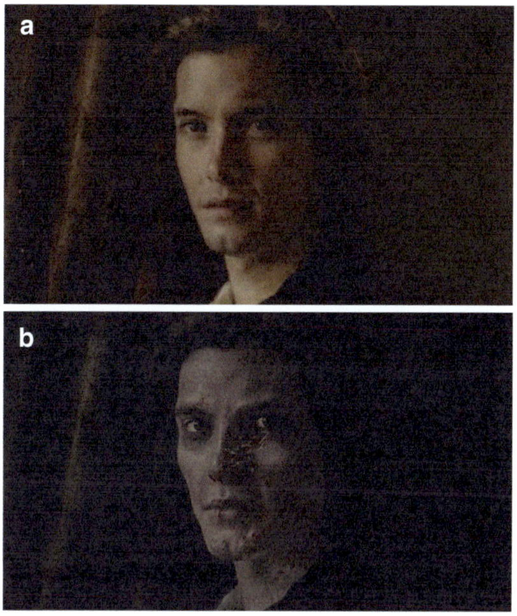

Fig. 5.8 A scene in the movie "The Picture of Dorian Gray." A, Portrait of young Dorian Gray. B, The portrait becomes old and ugly instead of the protagonist

corruption of time and nature and being unable and unwilling to mature, he gives his soul away, and his wish is granted. The oil portrait and protagonist represent the dyad of the person and the mirror. While the protagonist is virtuous and loves his girlfriend, his portrait remains beautiful—but when he abandons his lover and she commits suicide, his portrait becomes ugly and a larva comes out of the eye.

In a search of PubMed using the keyword "Dorian Gray Syndrome (DGS)," I found only one article. This article presents three diagnostic criteria: body dysmorphic disorder, narcissistic regression, and denial of the maturation process. Brosing suggested treatment strategies for DGS: psychodynamic therapy with properly motivated patients, additional medication with psychoactive drugs in serious cases of chronic body dysmorphic disorder, intensive psychotherapy, and cognitive-behavioral methods as an alternative to psychodynamic approaches [19].

As a plastic surgeon, I have a somewhat distinctive viewpoint on the novel. Humans have tried to maintain a youthful appearance using beauty treatments since long before the development of aesthetic plastic surgery. Descriptions of yearning for youth can be found even in ancient literature, as the Fountain of Youth was first described by Herodotus (484–425 BC). Spanish explorer Ponce de Leon (1460–1521) heard a legend about a fountain that made people young again, which provoked his curiosity and started a journey to find this mystical place. Through the long journey of Ponce de Leon, we can realize that humankind's quest for youth has been endless. A wrinkled face is the harshest expression of the reality of aging [14].

Psychodynamic therapy, medication, intensive psychotherapy, or cognitive-behavioral methods might help the syndromic symptoms of DGS. Nonetheless, suppressing patients' quest for youth is not possible by psychiatric methods.

Although many panaceas have been used, they could not help with the problem of a furrowed profile until the modern era. The only pragmatic alternative to the inevitability of aging is plastic surgery, the narrow path to the Fountain of Youth.

5.8 Why Do We Quest for Youth?

As plastic surgeons, patients frequently ask us, "How young will I look if I have facelift surgery?" or "Will I be more attractive after surgery?" These questions deal with the degree of perceived age change and improvement in attractiveness after aesthetic facial surgical procedures.

In an objective assessment study, the average reduction in apparent age after a facelift alone was 4.6 years. Laser resurfacing provided a 2.5-year reduction, while eyelid surgery and endoscopic forehead lift each contributed a 2-year reduction [20]. Another paper reported that the mean overall age reduction following aesthetic facial surgery was 3.1 years (range, −4.0 to 9.4 years). However, there was no significant increase in attractiveness scores in postprocedural photographs relative to preprocedural photographs [21].

Humans tried to maintain a youthful appearance using beauty treatments long before the development of aesthetic plastic surgery. Ranging from the Chinese emperor's search for the potion of eternal life to the wanderings of Ponce de Leon, mankin's quest for youth has been endless [14]. Facial wrinkles are the harshest expression of the reality of aging. Numerous panaceas could not aid furrowed profiles until the modern era. The only pragmatic alternative to the inevitability of aging is plastic surgery.

Why, then, does mankind quest for youth? Why do we prefer a young-looking appearance?

Infants have soft skin and hair, huge eyes, big pupils, chubby cheeks, and small noses. Infants would die without our care; therefore, their appearance must be irresistible. Although there is nothing intrinsically beautiful about huge eyes and small hands, the basic anatomical configuration of babies has a profound meaning for us and elicits tender feelings. Young humans have big heads and big eyes, chubby cheeks, and little noses that signal their helplessness. Jane Goodall found that baby chimpanzees were safe from attack as long as they retained a tuft of white on the tail, suggesting that white tail tufts are biological tags warning adult chimpanzees not to harm the little ones. Therefore, it can be said that a young appearance turns off aggression [22].

This leads to an interesting question: when do children acquire their preferences for beauty? A study examined the preferences of infants (2–3-month-olds and 6–8-month-olds) for attractive faces using a standard visual preference technique. The results showed that infants looked longer at attractive faces when the faces were presented in contrasting pairs of attractiveness (attractive/unattractive) [23]. This study shows that we are born with preferences and even a baby knows beauty when she sees it.

Attractive women have been found to have advantages over unattractive women. A researcher hypothesized that attractive ladies-in-distress would receive more offers of aid than unattractive ladies-in-distress. He used a "lady-with-a-manufacturing-car paradigm" and about 25 eligible vehicles were observed in each condition. The results showed that physical attractiveness played a part in inducing aiding behavior [24].

As a description of mortal beauty, I remember the scene in *A Portrait of the Artist as a Young Man*, where the Stephen Dedalus found perfect beauty in a girl [25].

> Her long slender bare legs were delicate as a crane's and pure save where an emerald trail of seaweed had fashioned itself as a sign upon the flesh. Her thighs, fuller and soft hued as ivory, were bared almost to the hips, where the white fringes of her drawers were like feathering of soft white down. Her slate blue skirts were kilted boldly about her waist and dovetailed behind her. Her bosom was as a bird's, soft and slight, slight and soft as the breast of some dark plumaged dove. But her long fair hair was girlish: and girlish, and touched with the wonder of mortal beauty, her face (Fig. 5.9).

On a late spring day, years ago, I also visited Martello Tower (James Joyce Tower and Museum) with my daughter. At the Sandy Cove beach, I saw several pretty girls swimming. My

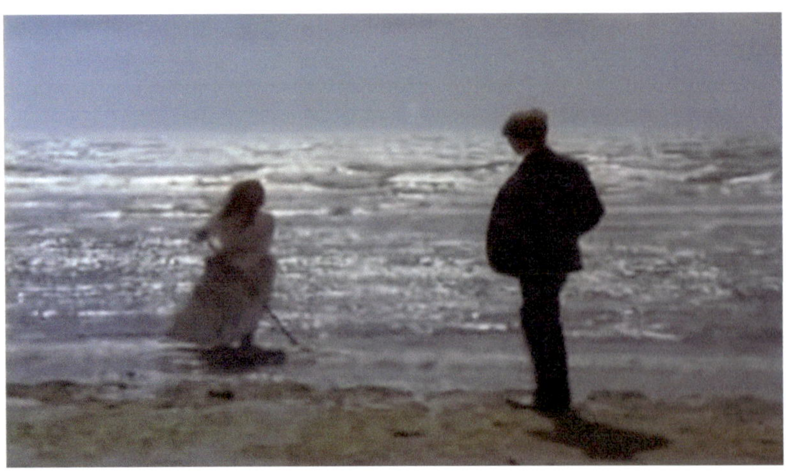

Fig. 5.9 A scene in *A Portrait of the Artist as a Young Man* where Stephen Dedalus finds perfect beauty in a girl at the beach

daughter was sitting on the dock and fell asleep, and I was looking at her. Like a porcupine loves her offspring's "soft" skin, I thought she was lovely. She was young.

References

1. Jacobus de Voragine. The Golden Legend (Aurea Legenda), 1275. Englished by William Caxton, 1483. https://sourcebooks.fordham.edu/basis/goldenlegend/. Accessed 30 Sept 2021.
2. Gao H, Liu J, Yu S, et al. A new polyester technique for sheet plastination. J Int Soc Plastination. 2006;21:7–10.
3. Sui HJ, Henry RW. Polyester plastination of biological tissue: Hoffen P45 technique. J Int Soc Plastination. 2007;22:78–81.
4. Hwang K, Sui HJ. Sheet plastination for understanding important structures in craniofacial surgery. J Craniofac Surg. 2021;32:e850. https://doi.org/10.1097/SCS.0000000000008097.
5. Hwang K, Sui HJ, Han SH, et al. The nasolabial area shown on histology and P45 sheet plastination. J Craniofac Surg. 2021;32:771–3.
6. Hwang K, Sui HJ, Kim H. Superficial fascia of the cheek shown in P45 sheet plastination. J Craniofac Surg. 2021;32:759–61.
7. Eliot TS. The waste land. https://www.poetryfoundation.org/poems/47311/the-waste-land. Accessed 15 Oct 2021.
8. Ahmed FF. Rejuvenation in T.S. Eliot's the waste land. Eur Sci J. 2015;11:159–68.
9. Sallis EK. Looking to death for what life cannot give: the Waste Land and F. H. Bradley; 1991. p. 1–163.
10. Hwang K. Portraits of two innovative plastic surgeons in the National Portrait Gallery. Plast Aesthet Res. 2017;4:15–7.
11. Skoog T. Plastic surgery: new methods and refinements. Philadelphia: Saunders; 1974. p. 302–30.
12. Mitz V, Peyronie M. The superficial musculoaponeurotic system (SMAS) in the parotid and cheek area. Plast Reconstr Surg. 1976;58:8088.
13. Hwang K, Choi JH. Superficial fascia in the cheek and the superficial musculoaponeurotic system. J Craniofac Surg. 2018;29:13781382.
14. Hwang K. Humankind's endless quest for youth. J Craniofac Surg. 2019;30:2303.
15. Hwang K. Why do we quest for youth? J Craniofac Surg. 2021;32:e848. https://doi.org/10.1097/SCS.0000000000007868.
16. Ahn SH. A study on Kangnoseonsaeng-Jeon of Lee Ok: focusing on the aging and autobiography. J Korean Lit Chin. 2016;45:253–76.
17. Song HS, Park CG. Masseter muscle atrophy after ostectomy of the mandibular angle in rabbits. Plast Reconstr Surg. 1997;99:51–60.
18. Zhang LD, Liu Q, Zou DR, et al. Occlusal force characteristics of masseteric muscles after intramuscular injection of botulinum toxin A (BTX-A) for treatment of temporomandibular disorder. Br J Oral Maxillofac Surg. 2016;54:736–40.
19. Brosig B, Kupfer J, Niemeier V, et al. The "Dorian Gray Syndrome": psychodynamic need for hair growth restorers and other "fountains of youth". Int J Clin Pharmacol Ther. 2001;39:279–83.
20. Swanson E. Objective assessment of change in apparent age after facial rejuvenation surgery. J Plast Reconstr Aesthet Surg. 2011;64:1124–31.
21. Zimm AJ, Modabber M, Fernandes V, et al. Objective assessment of perceived age reversal and improvement in attractiveness after aging face surgery. JAMA Facial Plast Surg. 2013;15:405–10.
22. Etcoff N. Survival of the prettiest: the science of beauty. Hamburg: Anchor Academic Publishing; 2000.
23. Langlois JH, Roggman LA, Casey RJ, et al. Infant preferences for attractive faces: rudiments of a stereotype? Dev Psychol. 1987;23:363–9.
24. Athanasiou R, Greene P. Physical attractiveness and helping behavior. In: Proceedings of the annual convention of the American Psychological Association. 1973:289–290
25. Joyce J. The portrait of an artist as a young man. https://www.gutenberg.org/files/4217/4217-h/4217-h.htm#link2HCH0001. Accessed 5 Feb 2021.

6 Plastic Surgeon as a Researcher

6.1 Gutenberg's Spirit in Today's World

Sola scriptura (by scripture alone)—Martin Luther

When writing papers, we cite articles and put them in references. If the content we want to cite or quote is derived from other articles, we have to consult the original source. By clicking on an inline citation, we reach the reference information, and we can easily get the abstract from PubMed. If the citation is from a journal to which our library subscribes, we can get the full text for free. If it does not subscribe to the journal, we can get the full text either through interlibrary loan or by sending a request to the corresponding author of the paper.

If a citation is from a book that I do not have, I first try to find it through a Google search. If it is not available, I have to order it from Amazon, which takes usually several weeks to deliver to me. After I get a book volume in my hands, it is easy to find the content I want to confirm if the pages are provided in the reference. If the title of the book is provided without specific pages, I have to look from beginning to the end of the book to find it.

Getting old books is not easy. Most rare editions are only occasionally available from most booksellers. I sometimes imagine how happy I would be if scientific books became widely available to the public 70 years after the death of the author, when copyright protection ends.

Recently, I learned about Project Gutenberg, a volunteer effort to digitize and archive cultural works through the creation and distribution of full texts of public-domain books. Releases are available in plain text, HTML, PDF, and other common formats. On their website, one can see the top 100 authors and their books: Mark Twain, Jane Austen, Conan Doyle, and Charles Dickens—that is, mostly classics of literature. I hope that old books on anatomy or surgery could be provided, as well as literary works.

During my stay in Germany for collaborative work, I had the chance to visit the Gutenberg Museum located in Mainz, where I saw Gutenberg's portrait (Fig. 6.1) and the famous Gutenberg Bible (42-line Bible). His mechanical movable type printing (press) started the Printing Revolution and played a key role in the Reformation started by Martin Luther ("*Sola scriptura*"), because these new technologies enabled the Bible to be widely read by the masses.

If old scientific books are made available to researchers, like Bibles to sixteenth-century Europeans, journal articles will become more accurate and contain deeper, error-free "original descriptions," which might be the beginning of another scientific revolution. Again, Gutenberg!

K. Hwang, *Good Physician, Good Plastic Surgeon*, https://doi.org/10.1007/978-981-97-1864-1_6

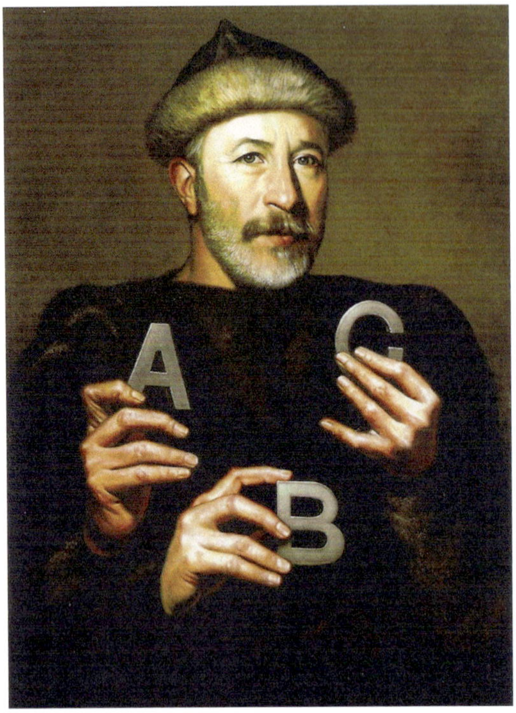

Fig. 6.1 "Gutenberg." 2001, Oel/Leinwand, 85 × 65 cm. (Reproduced with permission from artist Dietmar Gross and Gutenberg-Museum, Mainz, Germany)

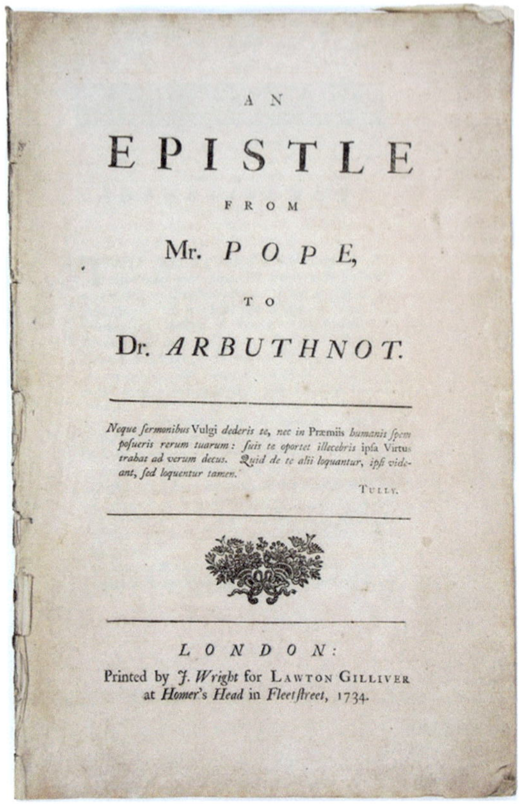

AN

EPISTLE

FROM

Mr. *POPE*,

TO

Dr. *ARBUTHNOT.*

Neque ſermonibus Vulgi *dederis te, nec in* Præmiis *humanis ſpem poſueris rerum tuarum: ſuis te oportet illecebris* ipſa Virtus *trahat ad verum decus. Quid de te alii loquantur, ipſi videant, ſed loquentur tamen.*

TULLY.

LONDON:

Printed by *J. Wright* for LAWTON GILLIVER at *Homer's Head* in *Fleetſtreet*, 1734.

Fig. 6.2 A book cover of "An Epistle from Mr. Pope to Dr. Arbuthnot" (first edition) written by Alexander Pope

6.2 Why Do Poets and Scientists Write? Why Then Publish?

In the novel *The Da Vinci Code* written by Dan Brown, Professor Langdon and Sophie interpret a verse reading "In London lies a knight A. Pope interred." At first, they think that "A. Pope" refers to the Catholic pope, but after searching, they realize that the actual meaning is, "Sir Isaac Newton's burial, attended by kings and nobles, was presided over by Alexander Pope, friend and colleague, who gave a stirring eulogy before sprinkling dirt on the tomb." Therefore, they travel to Westminster Abbey (Fig. 6.2).

Alexander Pope (1688–1744), a famous English poet, was moved by Newton's (1642–1727) accomplishments, and wrote the famous epitaph: "Nature and nature's laws lay hid in night; God said 'Let Newton be' and all was light." However, this was not allowed to be put on the monument in Westminster Abbey.

Alexander Pope had a friend who was a physician as well as a poet: Dr. John Arbuthnot (1667–1735). They were members of the Scriblerus Club, as was Jonathan Swift (1667–1745). In the year before the death of Arbuthnot, Alexander Pope wrote "The Epistle to Dr. Arbuthnot" as a memorial of their friendship, and it was published in a year later (1735).

In this poem, the answer appears to a question that I am frequently asked by my friends, or my pupils: "Why do you write? Why do you publish?"

Why did I write? What sin to me unknown
Dipp'd me in ink, my parents', or my own?
As yet a child, nor yet a fool to fame,
I lisp'd in numbers, for the numbers came.
I left no calling for this idle trade,
No duty broke, no father disobey'd.

The Muse but serv'd to ease some friend, not wife,
To help me through this long disease, my life,
To second, Arbuthnot! thy art and care,
And teach the being you preserv'd, to bear.
But why then publish? Granville the polite,
And knowing Walsh, would tell me I could write;
Well-natur'd Garth inflamed with early praise,
And Congreve lov'd, and Swift endur'd my lays;
The courtly Talbot, Somers, Sheffield read,
Ev'n mitred Rochester would nod the head,
And St. John's self (great Dryden's friends before)
With open arms receiv'd one poet more.
Happy my studies, when by these approv'd!
Happier their author, when by these belov'd!
From these the world will judge of men and books,
Not from the Burnets, Oldmixons, and Cookes.

As a plastic surgeon, I thought about the reasons why I write and publish.

In the field of plastic surgery, surgeons and researchers develop many new ideas and skills. Science is strengthened not by research alone, but by the publication of research articles in scientific journals that are read by the scientific community. Scientists write papers to share knowledge or skill with others or to receive promotions at universities [1]. "Publish or perish" is a phrase coined to describe the pressure in academia to publish work constantly to further or sustain one's career [2].

An author submits a manuscript to an editor, who decides to accept or reject it. The editor then sends the manuscript to reviewers for their opinion. Aside from the author, editor, and reviewer, publishers and subscribers play their role in scientific journals as well. These five stakeholders are all essential.

As an editorial board member, I am willing to be designated a "devil's referee," that is, a kind of devil's advocate with the responsibility of examining the originality of a manuscript, taking a skeptical view of the manuscript, and looking for holes in the methods and results of reported experiments. As an author, I have responsibilities to submit manuscripts with scientific integrity and have to be ready to take responsibility for my articles even long after publication [3].

I will be more than happy when my studies are approved by reviewers and beloved by subscribers, as "A. Pope" described.

6.3 Gender Bias in a Man's World

I never saw a wild thing sorry for itself. A small bird will drop frozen dead from a bough without ever having felt sorry for itself.—David H. Lawrence

I recently enjoyed a movie entitled "The Wife" (2017; Director Bjorn Runge, Writer Meg Wolitzer), in which a senior plastic surgeon (Dr. Mutaz Habal) recommended to me. This movie presents the story of a writer who receives the Nobel Prize for literature and his devoted wife.

In 1956, Joan Archer meets Joseph Castleman, a handsome young man married to a professor at a women's college, and falls in love with him. She was already an accomplished (but unpublished) writer. At a conference, Joan meets an alumna author, Elaine Mozell, who had self-published a book (only 200 volumes) and distributed it to her friends only.

They have the following conversation:

Elaine: The public does not tolerate bold prose from a woman. You must never imagine that you can get their attention.
Joan: Whose?
Elaine: The men who write the reviews, drive publishers, and publish the journals.
Joan: An author should write.
Elaine: An author should be read.

Elaine's cynical views on opportunities for female writers disheartened Joan. After Joseph's divorce from his ex-wife, his first attempt at writing a novel turns out very poorly. Joan agrees to fix Joseph's novel for him. As they live together, Joan works hard writing a novel, to be published under Joseph's name, while Joseph supports her by cooking, cleaning, and caring for their first child. She functions as a "ghostwriter" for her husband. On the evening of Joseph's Nobel Prize, Joan declares to him that she will leave him (Fig. 6.3). This movie awarded with 10 awards, including 76th Golden Globe Awards.

This impressive movie reminded me the story of Mileva Marić (1875–1948); Albert Einstein's college classmate and first wife. The question whether Mileva contributed to his work is still the subject of debate. Many professional historians

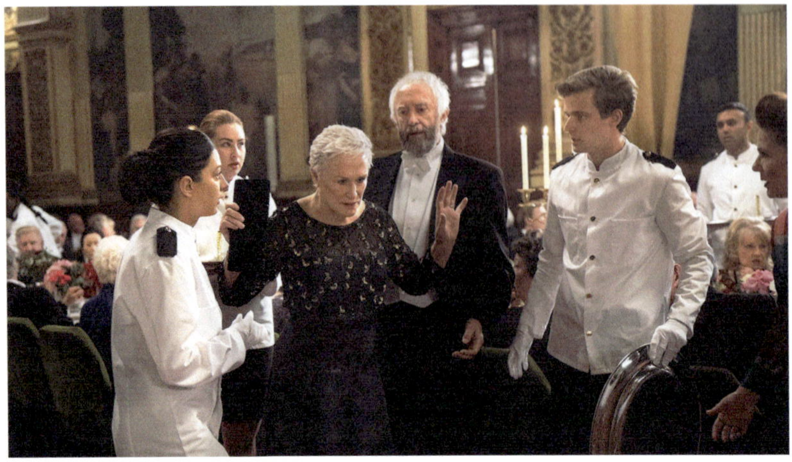

Fig. 6.3 "The Wife." On the evening of Joseph's Nobel Prize, Joan declares that she will leave him

of physics suggest that she was a supportive companion in science and may have helped him materially in his research. Einstein married again in the year they divorced (1919). She alone took care of their three children by teaching mathematics. From this story, I have learnt that there is always a help or even sacrifice of a greater woman hidden behind the achievement of a great man.

I searched the literature for studies on gender bias in the plastic surgery field. In a recent anonymous electronic survey distributed to the American Society of Plastic Surgeons, women were more likely than men to have experienced sexism or bias. Women were less likely to be married, be satisfied with work-life balance, or feel recognized for ideas, authorship, promotions, or raises. Women felt that their sex was a disadvantage in career advancement, with one exception: unlike men, women felt that many patients chose them because of their sex [4].

A systematic review reported that women plastic surgeons continue to be underrepresented in the United States, Canada, and Europe, with proportions ranging from 14 to 25.7%. Academic plastic surgeons are less frequently female than male, and women academic plastic surgeons score less favorably when outcomes of academic success are evaluated [5].

In residency and fellowship training, persistent gender bias is present, and it impacts female physicians. Several institutions have enacted successful interventions to identify and address gender bias [6].

After reading the above literature, I remembered a picture of a father and daughter pair of plastic surgeons who were not victims of gender bias: Dr. Alexander Limberg, who designed the famous rhomboid flap, and his daughter Dr. Ala Limberg, who took over her father's work. I also noticed that the author of two of the above articles is the daughter of a famous plastic surgeon, Dr. David W. Furnas, whose anthropometry book I have [4, 5].

Since I became a clinical faculty member in 1993, I have trained four female residents. During their training, in the depths of my heart, I regarded them as my daughters. Officially, however, I tried to make them into warriors, like G. I. Jane, and gave them the poem "Self-Pity" written by David H. Lawrence. They were all competent and talented and successfully completed their residency. Now they are doing well as clinical faculty and private practitioners.

¡Viva la Vida!
¡Vivan las Mujeres cirujanos plásticos!

6.4 The Privileges Enjoyed by Fellows

Don't be intimidated. Great knowledge comes from the humblest of origins.—John Edensor Littlewood

I enjoyed the film entitled *A Man Who Knew Infinity* (2015), directed by Matt Brown (Fig. 6.4).

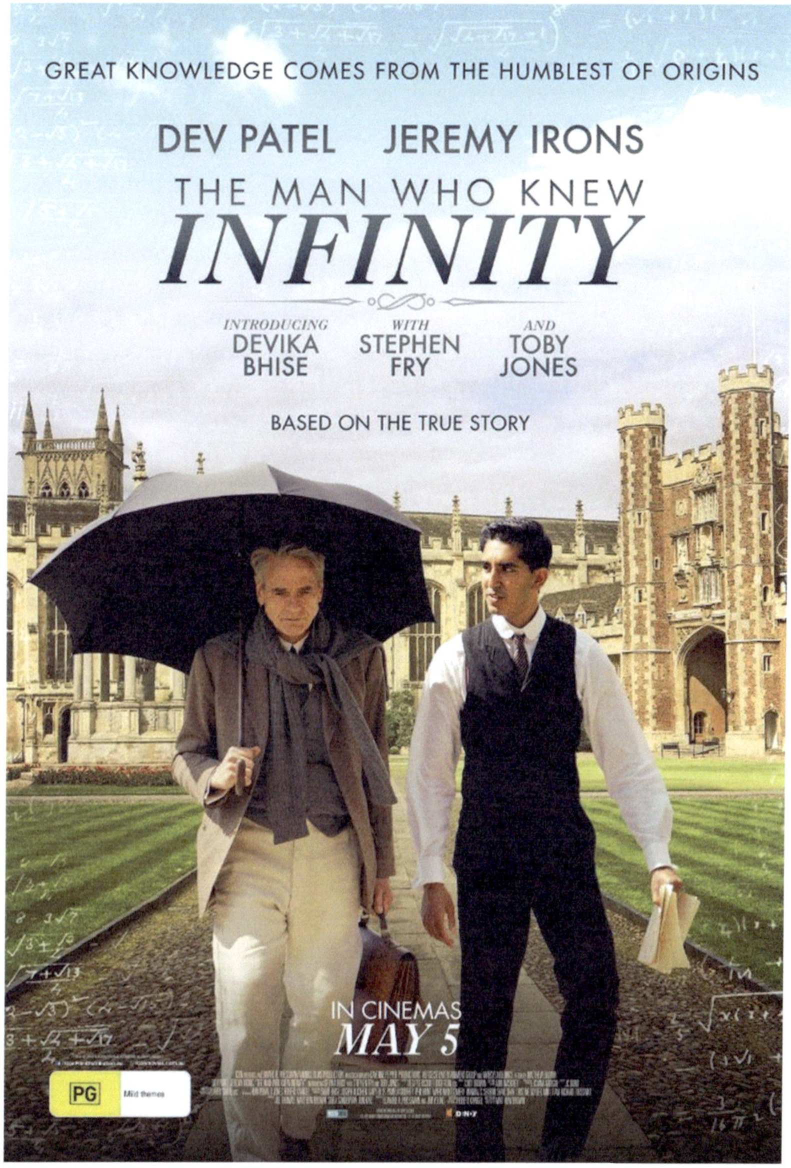

Fig. 6.4 Poster of the movie "A Man Who Knew Infinity (2015)," directed by Matt Brown

The story was so interesting that I had to order the book of the same name written by Robert Kanigel. It is the story of the life and academic career of the pioneer Indian mathematician, Srinivasa Ramanujan (1887–1920), and his friendship with his mentor, Professor Godfrey Harold Hardy (1877–1947).

When Ramanujan started his studies at Trinity College Cambridge, he unintentionally walked across the green from his dorm to the lecture room and was immediately stopped by a guard. The guard said "Only the fellows can walk across this green." As is well-known, Trinity College of Cambridge is governed by the Master and Fellows, across a very wide range of academic specialties, who are responsible for maintaining it as a place of education, learning, and research.

In the book, I found some thought-provoking quotes:

> *Hardy looked like a sort of White Rabbit hopping around the Fellows Garden at Trinity...* [7]

> *Ramanujan was a fellow of Trinity! He sat at the high table now, and the grave portraits of the founders and the illustrious dead looked down*

> *upon him approvingly. He wore his honours as he had worn his misfortunes, with becoming modesty, and was warmly welcomed by the grave, scholarly old Fellows who sat around the great horseshoe table in the Combination Room* [7].

From these quotes, I realized that fellows had several privileges: they could walk across the fellows' bowling green, have their own seat at the high table in the dining hall, and have a seat at the great horseshoe table in the Combination Room (Fellows' Hall).

I thought over the reasons why one of the best colleges in the world gave privileges to their fellows. First, these privileges are an expression of respect toward scholars who attain high distinction in academic or public life. Second, they are for the convenience of the researchers, allowing them to save time. Finally, they encourage discussions among researchers, which might lead to flashes of inspiration.

As plastic surgeons and researchers, we move from outpatient offices to the operating theater, from the lecturer's office to the laboratory. In hospital cafeterias, there is no "high table" for surgeons. We need time and space to engage in discussions with other qualified plastic surgeons.

Many qualified plastic surgeons have the qualifications of FRCS (Fellow, Royal Colleges of Surgeons, founded 1368) or FACS (Fellow, American College of Surgeons, founded 1912).

It has been just 100 years since the Queen's Hospital opened in 1917; in this hospital, Sir Harold Gillies developed many techniques of plastic surgery through more than 11,000 operations, mostly on soldiers with facial injuries.

It is time for plastic surgeons to gather together. My dream is to create a "College of Plastic Surgeons" for plastic surgeons worldwide. Conducting "horseshoe table" discussions through the Internet will give us inspiration.

6.5 You Will Be a Researcher, My Student!

> If you can trust yourself when all men doubt you, but make allowance for their doubting too; you'll be a man, my son!—Rudyard Kipling

I again received a decision letter from a journal office: "Major revision required—No guarantee of acceptance" for the revised manuscript which I recently submitted. Although I know that experiencing repeated major revisions or even rejections make a researcher more mature, this set heavily on me.

In order to overcome this feeling, I went to the theatre to watch the movie "Mission Impossible 6: Fallout" (2018), in which Tom Cruise stars as agent Eden Hunt. To follow the story, I had to rewatch the previous move in the series, "Mission Impossible 5: Rogue Nation" (2015). In this movie, agent Hunt kidnaps the British prime minister and hypnotizes him by an injection in order to get a password from him. As Hunt gives the prompt "Kipling" to the prime minister, the hypnotized minister releases the password: the beginning of Kipling's poem, which starts "If you can keep your head when all about you/are losing theirs and blaming it on you." After getting this password, Hunt unlocked the trove of secrets.

Rudyard Kipling (1865–1936) is well-known as the author of *The Jungle Book* (1894), which I read in elementary school about 50 years ago (Fig. 6.5). As I entered my 60s, I was reminded again of his work and enjoyed his poem "If-". "If you can trust yourself when all men doubt you, but make allowance for their doubting too; if you can wait and not be tired by waiting, or being lied about, don't deal in lies, if you can meet with triumph and disaster and treat those two impostors just the same; yours is the earth and everything that's in it, and—which is more—you'll be a man, my son!"

When writing scientific papers—either research articles or clinical studies—we plastic surgeons, including myself and my students, are frequently confronted with difficulties.

Grants are difficult to get. For clinical studies, the IRB process takes several months. Animals can die during experiments. The data cannot be collected as expected. Writing on a PC is tedious.

After submission, too early of a response from the journal office is usually bad news, beginning with "I regret to inform you that." A late response usually asks for a major revision, with no guaran-

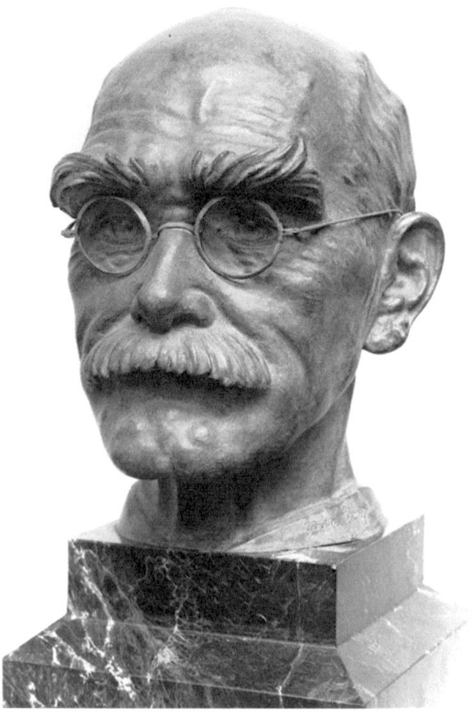

Fig. 6.5 Rudyard Kipling by Ginette Bingguely-Lejeune, bronze head, 1936–1937. NPG 2955. (Reproduced by permission from National Portrait Gallery, London)

tee of acceptance. In most cases, I can revise the manuscript according to the reviewers' reasonable suggestions. However, sometimes we might despair because of the referee's "merciless demands," which seems like a "mission impossible."

After struggling through several revisions, we receive a letter beginning "I am pleased to inform you that your manuscript is now accepted." We are delighted to receive this letter. But is not the end; in fact, it is just a beginning.

If the paper is published online before print, subscribers can read it, and if they have a difference of opinion, they can submit a letter to the editor or piece of correspondence beginning with "Comments on…" or "Questions on…," like a football player making a shot. Most readers ask genuine questions about what they really want to know, but some famous researchers can throw a "stone" at the author if the content of the article contradicts their previously published opinion. If the author fails to reply, it seems like the author is admitting that the objections in the letter are correct. Therefore, the author has the responsibility to respond.

Since Kipling's poem was a comfort to me. I would like to share it with my students, who are working hard in writing papers. I invited them a dinner and asked if they knew "Kipling." At first, they recognized "Kipling" as a brand of handbags or backpacks.

I substituted several words of a poem "If-" and gave it to my students:

> If we can wait and not be tired by waiting through the research and publication process; if we have to trust ourselves when readers might doubt us, but allow them to their doubting too; if we meet with acceptance, revision, or rejection, and treat these impostors just the same, we'll be researchers, my students!

This revised poem consoled my students who are depressed in repeated revisions and rejections. Experiencing these procedures make a researcher more mature because it produces endurance. If we treat acceptance, revision, or rejection just the same, we will not be negatively affected by rejection.

6.6 The Cowardly Lion's Medal of Courage

> The plastic surgeon can learn from his colleagues in the clinical fields and from research workers in basic sciences, thus enlarging the body of knowledge of the specialty.—John Marquis Converse, MD (1909–1981)

When I became a chief resident in 1990, the new textbook of plastic surgery edited by Joseph McCarthy had appeared. I bought it and read it thoroughly to prepare for the board certification examination. In the author list, I looked at the academic degrees of the contributors. Among them, two authors had special abbreviations: Paul W. Brand, CBE, and Bernard M. O'Brien, CMG. Later, I learned that these are kinds of orders. CBE stands for Commander of the Order of the British Empire, and CMG for Companion of St. Michael and St. George.

Today, 28 years later, I received an Order of Science and Technology Merit award from the Korean government for contributions to anatomical knowledge in the field of plastic surgery. From now on, I can write "OST" just before my academic degrees ("MD, PhD").

With this precious medal in my hand, I remembered a movie entitled "Wizard of Oz" (1939, with Judy Garland starring as Dorothy), which I loved a long time ago.

The scarecrow (Hunk) had no brain, the tin man (Hickory) had no heart, and the cowardly lion (Zeke) had no courage. The scarecrow received a brain (much like a PhD degree) from Oz, the tin man received a pocket watch, and the cowardly lion received a medal marked "courage." Although lions are supposed to be "the kings of beasts," the cowardly lion did not understand that courage means acting in the face of fear, which he did frequently. After receiving the medal marked "courage," he was no longer filled with fear.

When I turned 40 (1997), my first and second international articles appeared in the *Journal of Craniofacial Surgery* (*JCFS*) [8, 9]. The letter of acceptance from the editor became a "medal of courage" to me. Since then, I have not been filled with the fear of rejection. I owe a lot to the editor Dr. Mutaz Habal and reviewers of *JCFS*.

As researchers and surgeons, we should not shy away from submitting an article owing to the fear of repeated rejection. We should understand that courage means acting in the face of fear.

In case of major revisions, we should not give up on revising in response to so many difficult suggestions. We must be confident. We do not have to change our manuscript exactly according to the reviewer's comments. We should have the courage to respond "Regarding this suggestion, I cannot change my original manuscript because…," or "I would decline to revise rather than change the format to correspondence."

When submitting an article, we should remember we have a "medal of courage" in our heart (Fig. 6.6).

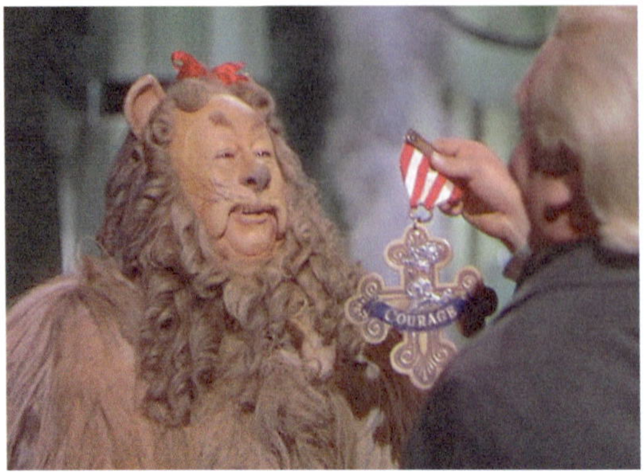

Fig. 6.6 Medal of courage in "Wizard of Oz"

6.7 Lost Music and Remaining Manuscripts

The most difficult step in research is to improvise a motif [10]. I usually find a motif at conferences of plastic surgeons or anatomists.

When listening to the presentations of other researchers and the subsequent question-and-answer sessions, I try to figure out what they found, what they want to convey, what they want to do next, and what blind spots might be present in their research. Because my memory is treacherous, I take notes in the margins of the abstract book or in a notebook before I forget my impressions.

When I return to my office, I read these notes and remind myself of the environment at the conference. When I feel that a topic is interesting, I search for the references and wonder about whether or not there is something new to be discovered on this topic (*etwas neues*).

If I think that I might embark upon the research immediately or in the near future, I start writing a rough draft of an introduction in three brief paragraphs, identifying the facts already known about the topic, what is lacking in the current knowledge, and why is it important to ask certain questions (i.e., the objectives of my study or the research question). In a draft of the methods section, I try to write out the possible materials I might use and details about the methods I would employ [11]. Once I write a draft, I save it—along with the references—in a specifically named folder on my PC. Of course, I also print each draft out and store it in paper form. Therefore, many paper drafts are stored on my bookshelves, as well as in folders on my PC.

If I have enough time and resources, I proceed with the research. If not, however, the files wait for me for months or even years.

As usual, at the end of last year, I reviewed the files waiting for me and classified them using a triage expected (abort), immediate, or delayed. When I was classifying them, a thought suddenly came to mind: I may not accomplish all these studies before my retirement, which is only 3 years in the future.

The very next day, I enjoyed a broadcast of the 2020 Vienna Philharmonic New Year's Concert at a music hall in Korea. This concert was conducted by Andris Nelsons from the Wiener Musikverein in Vienna, Austria. Between Part 1 and Part 2, we watched a video set to music entitled "Beethoven's Blätterwirbel: The Lost Music."

While a metronome is ticking, a musician is writing music on a blank sheet of music under candlelight. When a maid opens the door, the wind sweeps away the music sheets through the window. The sheets are scattered to the air and vanish. The maid goes out to search for the lost sheets, and on her way, she visits several places related to Beethoven, encountering several open-air concerts. She finds them in a tree, along a road, in a restaurant, in a small stream, and even in a florist's shop. Gathering up most of the lost music sheets, she eventually arrives at the Austrian National Library in Vienna. Standing in front of a large table in the stately hall, she hugs the sheets she gathered and places them on the table with a sigh. The front page of the sheets shows the title of the music: Symphony 10 for orchestra, 1826 L. van Beethoven (Fig. 6.7).

Symphony No. 10 in E$^{\flat}$ major is a hypothetical work, assembled in 1988 by Barry Cooper from Beethoven's fragmentary sketches. The sketches assembled were intended for the same symphony, following the Ninth Symphony, and a consensus exists that Beethoven intended to compose another symphony. It was first performed at a concert in 1988, about 150 years after Beethoven himself had proposed a new symphony in 1827.

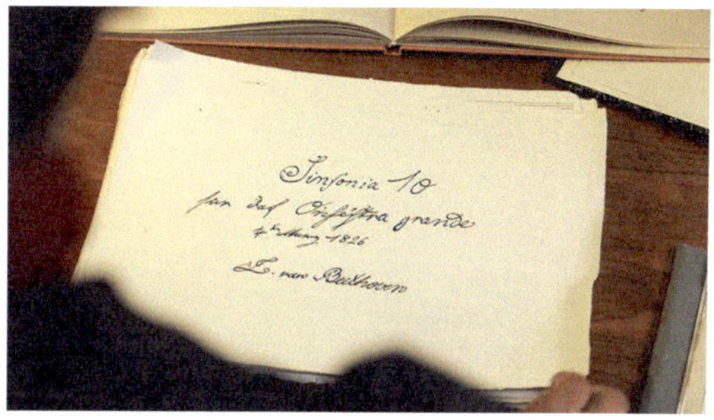

Fig. 6.7 A scene from "Beethoven's Blätterwirbel; The Lost Music"

On the second day of the new year, I started to work on one of the files I created years ago. I do hope that after my retirement, my students will be able to carry to completion the manuscripts I started.

References

1. Hwang K. How to write a scientific paper: three tips to remember. Arch Plast Surg. 2012;39:77.
2. Neill US. Publish or perish, but at what cost? J Clin Invest. 2008;118:2368.
3. Hwang K. Appropriate roles for the subscriber, publisher, editor, author, and reviewer in the archives of plastic surgery. Arch Plast Surg. 2013;40:663–5.
4. Furnas HJ, Garza RM, Li AY, et al. Gender differences in the professional and personal lives of plastic surgeons. Plast Reconstr Surg. 2018;142:252–64.
5. Bucknor A, Kamali P, Phillips N, et al. Gender inequality for women in plastic surgery: a systematic scoping review. Plast Reconstr Surg. 2018;141:1561–77.
6. Phillips NA, Tannan SC, Kalliainen LK. Understanding and overcoming implicit gender bias in plastic surgery. Plast Reconstr Surg. 2016;138:1111–6.
7. Kanigel R. The man who knew infinity: a life of the genius Ramanujan, vol. 110. New York: Washington Square Press; 1992. p. 125.
8. Hwang K, Kim JH, Baik SH. Thickness map of parietal bone in Korean adults. J Craniofac Surg. 1997;8:208–12.
9. Hwang K, Kim JH, Lee SI, et al. A thickness map of iliac bone of Korean adults. J Craniofac Surg. 1997;8:274–8.
10. Hwang K, Hwang SH. In the heart of the sea: how to get a motif? J Craniofac Surg. 2016;27:543.
11. Perneger TV, Hudelson PM. Writing a research article: advice to beginners. Int J Qual Health Care. 2004;16:191192.

7 How to Write a Paper? Plastic Surgeon as an Author

7.1 How to Write a Scientific Paper: Three Tips to Remember

In the field of plastic surgery, many new ideas and skills are developed by surgeons and researchers. "Publish or perish" is a phrase coined to describe the pressure in academia to publish work constantly to further or sustain one's career [1]. To share knowledge or skill with others or promote one's position in schools, they should write papers. However, it is not easy to gather and develop writing material.

I learned an invaluable lesson at the International Confederation of Plastic, Reconstructive, and Aesthetic Surgery meeting, which was held in Yokohama, Japan in 1995. At the opening ceremony, Dr. Joseph Murray, who performed the first successful human kidney transplant on identical twins and who shared the Nobel Prize in Physiology or Medicine, had the keynote lecture.

The elder retired plastic surgeon emphasized that scientists should remember three important words: curiosity, imagination, and persistence. Curiosity is an emotion related to natural inquisitive behavior, such as exploration, investigation, and learning. We can have curiosity in any basic research or about surgical procedures. Imagination is the ability to form mental images, sensations and concepts, in a moment when they are not perceived through sight, hearing, or the other senses. Lastly, persistence is the determination to do something even though it is difficult or other people oppose it.

Reading a book about swimming cannot guarantee the ability to swim. Likewise, there is no royal road to writing papers. However, it would be helpful to the surgeon to remember Dr. Murray's three words: curiosity, imagination, and persistence.

7.2 The Importance of Brevity in Scientific Writing

I recently enjoyed rewatching the movie "A River Runs Through It," directed by Robert Redford and starring Brad Pitt. It was based on a novel of the same name written by Norman Maclean in 1976. This semiautobiographical story tells how two sons (Norman and Paul) of a Presbyterian minister grow up and come of age in the Rocky Mountain area during a period of time approximately ranging from World War I to the early days of the Great Depression.

Early in the story, young Norman is shown writing and then rewriting a paper and having his minister father look it over for him.

(Norman is at his desk hard at work writing a paper, which he then turns in to his father for review. His father marks it up with a red pen and

K. Hwang, *Good Physician, Good Plastic Surgeon*, https://doi.org/10.1007/978-981-97-1864-1_7

simply says, "Half as long." Norman goes back to work, cuts the length of the paper in half, and turns it in for further review. His father marks it up once more and says, "Again, half as long." Following a final round of edits, his father looks over the finished product and says, "Good, now throw it away.") (Fig. 7.1).

When writing a paper, it is challenging to summarize the manuscript without losing its content. The minister father is training his first son, who later becomes a professor, on brevity in writing. He also emphasizes the process of writing, rather than the finished output.

In preparing an original article or case report, we follow the order IMRAD (introduction, methods, results, and discussion) or ICD (introduction, case, and discussion), respectively. After finishing the text, we must summarize it as a structured or unstructured abstract of about 250 words. A structured abstract requires the purpose, methods, results, and conclusion. Sometimes it is not easy to include important results within the limited space of the abstract.

Therefore, training on "half as long" is needed for writing scientific papers. We should eliminate redundancy (i.e., unnecessary repetition). As an author for whom English is not my mother tongue, I have to write each sentence as concisely as possible.

Summarizing the results for an abstract is particularly difficult for me. At this stage, I make it "half as long" and "again half as long" and finally submit it.

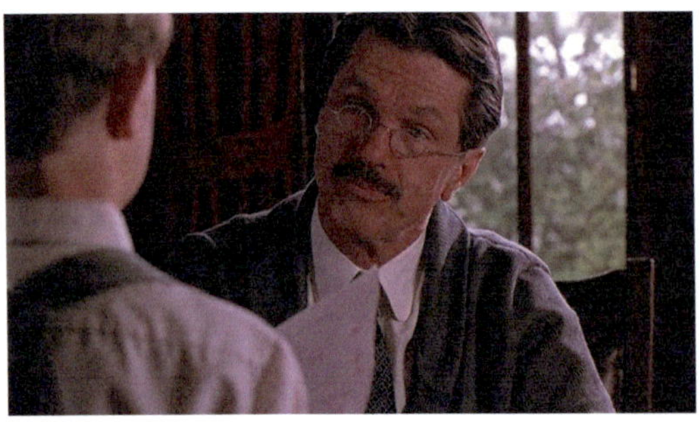

Fig. 7.1 "Half as long." The young son is shown writing and then rewriting a paper and having his minister father look it over for him

7.3 Festina Lente in Writing Papers

Ohne Hast, aber ohne Rast,—*Johann Wolfgang von Goethe and Friedrich Schiller (1796)*

When searching the literature, I sometimes happen to see two or more papers that have very similar content, including the surgical methods. Interestingly, the papers were sometimes published in the same year by different authors from different institutions [2]. When writing my manuscript, I usually cite both of them; however, I sometimes have to cite only one due to limits on the number of references. In such cases, I choose the paper that was published in the earlier month of that year. Worldwide, many different authors may be focused on similar surgical methods for procedures that they perform every day. This raises the question of who will be acknowledged as the originator of the procedure. Needless to say, the author who publishes first should receive this recognition. Therefore, we must make haste (in Latin, festina) in writing a manuscript and submitting it to a journal.

In letters to the editor in some journals, we frequently find questions from a reader and answers from the authors. However, some questions do not have accompanying answers, because the authors could not defend their position to the reader who raised the question. Furthermore, when I review papers as an editorial board member, I frequently encounter manuscripts that were written in a hurry. Sometimes, the reference style is different from the journal instructions, and the font and size of the letters are different. The most important point, however, is how authors cite similar papers that have been previously published. Some authors do not point to previously published papers and state that their findings are novel or even develop new nomenclature for a structure they believe to have found by chance in an operation or cadaver dissection [3]. The point of commonality of these papers, I suspect, is that they were written in a hurry.

When I am preparing a manuscript that will be submitted to a scientific journal, I remember the epigram that Augustus, the Roman emperor,

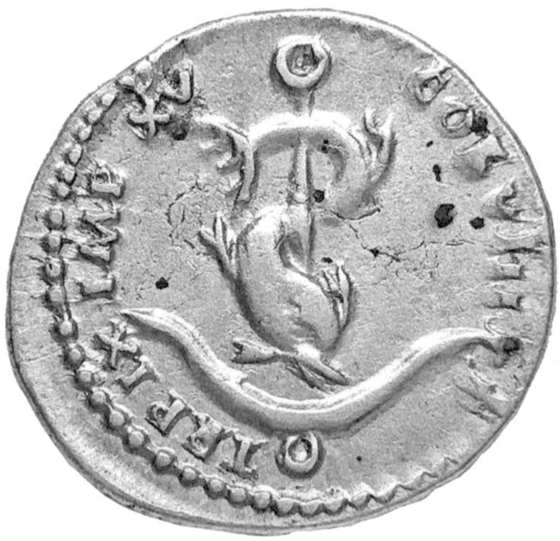

Fig. 7.2 Dolphin-anchor symbol, on an 80 A.D. Roman coin

loved: festina lente (make haste slowly; more haste, less speed). He disapproved of urgency and rashness among his officers and so encouraged them with the Greek saying σπεῦδε βραδέως (festina lente in Latin). The anchor-dolphin symbol in Erasmus's book is from a Roman coin: these components symbolize the slowness of deliberation and the speed of performance, respectively (Fig. 7.2) [4].

This motto was reused by Goethe and Schiller: "Ohne Hast, aber ohne Rast" ("without haste, but without rest") (Zahme Xenien [with Schiller, 1796] Sect. 2, no. 6, l. 281) [5].

If writing and submitting are rushed too quickly, they are prone to mistakes, and the long-term results may not be as good as expected. In Buddhist terms, writing is best achieved in a state of flow in which one is fully engaged and there is no sense of time passing (freedom from all thought and ideas, 無念無想). When I sit down in my desk for writing, I always reiterate to myself, "festina lente."

7.4 Writing Paper: Flash Inspiration or Arduous Effort?

They go from strength to strength; God of gods will appear in Zion.—*Psalm 84:7*

For me, the most difficult step of writing a new paper is in the first part of the introduction and the beginning of the discussion. Major revisions following reviewer's comments are stressful. Rewriting a rejected paper following the comments of referees, which have abandoned me, is even more distressing.

During the rewriting of a rejected paper or when going through major revisions, I sometimes feel I'm in front of a wall without an exit.

In those moments, I recall the picture "Saint Matthew and the Angel" by Caravaggio in 1602 (Fig. 7.3) [6]. Saint Matthew is holding a pen, and an angel is moving his hand to write the Gospel. It would be very auspicious if an angel would come to me and grant me flash inspiration or guide my hand to write the blocked part of a draft! I wish I were a genius and had creative brilliance like Mozart.

In the Oscar-winning film "Amadeus," Mozart was an idiot savant divinely inspired. He could envision pieces whole in his imagination and needed only time to write them down [7]. This tale was from the letter published in 1815, in which Mozart is said to have written to Baron von X. However, it was later discovered that this letter was markedly different from Mozart's actual descriptions, and it proved a forgery. The musical manuscripts of Mozart contained sketches or drafts of unrealized works, which were kept for possible completion by others, while curiously, those containing sketches or drafts of completed works could be discarded. This genius composer also needed arduous and intensive training and much practice and hard work in a lucid state [7].

In writing the first part of an introduction, I usually start with three sentences: something already known, what is still unknown and current controversies, and, finally, the question and purpose of my paper [8]. The easiest way to begin the discussion is to redescribe the purpose of the study and show that some previous studies support or at least do not contradict my results [9].

The referees with keen eyes usually point out deficiencies as part of the "answers." Thereafter, during the rewriting of the rejected paper or for major revisions, I have to explain and defend the

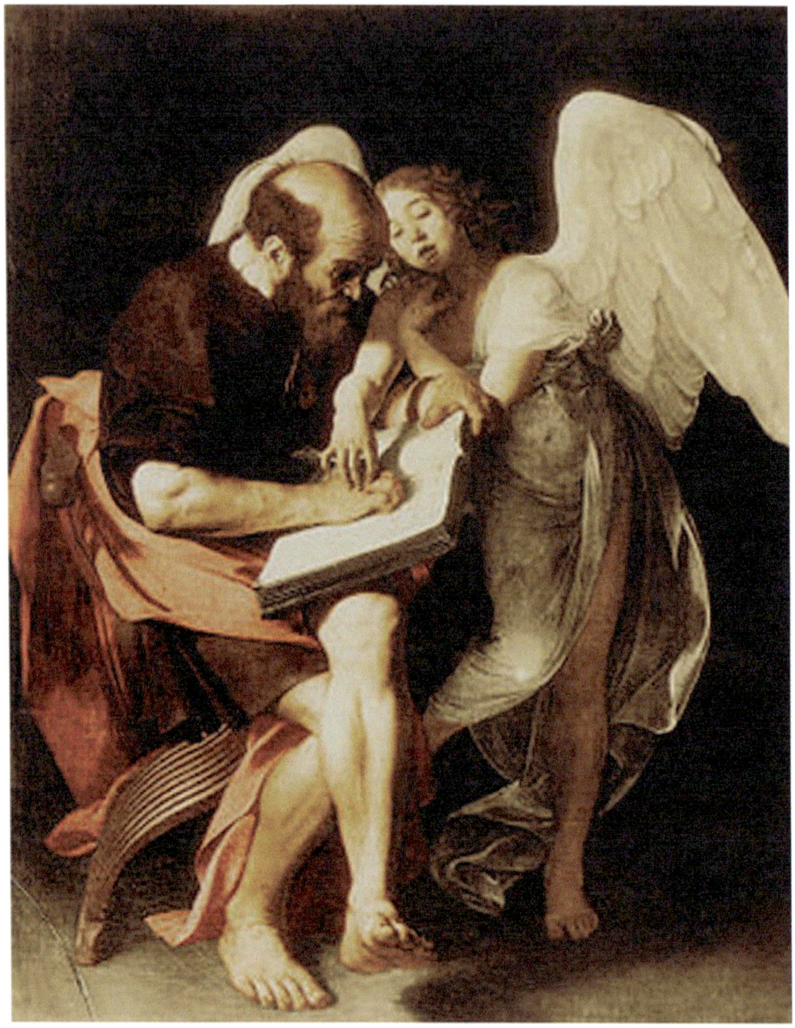

Fig. 7.3 "Saint Matthew and the Angel" by Caravaggio (1602)

answer, which is the result I found through my methods. I have to explain conflicting results or unexpected findings.

What shall I do when I have an uncompleted draft? Instead of waiting for an angel's hand, shall I find an angel's hand myself?

I believe that the more belligerent the referees' comments are, the more vulnerable points of my paper can be overcome through revisions. I ritually search previous literature with the keywords from the tenacious and sharp comments of referees who have reviewed my paper. The work of previous researchers will help to explain and defend my findings. By analyzing every detail of referees' comments and have consideration on them, the draft receives a new breath. Thereafter, referee's comments can be the hand of an angel and the literature discovered can be a whispering of God.

I hope to go "from strength to strength" by the comments of other researchers. If I revise section by section following "the hands" and "the whispering," I do believe the paper will ultimately be completed.

7.5 In the Heart of the Sea: How to Get a Motif?

> All visible objects, man, are but pasteboard masks [...] If man will strike, strike through the mask! How can the prisoner reach outside except by

thrusting through the wall? To me, the white whale is that wall, shoved near to me.—*Herman Melville in* Moby-Dick (1851)

The most difficult step in research is to improvise a motif. If the first line could not be written, there is my improvised ritual that will rectify the situation. I open the refrigerator in the kitchen, get out of the house, walk down the road, or sit peacefully on a bench in the park. However, there are times where the idea just simply would not come up in my mind.

With the purpose of finding a motif that is masked for me, I went to see the movie "In the Heart of the Sea," where the plot regards the loss of a ship in Essex written by Nathaniel Philbrick.

The movie started with the scene where Herman Melville, a writer who later became the author of *Moby-Dick*, knocks on the house door of old Thomas Nickerson in the rain. Mrs. Nickerson persuaded her husband to exhort his painful experiences to Melville. The story was regarding a whaleship from Massachusetts (Essex), which sank following an attack from a sperm whale in the Pacific Ocean in 1820. Having lost their ship, the crew underwent severe starvation, where most of the crew died, with only eight survivors.

Melville wrote down what Nickerson remembered, told, and confessed, after paying a sum of money. Toward the end of the encounter, Nickerson asked Melville whether he will write everything that was told to him. There was a consensus that a novel "inspired by the fact" will be written. This of course became *Moby-Dick*. In this novel, the only survivor of whaling ship narrates the tale of his captain's obsession to hunt the white whale, which gave him his crutch. Combining his experience as a whaleman and Melville's account, *Moby-Dick* was generated.

The compelling plot ended and I returned to my desk. I remembered that I in fact have a similar experience of gaining a motif from the discussion with a plastic surgeon, whom I had met in a conference. He consulted me whether the location of the mandibular branch of the facial nerve according to the neck position could be known. His curiosity was originating from his surgical regimen, where he moves the patient's neck from one side to the other. I answered him: "I cannot answer your question right now, but I will find it and let you know." A paper was published the following year [10], and a manuscript was sent to him. Of course, at the end of the paper, I acknowledged and thanked him for discussing the idea he had in mind.

Plastic surgeons, especially those who specialize in a specific area, may have abundant surgical experiences. A lot of them also would have curiosities to break through the masked anatomical structures that cannot be explained from studying orthodox anatomical textbooks. Their curiosities and imaginations can be a real motif for the research, "inspired by surgery." If persistence is added, I believe a paper could be published.

7.6 Selecting Trustworthy Papers

But while everyone was sleeping, his enemy came and sowed weeds among the wheat, and went away.—*Matthew 13:25*

First collect the weeds and tie them in bundles to be burned; then gather the wheat and bring it into my barn.—*Matthew 13:30*

It goes without saying that plastic surgeons need solid anatomical knowledge. Surgeons without anatomy are similar to the moles that dig mole hills in the dark [11]. Not every plastic surgeon has the opportunity to dissect cadavers. Of course, participating in a workshop with hands-on dissection cannot guarantee true learning. In any patient, most of us learn anatomy from published journal articles or book chapters. Given that the number of papers which describe the surgical anatomy of the face is growing, surgeons have to try to identify the papers that are most trustworthy and applicable.

And which anatomy papers are trustworthy and applicable? It is difficult to distinguish papers written just to meet publication requirements from the true gems; readers should open their eyes wide to distinguish the weeds from the wheat (Fig. 7.4). Papers that have not cited previous papers on similar topics (similar article not cited) [12] and insist on their originality should be filtered out in the review process; however, sometimes appear in publication. If a paper has provoked a letter to the editor and if the authors have not responded to this letter, it can be concluded that the authors were avoiding criticism and their paper should be disregarded.

Anatomical researchers' paper should do research provoked by their own curiosity arising from their surgical experiences or discussions with their colleagues. The structures should be located using topography relative to anatomical landmarks. Anatomic landmark is a morphologic feature of the anatomy that is readily recognizable and may be used as a reference point for other body features [13]. Structures should be demonstrated in layer-by-layer dissections, along the surgical plane same as real operation field. Additionally, the depth of the structure should be displayed using histology or tomography [14].

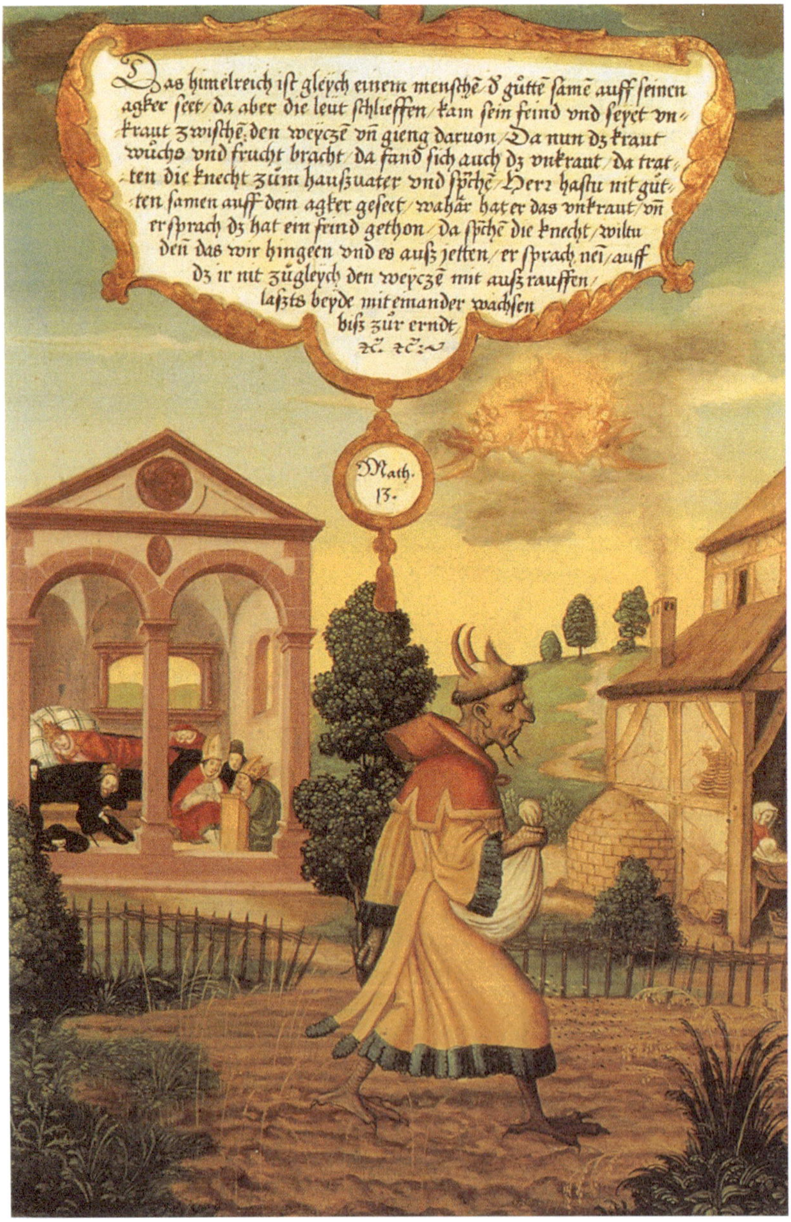

Fig. 7.4 Enemy sowing weeds. Heinrich Füllmaurer (1505–1546)

Since facial appearance varies in people of different ethnic origins, transracial anatomy may also be needed.

Systematic reviews and meta-analyses of the facial anatomy are encouraged. Through systematic reviews, readers can see the whole picture and cannot be shifted to a biased perspective. A well-written systematic review should be helpful for selecting trustworthy and applicable papers, removing the weeds from the wheat.

Writing the Discussion

Some residents and junior staff members have asked me how to write the "discussion part" of a scientific paper. In reviewing the manuscripts of original articles and case reports submitted to journals including the *Archives of Plastic Surgery*, I don't infrequently find or I frequently find that the authors have written summaries of references cited that are not directly related to the topic they are discussing. This paper is aimed at helping beginners easily start and end the discussion section of a journal article.

What do your findings mean? Why are they important? Discussion and conclusion sections exist to answer these questions [15]. Hess [16] summarized the tasks performed in the discussion as follows: state the study's major findings, explain the meaning and importance of the findings, relate the findings to those of similar studies, consider alternative explanations of the findings, state the clinical relevance of the findings, acknowledge the study's limitations, and make suggestions for further research. He also stated that elements to be avoided in the discussion are as follows: over presentation of the results, unwarranted speculation, inflation of the importance of the findings, tangential issues, and the "bully pulpit" [16].

Most authors agree that beginning the discussion is difficult. Huth [17] emphasized that the opening of the discussion should give the answer to the research question. In the first paragraph of the section, state concisely the central conclusion, or answer, to be drawn from the data presented in the results.

In my experience, the easiest way to begin the discussion is to redescribe the purpose of the study and show that some (about 40%) previous studies support or at least do not contradict my results. For example, "Results of this study 'correspond well with' those of an earlier study which…." Use phrases such as "be quite similar to; resemble; in agreement with; almost identical to; coincide with; be in accord with; show similarity to" instead of repeating "corresponds with" each time.

Then, I present a lesser number (about 25%) of previous studies that contradict my results. An example is "Our findings are in contrast to the results of Hwang et al." Use the phrases "differ from; be distinct from; do not correspond with; disagree with; be contrary to; be inconsistent with; be in disagreement with" as well.

The rest of the references (35%) were already described in introduction and do not appear in the discussion again. Lastly, I indicate what is new (etwas neues in German) in my results and describe its significance. If you are sure of your findings, use "prove"; in case you are less confident, use "demonstrate, or document." Usually "show or indicate" is stronger than "suggest, imply, suppose, or assume." I usually do not repeat the same content or same contents that already appeared in the introduction.

The most important thing, I think, in writing the discussion is "write the discussion for the reader," that is to say, be "reader friendly."

7.7 Missing Pieces of Surgery, Puzzle, and Systematic Review

> The plastic surgeon requires imagination for he must look into the puzzle of cleft. With this picture as transparency in his mind eye superimposed over the cleft patient, the surgeon is abetted in the sorting out and fitting together of the pieces of the puzzle.—*Ralph Millard Jr, 1919–2011*

In the systematic review/meta-analysis, the first step is finding papers and the accuracy for presenting data is essential. MEDLINE and EMBASE searches are usually used. If EMBASE is not available, a Scopus search can be used instead [18]. For the meta-analysis, it might be possible to combine the homogenous data from at least two papers. However, more than four papers are preferred to make a forest plot. In case I could not find sufficient full-text papers, I feel like I am trapped in a four-walled room without an exit. Shall I give up or continue searching? In such situations, I recall the front cover of Dr. Millard's "Cleft craft: the evolution of its surgery (1976) [19]" and reiterate to myself: "Find the missing pieces. They should be somewhere."

The front cover of the book is an unfinished jigsaw puzzle of a blond-haired boy with charming eyes. The central part of the face including his nose and mouth needed to be completed. In the preface of that book, Dr. Millard wrote "puzzle" and "piece" each four times and "normal" five times. He wrote this book to "find the missing pieces and fitting them carefully into the puzzle so that the final picture is complete, normal, and happy."

Usual jigsaw puzzle players first find a hard flat surface area large enough to accommodate the total number of pieces laid out individually face up. While turning all pieces face up, they first select all the edge pieces and put them to one side and construct the "frame" of the puzzle by assembling the edge pieces. They usually arrange all pieces into color groups and complete the different color groups of the puzzle after sorting. When daunted by what seems like an insurmountably difficult section, they are convinced that there are no missing pieces in the box, and if they applied one piece at a time, they finally conquer the challenge.

When I am on a systematic review, I arrange my pieces of references and data in a large table and classify and make a precise flow sheet using preferred reporting items for systematic reviews and meta-analyses [20]. Very frequently, I feel daunted by what seems like an insurmountably difficult situation. Sometimes, I am concerned if there are missing pieces in my results.

The missing pieces can be found in "the mined papers" that cannot be searched in the database but could be "mined" from the references of the papers.

Unpublished papers from the thesis or dissertation can be used for completion of the puzzle. Thereafter, the grey literature (gray literature) should be searched. The grey literature is a type of information or research output produced by organizations outside commercial or academic publishing and distribution channels. Examples of grey literature include technical or research reports, doctoral dissertations, some conference papers, and some official publications [21].

As in cleft surgeries or in jigsaw puzzles, missing pieces of systematic review can be found through the extensive and precise literature search. Of course, the "persistence" is necessary in all the procedures.

7.8 The Right to Heresy: Letters to the Editor

> Nothing whets the intelligence more than a passionate suspicion, nothing develops all the faculties of an immature mind more than a trail running away into the dark.—*Stefan Zweig*

When I receive a new issue of *The Journal of Craniofacial Surgery* (JCFS), I run my eyes over the titles. When I find an interesting paper, I read the abstract, then the methods.

When I disagree with the methods or results, I select the paper for my department's weekly journal club. A resident in training usually presents it using PowerPoint, and I ask for all the participants' opinions.

As the founding editor-in-chief declared in the first issue, JCFS is open to suggestions and comments from readers [22]. Letter to editor includes an interesting patient report or response to previous work published; however, too combative letters are not be welcomed.

If there are important questions for the authors, critiques, or disagreements with the article, I consider writing a letter to the editor.

When writing a letter to the editor with a difference in opinion regarding a published paper written by a famous author, I feel like a mosquito in front of an elephant. However, if there is something I really want to know from the authors and it would be of common interest for other readers, I start writing a letter to the editor.

After a letter has been submitted and, fortunately, accepted by the journal, I usually receive a sincere response from the authors. They are usually frank and kind and resolve most of my questions. However, sometimes, no answer follows, or the answer is even full of rage. I myself have had the experience of being asked to respond to a letter about a published paper of mine. I responded clause by clause to the question contained in the letter.

The recommendations of the International Committee of Medical Journal Editors (ICJME) state: "The authors of articles discussed in correspondence or an online forum have a responsibility to respond to substantial criticisms of their work using those same mechanisms and should be asked by editors to respond. Responsible debate, critique and disagreement are important features of science, and journal editors should encourage such discourse ideally within their own journals about the material they have published [23]."

The introduction of e-publications ahead of print can allow uninvited letters to the editor and the authors' replies to appear in the same printed issue, given the interval between the electronic publication and its appearance in print. I hope that journal readers do not hesitate to write a letter to the editor when they have questions or a difference of opinion.

Like many other journals, JCFS has "published ahead-of-print," that there will be interesting comments published online with responses from the authors. This will remove the obsolete publications and make it more dynamic with open time frame.

Finally, I must acknowledge the book *The Right to Heresy* written by Stefan Zweig (Fig. 7.5), who studied and summarized the story of three historical figures. First, John Calvin (1509–1564) was a reformer turned dreadful dictator. During his theocracy in Geneva, he expelled, and even killed, many people who opposed him. The second, Miguel Servetus (1511–1553), was a medical doctor who first described the function of pulmonary circulation and wrote a theological book to point out certain errors regarding the nature of the Trinity. Because Servetus argued for certain opinions that disagreed with Calvin's *Christian Religion*, Calvin became angry and demonized him. Servetus was rushed to judgment as a heretic and burned. Servetus did not withdraw the doctrine and kept his convictions. The third figure, Sebastian Castellio (1515–1563), was a humanist scholar, who studied and translated the Bible. He demonstrated that Calvin definitely did wrong to Servetus and defended the freedom of thinking and writing.

In the scientific field, we all have the "the right to heresy," even when it comes to disagreements with famous authors, just as Castellio argued against Calvin.

7.9 Finishing a Revision in Extreme Fatigue

Yes, I have had my vision.—*Virginia Woolf (1882–1941)*

It is painstaking work to respond to all of the reviewers' comments to a submitted article. Sometimes, there are two reviewers, sometimes three, and in rare cases even four or five.

Most reviewers hope to improve the manuscript, and their comments are truly helpful for polishing the paper. Usually, I agree with their keen insights into the weak points of my submitted manuscript.

However, because each reviewer has his or her own viewpoint; sometimes their opinions contradict each other. In those cases, I cannot follow all of their suggestions. If they want me to make extensive revisions, I cannot start to revise the manuscript immediately, or I become extremely fatigued during the revision process.

Usually, the time limit for a revision is 3 months, and no longer than 6 months. I have had the experience of not being able to complete the revision and abandoning the manuscript. Years later, I found that the manuscript had been removed from the journal's system, and I resubmitted the revised version to another journal.

When the deadline is approaching for completing a revision, I often become very nervous. In such moments, I will often open the refrig-

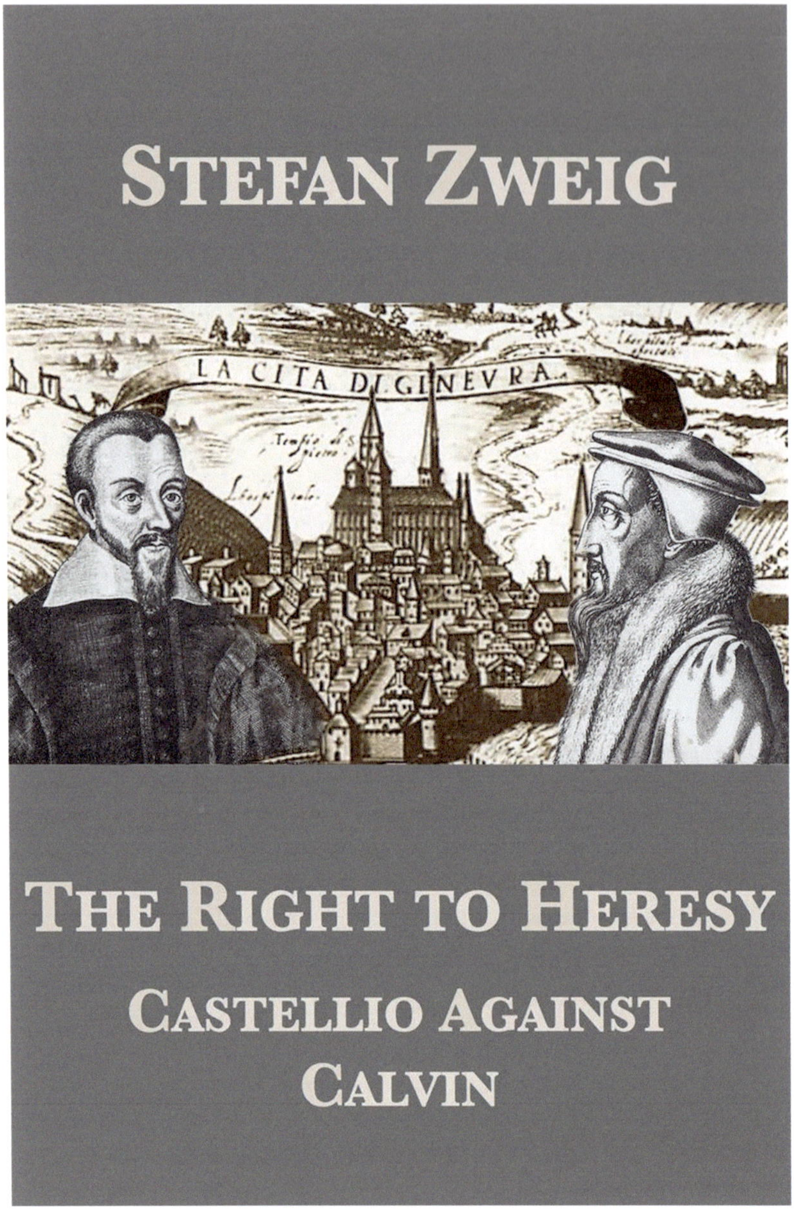

Fig. 7.5 Title page of The Right to Heresy written by Stefan Zweig

erator to get some food, even though I know that instant food is not good for me. If inspiration fails to strike even after I have a meal, I go out and walk along a trail near my home. If I have no idea of how to respond even once I return home, I watch a movie or read a novel. Under the heavy stress of two major revisions, to relax, I recently read and watched *To the Lighthouse*, written by Virginia Woolf (1882–1941) (Fig. 7.6).

In the first section ("The Window"), Mr. and Mrs. Ramsay, their eight children, and several guests are staying at the family's summer home. Just across the bay is a lighthouse. James, the youngest child, wants to go to the lighthouse the next day, but his father crushes his hopes by saying that the weather will not be pleasant enough for the trip. One of the houseguests, an unmarried artist named Lily, begins to paint a portrait of Mrs. Ramsay. In the second section ("Time

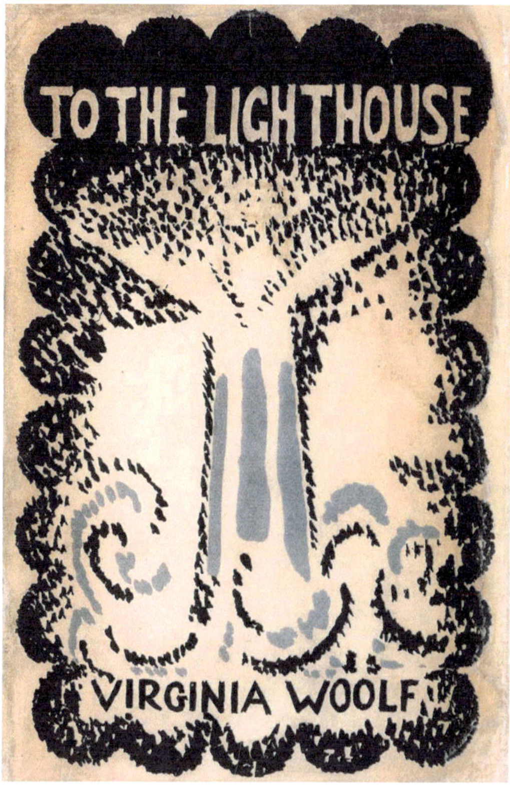

Fig. 7.6 Front cover of the To the Lighthouse (1st ed., 1927) by Virginia Woolf (1882–1941)

Passes"), Mrs. Ramsay unexpectedly dies one night and the house is abandoned for 10 years and falls into decay. In the third part ("The Lighthouse"), all of the living family and other guests (including Lily) return to the summer home. Mr. Ramsay decides that he and his sons will take the trip to the lighthouse. Lily decides to finally finish the painting that she started 10 years ago. As the boat reaches the island where the lighthouse is located, Lily paints the final stroke on her canvas and finally achieves her vision. The novel closes with the following paragraph: "Quickly, as if she were recalled by something over there, she turned to her canvas. There it was—her picture. Yes, with all its greens and blues, its lines running up and across, its attempt at something. It would be hung in the attics, she thought; it would be destroyed. But what did that matter? She asked herself, taking up her brush again. She looked at the steps; they were empty; she looked at her canvas; it was blurred. With a sudden intensity, as if she saw it clear for a second, she drew a line there, in the centre. It was done; it was finished. Yes, she thought, laying down her brush in extreme fatigue, I have had my vision."

After reading the book, I returned to my manuscript. I had to answer all the reviewers' comments. I reflected on how even if the paper were to be accepted after revisions, it would not be cited very often. But what does that matter? Only a few attentive and motivated readers are enough for me. I sat at the keyboard again and looked at the screen, which was blurry because I had stared at it for a long time. I focused my eyes on the key points of the revision and finally finished it in a state of extreme fatigue. Then, I was able to say, "I have had my vision."

7.10 A Lifetime of Rejection

Again, I received an email, "Major revision required—No guarantee of acceptance" for the revised manuscript, which was submitted recently. Each rejection still seems to disappoint me deeply. To overcome this feeling, I took my family to the theatre to watch the movie "The Intern." This was also a way to spend some time with my eldest son, who just completed his first year of medical intern in the UK and had to return to Korea for his 2-year military service.

In the movie, Ben Whittaker (Robert De Niro), a retired widower in his 70 s, applies for a senior internship position at an online fashion company, founded and run by 30-year-old Jules Ostin (Anne Hathaway). Initially, Jules was skeptical about bringing an old-timer like Ben into the mix. As she struggles juggling her business and a demanding home life of her husband and daughter, she finds Ben's wisdom and support very helpful. He provides advice and becomes her trusted friend over time.

I believe that wisdom, experience, and judgement come with age. More often than not, we miss the opportunity to utilize the qualities with early retirement. The movie provoked reflections on how I could reinvigorate the new generation of doctors, including my son who may face numerous uncertainties and challenges in the forthcoming future.

After coming home, I watched Robert De Niro's 2015 Commencement Speech, given at New York University TISCH School of the Arts [24]. He said: "You made it, and you're f***ed. A new door is opening for you; a door to a lifetime of rejection. It is inevitable. Rejection might sting, but my feeling is that often, it has very little to do with you. 'Next!' should be shouted when you didn't get that part."

I was surprised at his confession that even he, the famous actor and director, experiences numerous rejections until now. I had assumed that famous actors never get rejected according to the Matthew effect, which was derived from the Bible (Matthew 13:12 "For whoever has, to him shall be given, and he shall have more abundance: but whoever has not, from him shall be taken away even what he has."). In the case of academic publication, this effect means that manuscripts of famous researchers have a greater chance of being published even if they are inadequate, whereas unknown authors' work may be required to meet a higher standard or even rejected simply because of lack of an established reputation [25].

Several days later, I had a chance to talk to 250 young medical scientists for 40 minutes in a workshop on medical writing. The topic was as follows: how to refine the introduction, abstract, and title. I asked the audience to raise their hand, whether they had experienced rejection of their work. More than half raised their hand. Then, I asked whether any had experienced rejection of their work more than100 times, to which no one raised their hand. With conviction, I told them that experiencing repeated rejections makes a researcher more mature because it produces endurance. Once one acquires resilience to criticism, he will not be negatively affected by rejection. One can simply submit his manuscript to the next journal.

I sit at my desk to do "major revision" once again. I embark with the belief that as I revise section by section, the job will ultimately be accomplished.

7.11 Ephemeral or Timeless? The Brontë Sisters

> Life is so constructed, that the event does not, cannot, and will not match the expectation.—*Charlotte Brontë*

> "First study; then approve; then love."—*Anne Brontë.*

In my school days, I have read the Korean translated version of "Wuthering Heights," written by Emily Brontë, and "Jane Eyre," by Charlotte Brontë. Several years ago, I enjoyed the film of the latter, which reminded me of the touching impression I received 40 years ago.

Last week, I visited the National Portrait Gallery and watched a display "Celebrating Charlotte Brontë: 1816–1855." This exhibition explored the Brontës' life and literary career through the portraits and their handwritten manuscripts. All of their portraits look young. I could not find any middle-aged portraits. There was a colored portrait including the three sisters painted by their brother Branwell (Fig. 7.7). He painted himself among his sisters but later removed the

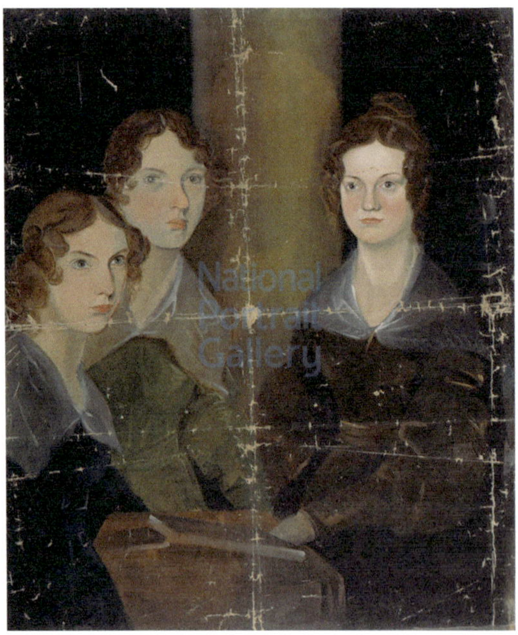

Fig. 7.7 Portrait of Brontë sisters (Charlotte, Emily, and Anne from left clockwise) by their brother Branwell (c. 1834). Reproduced with the kind permission from National Portrait Gallery (NPG 1715)

image so as not to clutter the picture. At the exhibit hall, I first noticed that they had all died before 40: Charlotte (1816–1855), Emily (1818–1848), and Anne (1820–1849).

Although Charlotte was ephemeral, her literary work is enduring, and thereafter, her 200th anniversary of birth is being celebrated. Although the Brontë sisters did not have any offspring, their literary DNA is still replicated because they inspire many readers.

Like the great writers, the Brontë sisters, surgeons must perish also. Then, how could we descend our academic DNAs as a surgeon and researcher? I believe our knowledge can get immortality through scientific papers.

If so, how can we write an everlasting paper? The ageless paper is an article that is loved and remembered by their readers for a long time. To be remembered and loved by the surgeons, it must be useful to surgeons. A useful paper is a paper that can help the surgeons take care of the patients in the "real field" (operating room, ward, or clinic). That is what the surgical literature is for: to help the patients.

The sequence of research (first, study; then, approve; then, write) is similar to that of love (first, study; then, approve; then, love). We should have curiosity and search for the previous work. If we cannot find the answer from the papers of other researchers, we can start. The papers have to approve something new (etwas Neues). A "Me-too paper" must be ephemeral. Of course, research is so constructed that the result does not, cannot, and will not match the expectations.

A logically written paper is easy to follow. A flight of ideas is not permitted in discussion. If we write "reader-friendly" papers, the readers feel comfortable in reading them, and we will have a better chance to be cited. Lastly, we should try hard to polish off the papers. Once it is published, we cannot revise it anymore.

The works of the Brontë sisters are being loved by readers for hundreds of years, because they create impressions to the readers. If our papers are helpful to the surgeons in the "real field," our papers will be remembered and cited for generations to come.

References

1. Neill US. Publish or perish, but at what cost? J Clin Invest. 2008;118:2368.
2. Hwang K. The origins of deltopectoral flaps and the pectoralis major myocutaneous flap. J Craniofac Surg. 2016;27:1845–8.
3. Hwang K, Huan F, Nam YS, et al. Location and tension of the medial palpebral ligament. J Craniofac Surg. 2013;24:2119–23.
4. Erasmus D. Adagiorum Chiliades Tres. Venice: Alldine Press; 1508. http://www.philological.bham.ac.uk/speude/ Assessed 5 Feb 2021
5. Von Goethe JW. Zahme Xenien. München, Germany: Verlag C. H. Beck; 2014.
6. Wikipedia. Saint Matthew and the Angel. https://en.wikipedia.org/wiki/Saint_Matthew_and_the_Angel. Assessed 3 Feb 2016.
7. Cornell University Library. Mozart and the Keyboard Culture of His Time. http://rmc.library.cornell.edu/mozart/intro.htm. Assessed 3 Feb 2016.
8. Hwang K, Chi JG. How to write an easily acceptable paper. J Korean Soc Plast Reconstr Surg. 2002;29:243–4.
9. Hwang K. Writing the discussion. Arch Plast Surg. 2012;39:183.
10. Hwang K, Huan F, Ki SH, et al. Location of the mandibular branch of the facial nerve according to the neck position. J Craniofac Surg. 2012;23:1488–90.
11. University of Heidelberg Digital Library. Friedrich Tiedemann. http://www.ub.uni-heidelberg.de/Englisch/helios/digi/anatomie/tiedemann.html. Assessed 7 Feb 2016.
12. Hwang K. Appropriate roles for the subscriber, publisher, author, and reviewer in the archives of plastic surgery. Arch Plast Surg. 2013;40:663–5.
13. Medical Dictionary for the Dental Professions. Anatomic landmark. http://medical-dictionary.thefreedictionary.com/anatomic+landmark.
14. Hwang K, Hwang SH. Surgeon-friendly anatomy. J Craniofac Surg. 2016;27:827.
15. Matthews JR, Bowen JM, Matthews RW. Successful scientific writing: a step-by-step guide for the biological and medical sciences. 2nd ed. Cambridge: Cambridge University Press; 2005.
16. Hess DR. How to write an effective discussion. Respir Care. 2004;49:1238–41.
17. Huth EJ. How to write and publish papers in the medical sciences. 2nd ed. Philadelphia: Williams & Wilkins; 1990.
18. Burnham JF. Scopus database: a review. Biomed Digit Libr. 2006;3:1–8.
19. Millard DR Jr. Cleft craft: the evolution of its surgery, vol. 1, 2. Boston, MA: Little Brown; 1976. p. 3.
20. Moher D, Liberati A, Tetzlaff J, et al. PRISMA group. Preferred reporting items for systematic reviews and meta-analyses: the PRISMA statement. PLoS Med. 2009;21:e1000097.

21. Alberani V, De Castro PP, Mazza AM. The use of grey literature in health sciences: a preliminary survey. Bull Med Libr Assoc. 1990;78:358–63.
22. Habal MB. Editorial. J Craniofac Surg. 1990;1:II.
23. ICJME. Correspondence. http://www.icmje.org/recommendations/browse/publishing-and-editorial-issues/correspondence.html. Accessed 25 Nov 2018.
24. New York Theater. Robert De Niro's Blunt, Inspiring Speech to NYU Arts Grads. https://www.youtube.com/watch?v=e6GFEfJtlnc. Assessed 29 Sep 2015.
25. Merton RK. The Matthew effect in science: the reward and communication systems of science are considered. Science. 1968;159:56–63.

8 Role of Editor, Reviewer, and Author in Plastic Surgery

8.1 The Need for a Reviewer to Play Devil's Advocate

It has been over a year and a half since the *Archives of Plastic Surgery* (APS) was listed in PubMed Central. As an ethics editor, I have encountered cases of "salami slicing," "imalas," and duplicate publication, as well as plagiarism. However, I cannot be certain that there is no plagiarism in the issues already published because I have not reviewed all of them.

Although there are several sites that check the similarity of papers [1], these search engines cannot detect "intelligently modified plagiarism" [2]. Thereafter the reviewer (referee) should read manuscripts in detail, look up the citations of the original paper, and identify missing papers that must also be cited.

The movie *The Devil's Advocate* (1997), in which Keanu Reeves and Al Pacino star as lawyers, comes to mind. The film's title is a reference to the commonly used phrase "devil's advocate." A devil's advocate is a person who expresses a contentious opinion in order to provoke debate or test the strength of the opposing arguments [3].

This terminology originated in the Roman Catholic Church tradition [4]: During the beatification or canonization process, the Church authorities appointed a lawyer to be the Promoter of the Faith (Latin: *promotor fidei*), popularly known as the devil's advocate (Latin: *advocatus diaboli*), to argue against the canonization of a candidate based on the candidate's character or other evidence at hand (Another advocate was appointed to argue in favor of the candidate.) [5].

Likewise, in the APS review process, an editor sends a manuscript to three reviewers,

and they fill out several checklists, make comments to the author as well as to the editor, and each make a recommendation (accept as is, accept with minor revisions, major revisions, or rejection). In the case where two or more reviewers accept the manuscript, the editor usually accepts it for publication. In the case where two or more reviewers reject the manuscript, the editor usually rejects it.

I would like to propose that the editor choose at least one reviewer from the reviewer pool to play the role of "devil's referee." Like the devil's advocate in Catholicism examines how accurate the inquiry is, a devil's referee could examine the originality of the manuscript. He or she should take a skeptical view of the manuscript, looking for holes in the results of the experiment, insisting that the paper contain *etwas neues* (something new).

In the Catholic tradition, once a person becomes 'Blessed' or the 'Saint' through the beatification or canonization process, he or she is recognized for having an exceptional degree of holiness, sanctity, and virtue. Similarly, after publication, a manuscript becomes an 'article' and is cited in the research databases (PubMed, Scopus, etc.). In both cases, it is the consistent

K. Hwang, *Good Physician, Good Plastic Surgeon*, https://doi.org/10.1007/978-981-97-1864-1_8

rigor of examination that lends value to the final status.

If unhappy cases of withdrawal after publication occur, the author is to blame. However, the editor and reviewers also hold some responsibility for preventing such cases in advance, to the best of their ability to detect irregularities. Creating a "devil's referee" role among the reviewers would strengthen the ethical publication standards of APS by ensuring that at least one person always evaluates each paper from a skeptical perspective.

8.2 A Periodical Article Reviewer as Gottfried: The Uncle of Jean-Christophe

> You want to make beautiful songs, so as to be a great man; and you want to be a great man, so as to make beautiful songs. You are like a dog chasing its own tail—*Romain Rolland*

Several months ago, I submitted a paper for publication, entitled "Two parallel papers for the pectoralis major myocutaneous flap for head and neck reconstruction." Many weeks later, I received a decision letter: major revision with no guarantee of acceptance.

The decision letter contained a list of previous studies I missed in my review and their significance. The reviewer's comments concluded as follows: "So, rather than reject I am going to ask you to rewrite. Have a focus that you really want to transfer to the readers and let us know of the value of bringing this back after 100 years."

The decision letter reminded me of a novel I read years ago: *Jean-Christophe*, written by Romain Rolland and translated into English by Gilbert Cannan [6]. The author depicted the life of a genius German composer, Jean-Christophe Krafft, a fictionalized version of Beethoven.

In his early life, Jean was influenced much by his uncle, Gottfried, as illustrated in the following quotes from the novel's characters.

Young Jean composed music and submitted it to his uncle. After listening to young Jean's compositions quietly, Gottfried questioned his nephew about why he needed to add more songs to the world's repertoire.

Uncle: "Why make them? There are enough [songs] for everything."

Nephew: "To be a great man!"

Uncle: "You want be a great man?"

Nephew: "Yes."

Uncle: "What for?"

Nephew: "To make beautiful songs!"

Uncle: "You want to make beautiful songs, so as to be a great man; and you want to be a great man, so as to make beautiful songs. You are like a dog chasing its own tail."

Jean wanted to show his uncle what an artist he was and showed him his compositions.

"Why did you write them?"

"I don't know. I wanted to write something pretty," the young nephew replied.

"There you are! You wrote for the sake of writing. You wrote because you wanted to be a great musician, and to be admired. You have been proud…. Music must be modest and sincere—or else, what is it? Impious, a blasphemy of the Lord, who has given us song to tell the honest truth." And later, "It is well enough written, but it says nothing…. You see, my boy, everything that you write in the house is not music. Music in a house is like sunshine in a room. Music is to be found outside where you breathe God's dear fresh air (Fig. 8.1)."

In the paper, I submitted that was sent back for revisions, I just compared two papers about the pectoralis major myocutaneous flap by Aryan (1979) and Baek (1979). Like the young Jean, I just wanted to write something interesting by comparing similar papers published in the same year (1979).

However, after the reviewer's sharp critique, I took up the reviewer's challenge to revise my paper extensively. Instead of consulting only the limited selection of references in the usual databases, I located some references that were outside of PubMed, like Gottfried's exhortation to his nephew to compose outside in God's fresh air; in fact, I added 12 new references. Finding and obtaining Aymard's 1957 paper in the *Lancet* and Conley's in *Surgery* (1954) meant drawing out my revision time to a couple of months. I changed the

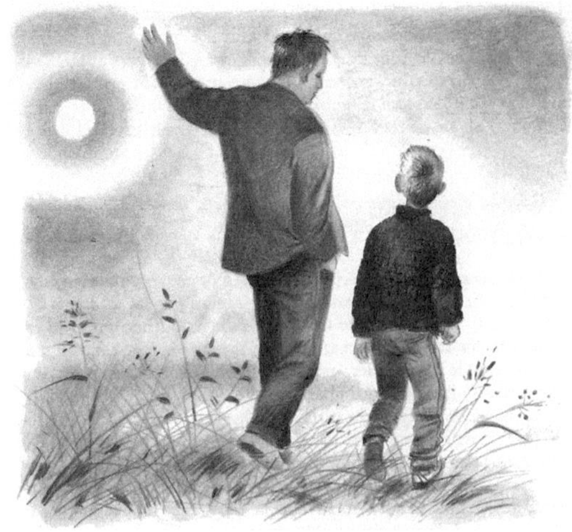

Fig. 8.1 Jean-Christophe and his uncle Gottfried are breathing fresh air in the sunshine. Available at: https://www.google.co.kr/search?q=jean-christophe+romain+rolland&biw=738&bih=364&source=lnms&tbm=isch&sa=X&ved=0ahUKEwiz66fFtYLQAhUCTLwKHfvDA8EQ_AUIBigB#imgrc=5V_5ibY2oG0LjM%3A. Assessed October 30, 2016

paper's title, completely rewrote the text, included 3 figures with permission, and prepared 1 chronological diagram. In the end, the revised version was published as a review paper [7].

After completing the publication process, I contemplated the role of the reviewer in the academic journal. The reviewer's responsibilities include protecting the integrity of a specialty, the reputation of the journal, and the welfare of human and animal subjects, as well as treating the author's manuscript with respect, fairness, and impartiality [8]. Sometimes a devil's advocate is needed, who takes a skeptical view of the manuscript, looking for the weaknesses in the paper and investigating whether the paper has etwas neues (something new) or not [9].

Once I achieved my revisions and produced a much better paper and a more worthwhile contribution to the literature, I was truly grateful to the reviewer who shows me the direction for my revision. Like Uncle Gottfried inspired young Jean-Christophe, we need "mentor–reviewers" who point out the stupidity of "a dog chasing its own tail" (writing for the sake of writing) and enlighten less experienced authors by "inducing focus" that they "really want to transfer to readers."

8.3 Good Surgical Illustrations

> When you look at an image and get the message immediately, then it works.—*Cassio Lynm*

As a subscriber, when I receive the table of contents of a new issue of the *Journal of Craniofacial Surgery*, I usually look through the titles. When I find an intriguing title, I read the abstract. When I receive a letter asking me to review a manuscript, I also read the attached abstract, and then I must decide whether to agree to review the manuscript. In both cases, if the abstract is interesting, I download the full text as a PDF file. After opening the full text, the first thing I do is scroll to the bottom of the manuscript, until I find the figures, illustrations, and their legends.

When reviewing a paper, if I can get the message immediately when I look at an illustration, the probability is very high that I will write a favorable evaluation. Looking at the illustrations helps me understand the core content that the author intends to communicate. As such, I agree with the saying "An illustration is worth a thousand words." However, not all illustrations are created equal; some are very good, some are confusing.

As a historical example, Vesalius's *De Humani Coporis Fabrica* (1543) contained exquisite woodcut illustrations based anatomic dissections. *Gray's Anatomy* (1858) contains the drawings of Henry Vandyke Carter. Nicolas Jacob's spectacular hand-colored lithographs in Bourgery's *Traité complet de l'anatomie de l'homme comprenant la médecine operatoire* (1866–1871) are anatomically correct and reflect a combination of direct laboratory observations and illustrative research (Fig. 8.2). Max Brödel (1870–1941) created illustrations for famous surgeons (Harvey Cushing, William Halstead, and Howard Kelly). I studied using the CIBA atlases drawn by Dr. Frank Netter (1906–1991),and still have them.

I thought about the virtues that good surgical illustrations should have:

1. They should be anatomically correct with precise proportions and should include prominent anatomical landmarks to enable easy orientation.

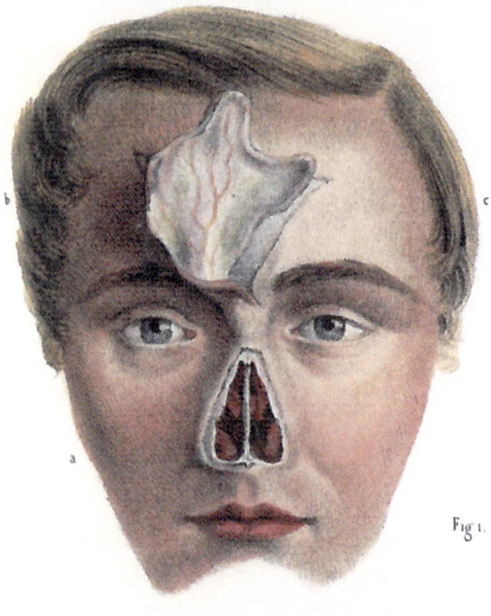

Fig. 8.2 Illustration of nasal reconstruction using forehead flap drawn by Nicolas Jacob. Reproduced from "Traité complet de l'anatomie de l'homme comprenant la médecine operatoire (1866–1871)" Vol. 7, Plate 14, Fig. 8.1

2. They should eliminate visual distractions; the goal should be to emphasize the key message and leave out the unnecessary parts.
3. They should show the structures behind the scene since viewpoints that the human naked eye could not achieve in the operative field are unrealistic.
4. They should simplify the key structures by using unrealistic colors to ensure that they do not blend into the background.

Surgeons are clients of medical illustrators. Surgeons are scientists and illustrators are artists. Therefore, there might be a gap between a client and an illustrator. Science pursues the state of art, and art seeks the state of science. If we "mind the gap," we can find the intersection of these 2 sets.

To receive a good illustration, clients should give the illustrator their intended ideas—that is, what they really want to show to the reader. Surgeons should provide the illustrator with quick sketches, sound information for all relevant points, and references that might be helpful.

Good communication between surgeons and illustrators will lead to reader-friendly illustrations—that is, to good illustrations.

8.4 Appropriate Roles for the Subscriber, Publisher, Editor, Author, and Reviewer in the Archives of Plastic Surgery

8.4.1 Introduction

Science is strengthened not by research alone but by publication of original research articles in international scientific journals that are read by a global scientific community. The publication process involves author-editor interaction, for which both get credit once the article gets published-the author directly, the editor indirectly [10]. Authors submit a manuscript to the editor, who decides to accept or reject it. The editor then sends the manuscript to the reviewers for their opinion. Aside from the author, editor, and reviewer, publishers and subscribers play their role in scientific journals as well. These five stakeholders are all essential to a journal's success.

It has been about 2 and a half years since the first issue of the *Archives of Plastic Surgery* (APS) appeared, and so it is worth taking stock of these five stakeholder roles, how they are playing out in APS, and what responsibility each stakeholder might have to participate more effectively. Thus, in this paper, I, firstly, briefly summarize the role and aims of each journal stakeholder. Secondly, I consider the current status of each APS participant. Finally, for each type of stakeholder, I propose an appropriate role and suggested future direction.

8.4.2 Subscribers (Readers)

Subscribers pay the journal to access new information. They may usually take what is written in a published paper at face value. However, the research experience and clinical expertise of the author do not guarantee validity and relevant recommendations. Uncritical acceptance of information by subscribers potentiates the dissemination of misinformation [11].

My fear is that APS readers do not read each issue carefully and critically because of the relatively small number of submissions of letters to the editor offering opinions, addenda, or critiques of published papers. Letters to the editor should be welcomed by all APS stakeholders for their insight into and relevant critiques of published papers. Both the authors and subscribers should take responsibility for their roles in producing clinical and scientific knowledge, and this partnership can improve patient care [11].

8.4.3 Publishers

A publisher is a kind of businessperson who sells knowledge to a limited number of subscribers, including libraries. The publisher is motivated to increase the number of subscribers and sometimes to improve the publication quality.

The publisher and editor both have considerable power to shape the content and form of the final publication. It is important that a system of checks and balances is maintained, such that the publisher cannot have undue influence on journal content because it is the editor-in-chief who brings clinical and technical knowledge to the table without a profit motivation. One way to accomplish this is to ensure that the editor-in-chief has a sufficient length of tenure and that the incoming editor-in-chief is already familiar with the practicalities of journal publication by serving in the associate editor role or another key role in the editorial board. Currently, APS is working toward this goal by maintaining the same editor-in-chief and associate editor for the third year.

Publishers have other responsibilities in the journal ecosystem. They should develop new products that will both help scientists in their work and enable publishing to remain a viable economic business model so that publication companies can continue to prosper in the future [12]. The publisher must also trust the editor and allocate appropriate levels of financial support to build journal quality on an ongoing basis.

8.4.4 Editors

The editors select manuscripts suitable for publication while rejecting unsuitable manuscripts. Most journals use peer review to raise the quality of published content. However, since the process of peer review can be prone to biases toward ideas that affirm the prior convictions of reviewers and against innovation and radical new ideas, a system of editorial review should also be established [13]. In both systems, the editor is responsible to and communicates with the readers, the publisher, as well as the authors and reviewers.

Editors are central stakeholders in a number of ways, having responsibilities to and simultaneously depending on all of the other journal participants. For the readers to easily locate papers of interest, the editor must attempt to get the journal listed in as many databases as possible. At the same time, the editor depends on authors to submit quality papers of interest to readers. The editor welcomes papers that have originality and that may be likely to be cited in other papers. A key goal of the editor is to have the articles in his or her journal cited by other authors, thereby increasing the journal's impact factor. The editor also wants papers from other journals to cite his or her own journal, which can also increase the impact factor.

The editor also has a responsibility to increase the author pool through personal and professional connections. Section editors share this responsibility. The editor may also find it helpful to designate a "devil's referee," a sort of devil's advocate who is responsible for examining the originality of a manuscript. The "devil's referee" should take a skeptical view of the manuscript, looking for holes in the methods and results of the experiment and insisting that the paper contain *etwas neues* (something new) [9].

The editor of a new journal may face a limited author pool since a journal is not well-recognized internationally. The present editor-in-chief of APS has successfully listed APS in PubMed, PubMed Central, and Scopus but not yet in Science Citation Index (SCI). He is in his third year, with one more year of his term remaining. It is not certain he can continue after 2014, given the time commitment and budget limitations. The other stakeholders must rally around the editor-in-chief to ensure that he has the proper resources.

8.4.5 Authors

The authors' primary goal is to have their paper read by many readers and cited by other authors. Authors should carefully read the aim and scope section of the journal before selecting a journal for manuscript submission. Authors want their manuscript to be accepted to a journal listed in high-profile databases and one with a high-impact factor. The higher the impact factor is, the greater possibility of the article being cited.

Since APS is not listed in SCI, it seems likely that Korean authors at university hospitals do not choose APS as their first journal for submission. As an ethics editor over the past 2 years, I have encountered cases of "salami slicing," "imalas," and duplicate publication, as well as plagiarism. In addition, a few thoughtless authors have made strong protests to the editors when their manuscripts were rejected.

Authors have an important responsibility of submitting manuscripts with scientific integrity. They must be aware that they continue to be responsible for their article's contents even long after publication. It is recommended that in cases in which a paper has been rejected by APS, especially when legitimate problems have been identified with the manuscript, the authors not argue with the editor but revise their manuscript and find another journal to which to submit their paper.

8.4.6 Reviewers

The peer review system is an important component of modern scientific publishing, and it is a great help to editors in deciding whether or not a submitted manuscript is suitable for publication. The manuscript reviewer is a key player in the manuscript processing system and journal publication process. The reviewer's responsibilities include protecting the integrity of a specialty, the reputation of the journal, and the welfare of human and animal subjects, as well as treating the author's manuscript with respect, fairness, and impartiality [8].

In APS, the quality and rigor of the reviewers has not yet been standardized. Some are prone to accept most papers, while others tend to reject more papers. Some recommend too many revisions, while others make too few suggestions. Most of the reviewers do not take sufficient time to seek out similar articles which are not cited (SANC).

In APS, the standardization of reviewers is needed through training in reviewers' workshops. In my case, when I have a manuscript to review, I hold a journal review club (JRC) session to gather the opinions of colleagues in my department. SANC is usually uncovered during a JRC.

In APS, reviewers are welcome to write a discussion on the article which they reviewed. This is a short response making public the kind of feedback that reviewers typically provide the authors during the review process. A quality discussion is of benefit not only to the authors but also to readers, who can discover different perspectives on the research presented, and particularly newer scholars, who are still learning to read critically.

8.4.7 Conclusions

The responsibilities mentioned here are only a few of those required of each stakeholder in the APS journal publication process. However, they are representative of the many other responsibilities that form the role of each participant in the journal publication ecosystem, all of which depend on and reinforce each other. All of the stakeholders should take pride in meeting their obligations to the scholarly community, because these seemingly mundane tasks all contribute to spreading clinical knowledge that raises the quality of care for our patients.

8.5 The Editor's Role as a Harriet Shaw Weaver

Two weeks ago I visited Dublin, Ireland, where the summer meeting of the Anatomical Society was held. A literary walk was included in the conference program, and it began just after the poster session. About 50 participants attended in two groups. It started at a famous pub on Duke Street, and an actor guided each group. In the pub, we were guided to a small private hall where I found a picture of James Joyce and a framed letter he had written (Fig. 8.3).

The actor told us that the letter was written to a magazine editor, Harriet Shaw Weaver, and when Joyce could not find anyone to publish his major work, *Ulysses*, Weaver set up the Egoist Press for this purpose at her own expense. It is thought that without the editor's help, the great novel would never have been published, and thereafter Joyce would not have become a world-famous writer.

On my way home, I thought about how much the reviewer's recommendations to a journal editor should be taken into account. Should the editor rely upon a reviewer's opinion or does he have the right to accept or reject the paper against the reviewer's recommendation? Should he play the role of one who 'plucks a pearl from the mud' as Weaver did?

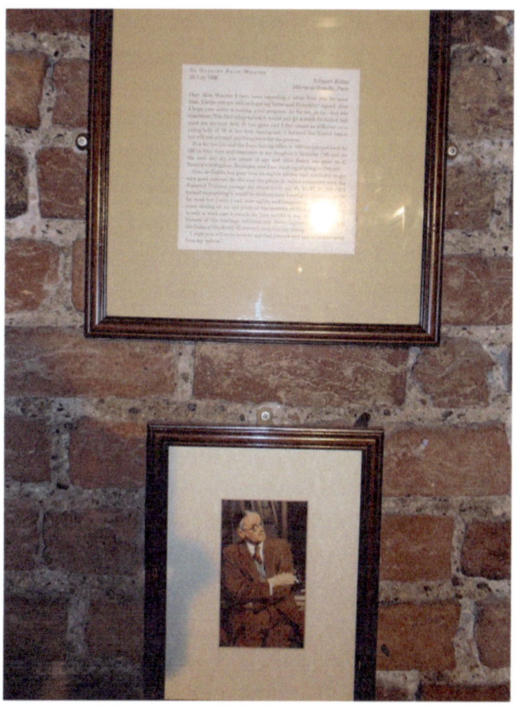

Fig. 8.3 Photograph of James Joyce and his letter to Harriet Shaw Weaver. Taken at "The Duke" in Dublin Weaver was the magazine editor and arranged the publication of Joyce's book

A recent paper shows that journal editors tend to place considerable weight on reviewers' recommendations. If all reviewers recommended not rejecting an article, editors still rejected the manuscript 20% of the time. If all reviewers recommended rejection, the editors rejected the piece 88% of the time. Further, if the reviewers were divided, the editors rejected the manuscript 70% of the time ($P = 0.001$) [14]. It is noteworthy that if all of the reviewers recommended rejection, the editors still accepted the paper 12% of the time.

The publication process involves author-editor interaction for which both get credit once the article gets published-the author directly, the editor indirectly [10]. However, the process of peer review can be prone to biases toward ideas that affirm the prior convictions of reviewers and against innovation and radical new ideas [13].

In the reviewing process, peer reviewers should avoid intellectual suppression due to the Matthew effect and Heider's assimilation-contrast theory. The Matthew effect is the phenomenon in which "the rich get richer and the poor get poorer." In the case of academic publication, it means that manuscripts of famous researchers have a greater chance of being published even if they are inadequate, while unknown authors' work may be required to meet a higher standard or even rejected simply due to lack of an established reputation [15]. Heider proposed the distinction between two types of affective reactions in relation to the emotional expressions of others. He argued that we experience concordant affective reactions to the ideas of persons who belong to our in-groups and discordant affective reactions to those with whom we do not identify [16].

The role of editors is to comprehend the degree of concordance of reviewers and determine whether to accept or reject an author's work on its own merits. Sometimes they should be a "devil's referee" [9], and sometimes they should be a Harriet Shaw Weaver.

At the pub, two actors performed a portion of "Waiting for Godot" by Samuel Beckett. Two characters, Vladimir and Estragon, waited endlessly and in vain for the arrival of someone named Godot. Godo's absence has led to many different interpretations. For me, as an author, after submitting a manuscript to a journal, the decision letter can be a figurative "Godot" that I feel I am waiting for endlessly. Until that letter finally arrives, I wonder whether the editor will truly be my advocate.

Editors should remain sympathetic to the fact that authors who have submitted a manuscript to a journal are waiting for a letter that begins "I am pleased to inform you that..." While enforcing strong standards of rigor and ethics, the best editors will be on the lookout for unconventional ideas that should be published. It is such ideas that will move science and clinical practice forward the most.

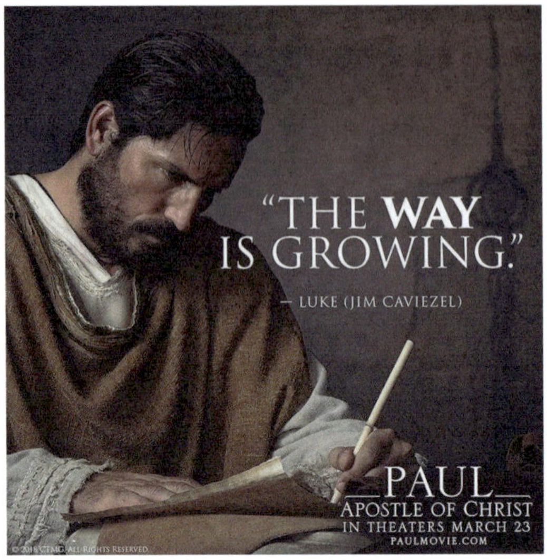

Fig. 8.4 St. Luke writing down the conversations of St. Paul, which became the "Acts of the Apostles" by Hye Won Hu, M.F.A. (1986–)

8.6 Importance of Narratives in Scientific Discussion

> Paul said "As soon as I shall be beheaded, true men shall take away my body; mark ye well the place, and come thither tomorrow, and ye shall find by my sepulcher two men, Luke and Titus, praying. To whom when ye shall tell for what cause I have sent you to them, they shall baptize you and make you heirs of the kingdom of heaven."—*Golden Legend* (1260)

I recently enjoyed a movie entitled *Paul, Apostle of Christ* (2018), directed by Andrew Hyatt. The plot is thought to be based on *Golden Legend* (1260), written by Blessed Jacobus de Varagine (1230 to 1299), rather than the New Testament.

After the Great Fire of Rome (ad 64), Emperor Nero persecuted Christians. Their most prominent leader, Paul (James Faulkner), was arrested, tried, and condemned to death, and awaited execution in a prison. Luke (Jim Caviezel) took a risk by visiting Paul in his cell at the jail. There, Luke wrote down a narrative of the conversions they performed and their missionary travels together, which would become the "Acts of the Apostles" (Fig. 8.4). This narrative eventually offered encouragement to Christians who were facing possible martyrdom.

If Luke did not record these conversations on parchment or if his followers did not copy the text ("Acts of the Apostles"), the New Testament would have 26 books instead of 27, and we could never know about the ministry and activities of the apostles after Christ's resurrection.

At international conferences, so many new ideas are presented. We can take a picture of the posters presented, but at oral presentations, taking pictures is strictly prohibited. In abstract book for free papers, some authors kindly provide the content precisely within the word limit (usually 250 words). However, the abstracts of some panel discussions or invited lectures usually contain only an introduction to the presentation. They are not usually very kind in sharing their "secrets," rather than "knowledge" about the topic.

Following the presentation, the discussions are usually opened to the floor, and these discussions generally involve good questions, comments, and answers. At that moment, we understand the point of the discussion and how various opinions converge. After the session, however, we cannot remember all of our insights. Even if we jot down some notes to capture the ideas, they are fleeting because our memory is treacherous.

If the scientific committee could provide a full video or transcript of the discussions, and the presentations, this would encourage registered participants to perform their activities more diligently, as in the operating room. The ability to rewind and repeatedly watch crucial parts of the presentation could make it more likely for audience members to write a letter to the editor when the material is published in a journal. Such innovations would be very valuable to the progress of knowledge in the field of plastic surgery.

8.7 Sine Qua Non Conditions for Research

Research is creating new knowledge.—*Neil Armstrong*

Research has been defined as a "creative work undertaken on a systematic basis in order to increase the stock of knowledge, including knowledge of humans, culture and society, and the use of this stock of knowledge to devise new applications [17]."

In the field of plastic surgery, research is carried out by many surgeons. Several residency training programs require that residents take time away from their clinical activities to focus solely on research, but the amount of time as well as the format of this research time vary considerably. Levi and Longaker insisted dedicated nonclinical research time at least a year would greatly benefit in the training of plastic surgeons [18]. He proposed several types of research for resident training: basic science, translational, outcomes, education, innovation/entrepreneurship, and public health/public policy.

Among them, translational research is increasing in plastic surgery field. Translational research implements a "bench-to-bedside," from laboratory experiments through clinical trials to point-of-care patient applications, model.

Ten qualities have been suggested to be necessary for a good researcher: interest, motivation, inquisitiveness, commitment, sacrifice, excellence, knowledge, recognition, a scholarly approach, and integration [19].

Then what are the prerequisites (sine qua non conditions) for research itself? In a forum, a retired professor (YO Ahn) of preventive medicine suggested that all research should exhibit professionalism, scientific integrity, logicality, autonomy, and ethics. I strongly agree with him and therefore conducted research into each of these conditions.

Professionalism is a pattern of behavior identified with scientific integrity that, in turn, gives certain privileges. Scientists are expected to behave with intellectual honesty and to exhibit excellence in their thought and behavior.

Scientific integrity is the quality of being honest and having strong moral principles. It generally reflects a personal choice to hold oneself to standards of morality and ethics. This includes values such as honesty in research and publishing, avoidance of plagiarism or cheating, and maintenance of academic standards.

Logicality is the condition of being logical, which means being in agreement with the principles of logic. Logic is a method of human thought that involves thinking in a linear, step-by-step manner about how a problem can be solved.

Autonomy refers to voluntary participation and is based on informed consent. An exception from the principle of voluntary consent can be made when research is conducted using published and public information and archived materials. Research concerning official registries and documents that is carried out without the consent of the research subjects is governed by legislation. Research subjects can provide consent orally or in writing, or their behavior can otherwise be interpreted to mean that they have given consent to participate [20].

Research ethics refers to the application of fundamental ethical principles to scientific research, including the design and implementation of research involving human experimentation, animal experimentation, and various aspects of academic scandals, including patients with scientific misconduct. The key ethical standard regulating medical research is the Declaration of Helsinki (1964).

In the bronze door of the Thomas Jefferson Building of the Library of Congress, the figure of "Research" is carved in relief in a panel of a sculpture by Olin Warner (Fig. 8.5). In the allegorical figure of the goddess with her head turned to the right in three-quarters profile, her left arm is holding the torch of knowledge, and her right arm is holding a sprig of laurel. The interpreta-

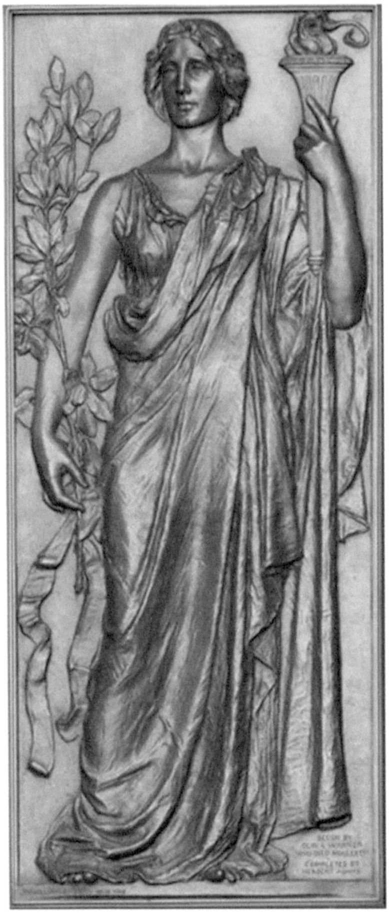

Fig. 8.5 Goddess of Research at the Library of Congress Thomas Jefferson Building by Olin Warner (1896). The left hand of the goddess is holding the torch of knowledge and her right hand is holding a sprig of laurel

tion of the allegory of "research" may be up to the viewer. I think that the researcher enlightens the world with the torch of knowledge and that the act of research itself is an honor.

To obtain the torch and laurel in both hands, professionalism, scientific integrity, logicality, autonomy, and ethics are needed.

8.8 Scientific Integrity and Mr. He's Jade

When I am carrying out research or writing a scientific paper, I always try not to forget scientific integrity and to make my paper flawless.

The term *flawlessness* originates from an episode of ancient Chinese history.

In the middle of the eighth century BCE, Bian He of Chu discovered a valuable piece of unworked jade and presented it sequentially to two kings, both of whom considered it be a worthless stone and punished what they perceived as deception by amputating his heel. When the jade was eventually cut and polished to make a ritual *bi* (jade-disk with a round hole in the center) it was acknowledged to be a priceless treasure, a perfect jade. Thus, Mr. He's jade became the most famous jade in Chinese history.

In the fourth century BCE, in the Warring States period, the state of Zhao acquired this jade. At this time, Qin was the most powerful state. One day, emissaries from King Zhao-Xiang of Qin (325–251 BCE) came to the Zhao court and offered 15 cities in exchange for the sacred Heshibi jade disk. The King of Zhao did not trust the King of Qin because he had been untrustworthy historically.

Lin Xiangru volunteered to go to the Qin court with Mr. He's jade. At the Qin court, the King of Qin passed Mr. He's jade among his ministers and concubines, making no mention of the promised 15 cities. Lin thought that the King of Qin did not intend to keep his word. Therefore, he tricked the King of Qin by claiming that there was a tiny "flaw" in the jade, and when the King of Qin returned the jade to him so that he could point out the flaw, Lin threatened to smash both the jade and his head (i.e., to commit suicide himself) against a pillar if the King of Qin tried to take it back by force (Fig. 8.6). The King of Qin, unwilling to see the jade ruined, agreed. That night, still not trusting the King of Qin, Lin ordered his henchman to take the jade back to Zhao in secret (returning the jade intact to the State of Zhao) [21].

As my teacher (Prof. Key June Seong, anatomist, 1926–1988) emphasized the importance of "flawlessness" when I was preparing my master's thesis, I think that scientific papers need scientific integrity.

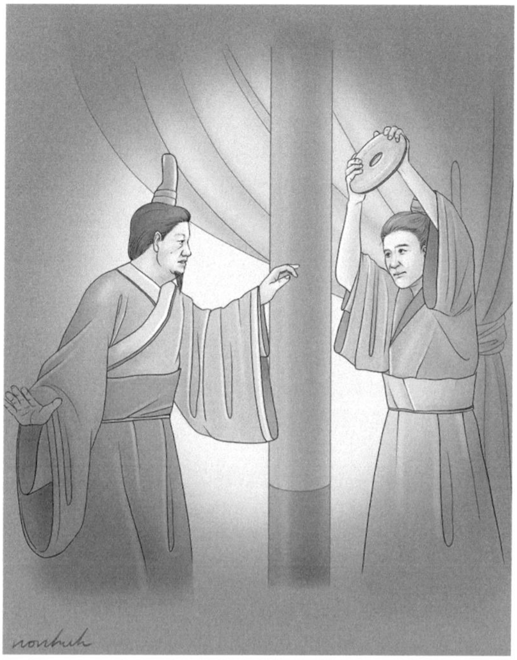

Fig. 8.6 Lin Xiangru threatens to smash both the jade and his head (i.e., to commit suicide himself) against a pillar if King Zhao-Xiang of Qin tries to take the jade back by force. Illustration by Hye Won Hu

Scientific integrity is the quality of being honest and having strong moral principles. It generally reflects a personal choice to hold oneself to standards of morality and ethics. This includes values such as honesty in research and publishing, avoidance of plagiarism or cheating, and maintenance of academic standards [22].

Since I strive for my papers to be flawless, I published a poem entitled "Scientific integrity [23]."

Tigers leave hides when they die,
I will bet on my proud name.
The messenger offered the famed jasper to the king,
and yet he nearly lost his neck by treachery.
In my papers, I will write truth and nothing but truth.
With the spirit of losing life at the cross,
I would place myself across the creek,
and become a stone bridge.

Now when I write a paper, I rub my heels with my fingers and reflect on the meaning of flawlessness.

8.9 My Scalpel Stops Here

If you can't stand the heat, get out of the kitchen.—*Harry Truman*

Recently, I participated in an annual conference held by the hospital where I was trained. The theme of the conference was "Advances in Facial Plastic Surgery," and the last session focused on revision rhinoplasty.

A presenter introduced his personal principle for revision rhinoplasty, in which the capsule is removed completely, followed by release and a septal extension graft. The most important point he made related to the attitude underlying this surgical technique: "It stops here." This meant that this operation should be the last one for the patient's nose.

This phrase reminded me of Harry Truman's farewell address in 1953. "The President—whoever he is—has to decide. He can't pass the buck to anybody. No one else can do the deciding for him. That's his job." This metaphorical expression, "passing the buck," is derived from the game of poker.

In the middle of the nineteenth century, the integrity of players was unreliable. Because the dealer has the greatest opportunity to cheat, players would take turns in the dealer role. To avoid arguments about whose turn it was, the person who was next would be given a marker, commonly a knife. The marker became known as a "buck," because the handles of many knives were made from buck (stag) at that time (Fig. 8.7).

Like President Truman, surgeons must choose the surgical plan based on his or her own decision. The surgeon must take the patient's history, perform a physical examination, and then sleep on the choice of the best option for the patient. If the patient is dissatisfied with the result, he or she will complain and perhaps even sue the surgeon who performed the operation. Surgeons must keep in mind the principle, "My scalpel stops here."

At that conference, I also gave a presentation, entitled "Anatomy for blepharoplasty." After my presentation, the chairperson asked me about the difference between the motor innervation of the

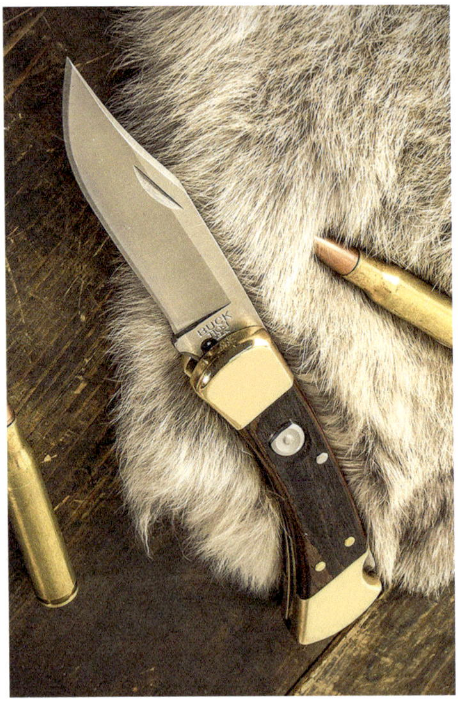

Fig. 8.7 A buck knife for designating the person who will be the next dealer

lower eyelid that I described in a publication years ago and a new publication by another author. I replied that the difference is due to the dissection method: from the skin or from the periosteum. I added that I had already submitted a letter to the editor on the topic, which has been published. An audience member asked me about the terminology of the layers of the orbital septum. I used the term "levator sheath" because Dr. Whitnall used it one hundred years ago. The audience member was confused because a Japanese ophthalmologist has been creating new terms for existing structures without searching the older literature.

On my way home I thought about the role of authors, especially the corresponding author. According to the International Committee of Medical Journal Editors (ICJME), the corresponding author is the individual who takes primary responsibility for communication with the journal during the manuscript submission, peer review, and publication process. The corresponding author should be available after publication to respond to critiques of the work and cooperate with any requests from the journal for data or additional information should questions about the paper arise after publication [24].

The buck also stops in front of the corresponding author of a manuscript, just like politicians and surgeons. They all have responsibilities that last as long as they breathe and will only perish when they pass away.

8.10 The Ajax Dilemma in Authorship

> For if they had been able to see the truth, then mighty Ajax, in anger over the arms, would never have planted in his chest the smooth sword—Ajax, who was the most powerful in battle, except for Achilles, and whom the breath of the unswerving Zephyr conveyed in swift ships, to bring back the wife of golden-haired Menelaus from the city of Ilus.—*From Nemean 7, by Pindaros* 518–438 BC

When I visited Rome before the coronavirus pandemic, I saw a fragmentary marble statue of a nude male (Fig. 8.8, left) in the Museo Pio-Clementino of the Vatican Museums. Because it was very similar to the torso showing visceral anatomy in the *Fabrica* of Vesalius (Plate 59, Fig. 8.8, right) [25], I read the text of the exhibition. The torso, which is named the "Belvedere Torso," is believed to have been made by Apollonios, an Athenian, during the first century BC. According to the Vatican Museum website, "the most favored hypothesis identifies it with Ajax, the son of Telamon, in the act of contemplating his suicide." The statue later came to be admired by Michelangelo, for which reason it came to be known as the "*Torso of Michelangelo*" and the "*School of Michelangelo.*"

In Homer's *Iliad*, Ajax was notable for his abundant strength and courage, shown particularly in two fights with Hector. After Achilles is killed by Paris, Ajax and Odysseus are the heroes who fight against the Trojans to retrieve the body and bury it. After the burial, each claims Achilles' armor, which had been made by the smith-god Hephaestus. A competition is held to determine who deserves the armor. To whom would the king, Agamemnon, give the

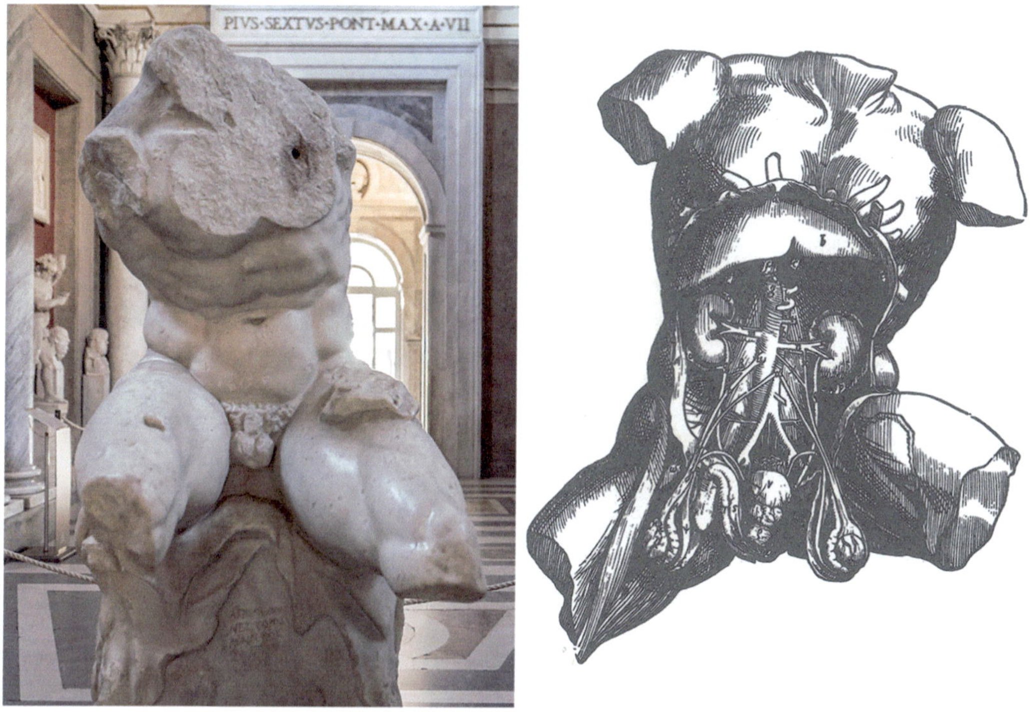

Fig. 8.8 The Greek hero Ajax depicted in a sculpture of his torso and in a drawing. Left: "Belvedere Torso" (first century BC, Athenian sculptor Apollonios) in the Museo Pio-Clementino. Right: Plate 59 of "*De humani corporis fabrica libri septem*" ("*On the fabric of the human body in seven books*," 1543) of Andreas Vesalius

gorgeous armor? Which soldier is more valuable: Ajax the magnificent, loyal, always in the thick of the fighting, always saving lives, or Odysseus the strategist, the trickster? The king arranges an oratorical contest to decide the issue. Odysseus proves to be more eloquent and, with the aid of Athena, the council gives him the armor. Ajax, the loyal workhorse, loses the contest. Ajax, "unconquered" and furious, becomes crazy and slaughters the Achaeans' herds of captured livestock, believing them to be his enemies through a trick of Athena. Unable to deal with this dual dishonor, he falls upon his own sword, "conquered by his [own] sorrow", and commits suicide.

Drawing inspiration from this ancient conflict between Ajax and Odysseus over the armor of Achilles, a book entitled *The Ajax Dilemma* was written by Paul Woodruff in 2011 [26]. This book deals with one of today's most pressing moral issues: how to distribute rewards and public recognition without damaging the social fabric. How should we honor those whose behavior and achievement is essential to our overall success? Is it fair or right to lavish rewards on superstars at the expense of the hardworking rank-and-file? How do we distinguish impartial fairness from true justice?

Reading this book, I reflected on coauthor meetings just before submitting a manuscript to a certain journal. Sometimes, everybody is happy in those meetings, but sometimes this is not the case. Of course, we have to verify our authorship during the submission process or just after the submission before the review process starts. This led me to wonder whether we also face the "Ajax dilemma" when determining the authorship of papers.

According to the "Recommendations for the Conduct, Reporting, Editing, and Publication of Scholarly Work in Medical Journals," the International Committee of Medical Journal Editors (ICMJE) [27] recommends that authorship be based on the following four criteria:

1. Substantial contributions to the conception or design of the work or the acquisition, analysis, or interpretation of data for the work.
2. Drafting the work or revising it critically for important intellectual content.
3. Final approval of the version to be published.
4. Agreement to be accountable for all aspects of the work in ensuring that questions related to the accuracy or integrity of any part of the work are appropriately investigated and resolved.

This recommendation states that all individuals who meet the first criterion should have the opportunity to participate in the review, drafting, and final approval of the manuscript. It furthermore specifies that the criteria used to determine the order in which authors are listed on the byline may vary and are to be decided collectively by the authors and not by editors.

As the recommendation states, the determination of the order of authors should be decided by the authors as a group. The corresponding author, like the king Agamemnon, can be the chairperson of the coauthors' meeting. However, it is not always easy to determine who will be the first author—analogous to the question of who is deserving to take Achilles' armor. Like the Greek army that won the Trojan War, we also are facing the "Ajax dilemma."

At this moment, we should remember a story from the Talmud, describing three brothers, who, respectively, had a magic telescope, a magic carpet, and a magic apple.

A king had a beautiful, beloved princess, but she was at the verge of death due to an illness. Many doctors prescribed and applied all kinds of medicines, but none worked. Becoming very desperate, the king proclaimed that whoever heals the princess will marry the princess and will eventually become the next king as the reward. Three brothers who lived far away from the palace heard that the princess was ill and discussed how to heal her. Each of these brothers had a magical item: the first brother had a magic telescope that could see anywhere; the second brother had a magic carpet that could fly anywhere; and finally, the third brother had a magic apple that could heal any illness. Therefore, they verified the proclamation with the magic telescope, and then they flew out to the palace on the magic carpet and gave the princess the magic apple. The princess got better immediately. The king could not decide which one to give his daughter to, because they all took part in healing her.

Here is the question: who would you accept as the bridegroom of the princess if you were the king and why? I would suggest accepting the third brother, because he gave up his magic apple, which the princess ate. I believe that we all have the wisdom to give credit for authorship according to the contribution that each researcher makes.

8.11 Archives of Korean Plastic Surgery

While I was in London for 3 months in 2016, I visited the British Association of Plastic, Reconstructive, and Aesthetic Surgeons (BAPRAS) archives located at the Royal College of Surgeons in London.

The palatoplasty method I have been using for almost 30 years (V-Y pushback) was derived from Dr. Kilner via Dr. Calnan, so I wanted to see some relics belonging to Dr. Kilner.

I contacted the Hunterian Museum and made an appointment with the curator. There, I met the honorary archivist Dr. Roger Green and was shown three boxes of Dr. Kilner's relics: drafts of papers, pictures of the patients he operated on, schemas submitted to journals, and his handwritten notes. While in the room, I wore gloves on my hands to protect the papers. As I read Dr. Kilner's lecture draft written 68 years ago, I felt as if I was listening to him give the lecture in the lecture room downstairs.

The records of plastic surgery go back to at least 500 BC. However, the modern discipline as we know it has its origins in the First World War. The BAPRAS archives were founded in the 1980s by Antony Wallace and are known as the Antony Wallace Archive. The current honorary archivist is Roger Green, who succeeded Brian Morgan, who retired from the post in 2014, having spent 15 years overseeing and expanding the archive. Mr. Morgan followed Phil Sykes and Charles Chapman in this role.

The BAPRAS archive holds a number of photographs, some of which depict staff and treatment procedures from the World War I, although the majority of the items are from plastic surgery personalities from the 1930s and the World War II. The BAPRAS archive has a collection of plastic surgery instruments, for example, that belonged to Professor Joseph, who was the pioneer of cosmetic rhinoplasty. All BAPRAS-archived instruments are available for viewing and can be accessed online (http://surgicat.rcseng.ac.uk/).

On my way back to Korea, I thought about the history of Korean plastic surgery. The Korean Society of Plastic, Reconstructive, and Aesthetic Surgery (KSPRS) was founded in 1966, and the first volume of the *Journal of the Korean Society of Plastic and Reconstructive Surgery (Taehan Sŏnghyŏng Oekwa Hakhoe chi)* appeared in October 1974 (Fig. 8.9). Starting with Vol. 39 (2012), it was continued as *Archives of Plastic Surgery (APS*). We marked our 50th anniversary in 2016. The KSPRS has its own office with sample space, and the pioneers of the KSPRS are getting very old; some of them have even passed away.

It is time to create our archives: the Archives of Korean Plastic Surgery. We should gather all our experiences and knowledge of plastic surgery in the past, including memories of working with or being a patient of the pioneering Korean plastic surgeons. When pioneers retire, the KSPRS should try to persuade them to donate their relics. A room should be dedicated as a space for the archives, and famous instruments and relics should be photographed and exhibited online.

There is an Oriental saying that "Tigers die and leave their skins; people die and leave their

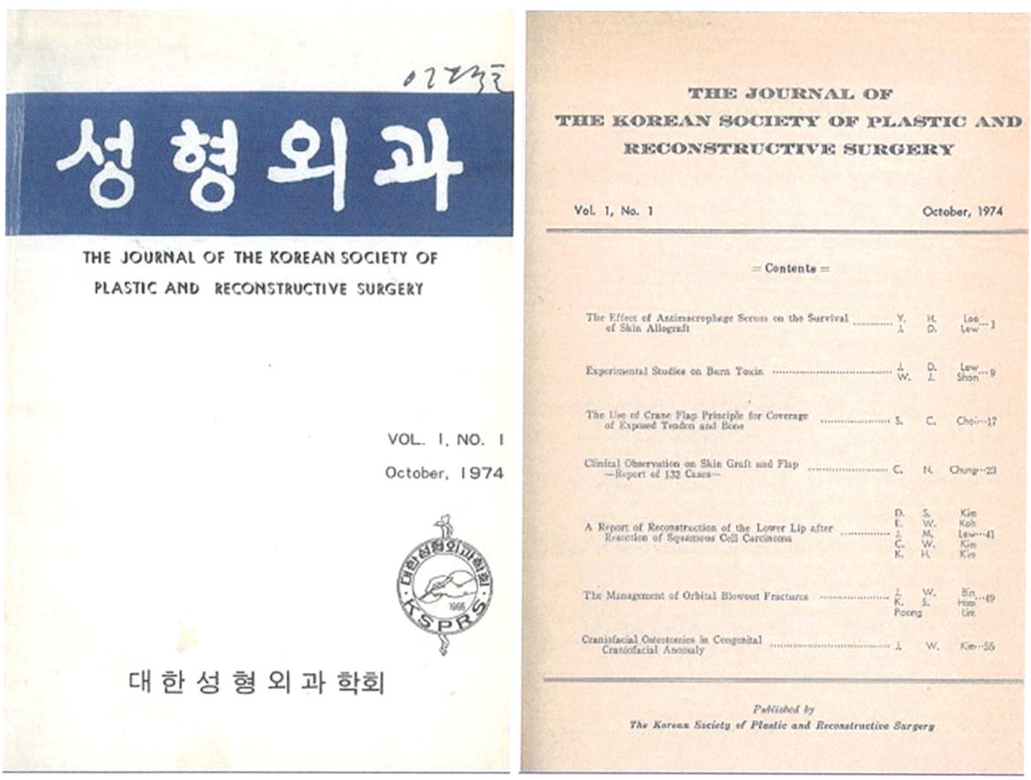

Fig. 8.9 The first issue of JKSPRS The first issue of the Journal of the Korean Society of Plastic and Reconstructive Surgery (Taehan Sŏnghyŏng Oekwa Hakhoe chi), vol. 1, no. 1, October 1974. Left, cover; right: table of contents. Donated from Dr. Lee Taik Ho (Board No. 9)

names." We should preserve our ancestors' relics and the spirits that are inside of them.

8.12 They are Analyzing Us: Our Own Survey is Needed

When I searched for a paper written by a plastic surgeon colleague of mine, I found that it had been cited four times [28]. Interestingly, one of the citations was from a paper that had been published in a journal in the field of management, not in a medical journal [29].

Because the title contained the intriguing words "cosmetic surgery" and "Seoul," I read the linked article. It was written by researchers in the fields of business and accounting from Malaysia and China, and the journal was published in the United States.

In order to collect market data on women's willingness to undergo cosmetic surgery in Seoul, the authors interviewed 400 women aged 19–40 years in Seoul using a self-administered questionnaire. These researchers in the fields of business and accounting used the theory of reasoned action, which analyzes factors such as attitudes, subjective norms (celebrities and the media), and psychological attributes (social status and self-esteem) that influence patients' intention to undergo cosmetic surgery. They found generally positive attitudes toward cosmetic surgery among women living in Seoul, with favorable intentions towards cosmetic surgery, as manifested by the belief among Korean women that undergoing cosmetic surgery is the most effective way to improve their appearance and social status. Their results revealed that celebrities and the media played an important role in influencing women to undergo surgery.

The authors approached this topic from the perspective of marketing and management and suggested that their results provided important information for designing effective strategies to advertise and promote cosmetic surgery. They also discussed psychological attributes, such as self-esteem and social status.

Reading this article, I was surprised that researchers in the field of business and accounting wrote this paper and that they were interested in cosmetic surgery marketing in Seoul. Although there are only about 51 million Koreans living in South Korea and 7.4 million Koreans living outside of the Korean Peninsula, accounting for roughly 1% of the world population [30], the authors were clearly aware that South Korea is ranked third in the world in the number of cosmetic procedures, with 1,156,000 Koreans undergoing such procedures in 2015 [31], and the Korean cosmetic surgery market has a 24% market share of the total world market [32].

I think that the authors of this article regard the Seoul cosmetic surgery market as a wide-open field (blue ocean) for future business initiatives.

The Korean Society of Plastic and Reconstructive Surgeons (KSPRS) has been gathering data from all training hospitals for many years. At any training hospital, we must report daily information on the operations performed and the number of patients in our department. However, I have not seen any articles based on the prospective data collected by our society.

As the authors in the field of business and accounting suggested, additional research is needed to determine patients' satisfaction with non-core and post-cosmetic surgery services (after-sales services), such as the doctor's skills and knowledge, the environment of the clinic, and other factors that collectively define the total or augmented product.

The KSPRS has recently been making efforts to internationalize itself as a society [33]. We, as members of the KSPRS, should have a prospective analysis of our market before our possible rivals. We should analyze the market ourselves, instead of letting further surveys be done by marketing managers from countries that compete with us. For this, a survey supported by the Korean Society of Aesthetic Plastic Surgeons of the KSPRS is needed. Remember that our city, Seoul, is the "center of cosmetic surgery."

References

1. Kim JT. The value of originality and proper quotation. Arch Plast Surg. 2012;39:279–80.

2. Huh S. How should authors address copyright issues before submission of manuscripts? Arch Plast Surg. 2012;39:445–7.
3. Oxford dictionaries. Devil's advocate. Oxford: Oxford University Press; 2013. http://oxforddictionaries.com/definition/english/devil%27s%2Badvocate?q=devil%27s+advocate.
4. Wikipedia. *Devil's advocate [internet].* Wikimedia Foundation Inc.; 2013. http://en.wikipedia.org/wiki/Devil%27s_advocate.
5. Fanning W. Promotor fidei [Internet]. New York: Robert Appleton Company; 1911. [cited 2013 Apr 7]. Available from: http://www.newadvent.org/cathen/12454a.htm
6. Rolland R. Jean Christophe, Cannan G. translator. Whitefish, MN: Kessinger Publishing; 2004.
7. Hwang K. The origins of deltopectoral flaps and the pectoralis major myocutaneous flap. J Craniofac Surg. 2016;27:1845–8.
8. Peh WC, Ng KH. Role of the manuscript reviewer. Singapore Med J. 2009;50:931–3.
9. Hwang K. The need for a reviewer to play Devil's advocate. Arch Plast Surg. 2013;40:171–2.
10. Kachewar SG, Sankaye SB. Reviewer index: a new proposal of rewarding the reviewer. Mens Sana Monogr. 2013;11:274–84.
11. Shaughnessy AF, Slawson DC. Getting the most from review articles: a guide for readers and writers. Am Fam Physician. 1997;55:2155–60.
12. Heller S. The changing role of a publisher and the publisher of the future. Drug News Perspect. 2007;20:413–5.
13. Steinhauser G, Adlassnig W, Risch JA, et al. Peer review versus editorial review and their role in innovative science. Theor Med Bioeth. 2012;33:359–76.
14. Kravitz RL, Franks P, Feldman MD, et al. Editorial peer reviewers' recommendations at a general medical journal: are they reliable and do editors care? PLoS One. 2010;5:e10072.
15. Merton RK. The Matthew effect in science: the reward and communication systems of science are considered. Science. 1968;159:56–63.
16. Epstude K, Mussweiler T. What you feel is how you compare: how comparisons influence the social induction of affect. Emotion. 2009;9:1–14.
17. OECD. *Frascati manual: proposed standard practice for surveys on research and experimental development.* 6th ed; 2002. http://www.oecd.org/sti/frascati-manua. Accessed 27 May 2012.
18. Levi B, Longaker MT. Research training in plastic surgery. J Craniofac Surg. 2011;22:383–4.
19. Toledo-Pereyra LH. Ten qualities of a good researcher. J Investig Surg. 2012;25:201–2.
20. Finnish Advisory Board on Research Integrity. Ethical principles of research in the humanities and social and Behavioural sciences and proposals for ethical review. http://www.uta.fi/english/research/ethics/guidelines/autonomy.html. Accessed 9 Oct 2016.
21. Hwang K. Sine qua non conditions for research. J Craniofac Surg. 2017;28:594–5.
22. Qian S, Shiji (History) Biographies of Lian Po and Lin Xiangru. Seoul. Korea: Samsung Press; 2019. p. 218–29.
23. Clayware HK, a potter. Seoul. Korea: Jaenam; 2020. p. 140–1.
24. International Committee of Medical Journal Editors. Defining the role of authors and contributors. http://www.icmje.org/recommendations/browse/roles-and-responsibilities/defining-the-role-of-authors-and-contributors.html. Accessed 14 Jun 2019.
25. Saunders JBdeCM, O'Malley CD. The anatomical drawings of Andreas Vesalius. New York: Bonanza Books; 1982.
26. Woodruff P. The ajax dilemma: justice, fairness, and rewards. Oxford: Oxford University Press; 2011.
27. International Committee of Medical Journal Editors (ICMJE). Recommendations for the Conduct, Reporting, Editing, and Publication of Scholarly Work in Medical Journals (Updated Dec 2019). http://www.icmje.org/icmje-recommendations.pdf. Accessed 26 May 2020.
28. Choi J. Cosmetic surgery: is it science or art? Arch Plast Surg. 2015;42:672–4.
29. Teng PK, Ling TJ, Seng KW. Propensity to undergo cosmetic surgery and services in Seoul. Int J Commun Dev Manag Stud. 2019;3:1–16.
30. Chang DW. Plastic surgeons of Korean heritage: why it matters to me. Arch Plast Surg. 2019;46:1–2.
31. International Society of Aesthetic Plastic Surgeons (ISAPS). ISAPS international survey on aesthetic/cosmetic procedures performed in 2015 [internet]. Hanover, NH: ISAPS; 2019. [cited 2019 Jul 15]. https://www.isaps.org/wp-content/uploads/2017/10/2016-ISAPS-Results-1.pdf.
32. Seoul Touch Up. Korean plastic surgery statistics. Seoul: Seoul Touch Up; 2012. https://www.seoultouchup.com/korean-plastic-surgery-statistics/.
33. Kim KS. Into a global future with our members to serve the people. Arch Plast Surg. 2019;46:99–101.

9 Praising the Pioneers

9.1 Viewed Relics Belonging to Abraham Colles in Dublin

A majority of medical professionals will most likely remember learning about Colles' fracture, a fracture of the radius in the wrist associated with a characteristic backward displacement of the hand [1]. However, I realized that my knowledge of Abraham Colles himself seemed limited. Colles, who first described his fracture as "taking place at about an inch and a half (38 mm) above the carpal extremity of the radius and the carpus and the base of metacarpus appears to be thrown backward" [2], is relatively unknown to many. After some research, it became apparent to me that he was an anatomist as well as a surgeon. This article is written in memory of Abraham Colles, a great anatomist and surgeon, and in this article, his contributions to the field of surgical anatomy are discussed.

Abraham Colles was born in 1773 in Ireland and completed his medical education at Trinity College, University of Dublin, and Edinburgh University. In 1804, he became a professor of Anatomy and Physiology, Royal College of Surgeons, Ireland (RCSI). In 1811, he wrote an important treatise on surgical anatomy, and some terms that he introduced, such as Colles' fracture, have survived in surgical nomenclature to this day. He also described the membranous layer of the subcutaneous tissues of the perineum, which came to be known as Colles' fascia [3]. He passed away in 1843 and was buried in Mount Jerome Cemetery, Dublin.

Recently, we participated in the summer meeting of the Anatomical Society of Great Britain and Ireland, which was held at RCSI. At that time, Professor Cleve Lee, who has been a Professor of Anatomy since 2002, showed me some relics that had belonged to Abraham Colles. Colles was a Professor of Anatomy and Physiology of RCSI from 1804 to 1827. A portrait of Abraham Colles was hanging on the wall of the College Boardroom (Fig. 9.1). A conference room that was named after the famous professor was in use (Fig. 9.2), and a board printed with the names of former professors was displayed in the dissecting room of the college (Fig. 9.3). A trip to his dissecting room suggested the thought, which seems convincing to us, that only Colles' sound knowledge of gross anatomy, obtainable only through cadaver dissection, could have enabled his great achievements.

Abraham Colles should be remembered as a pioneering surgical anatomist as well as a proficient surgeon. There is a South Korean saying, "Tigers leave fine hides when they die, and people leave their names upon their departure." Professor Colles has left us his famous name—a name that will be remembered, thanks to "Colles' fracture."

K. Hwang, *Good Physician, Good Plastic Surgeon*, https://doi.org/10.1007/978-981-97-1864-1_9

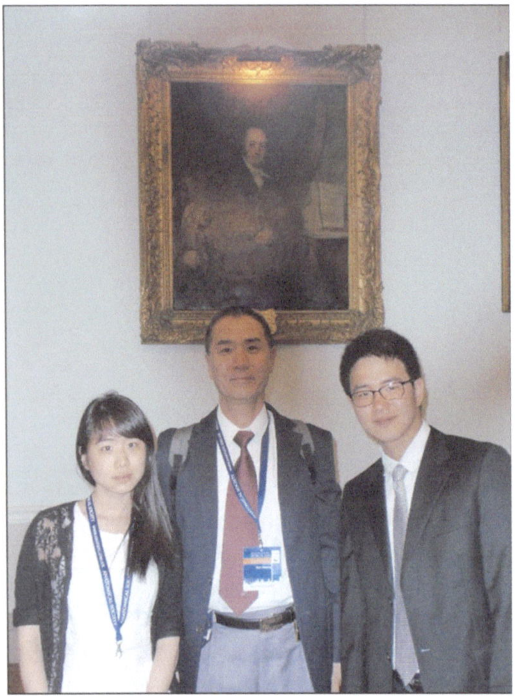

Fig. 9.1 The portrait of Abraham Colles in the College Boardroom of Royal College of Surgeons, Ireland

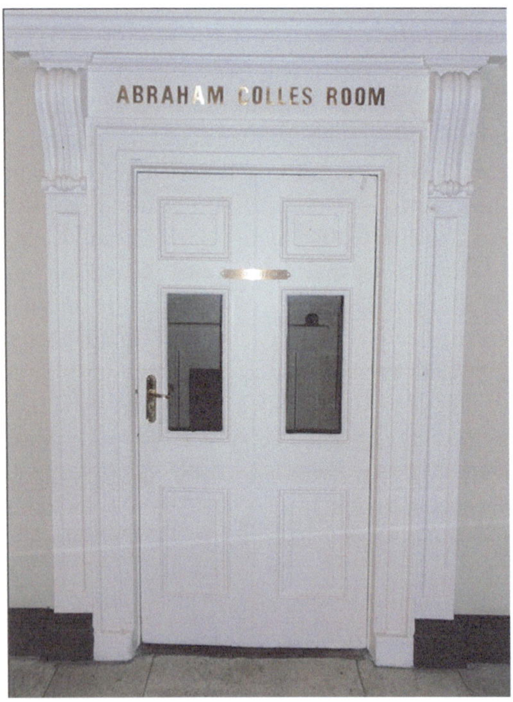

Fig. 9.2 Abraham Colles Room: conference room

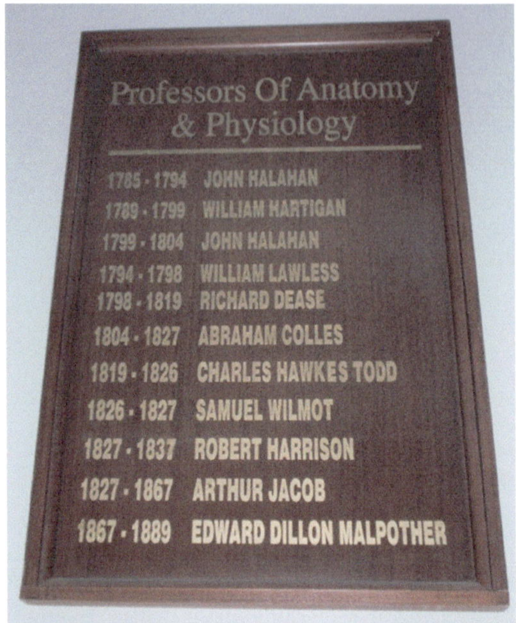

Fig. 9.3 Board in the dissection room showing the names and the dates of service of former professors of Anatomy and Physiology. Note Abraham Colles 1804–1827

9.2 Trench Coats, Cushing, and Gillies

In early spring and in late autumn, stylish dressers love to wear trench coats. Trench coats are raincoats made of waterproof heavy-duty cotton gabardine drill, leather, or poplin. Dandies wear trench coats, which are popular in Seoul and in London. This coat was developed prior to the war but was adapted for use in the trenches of the World War I (WWI). It was an item of clothing worn by Army officers. I vividly remember Robert Taylor and Vivien Leigh wearing stylish trench coats in "Waterloo Bridge" (1940) (Fig. 9.4), as well as Humphrey Bogart in "Casablanca" (1942).

The most famous instance of trench warfare was the Western Front in WWI. In this war, the machine gun first appeared. Soldiers stayed in trenches, in which troops were well-protected from the enemy's fire and sheltered from artillery. In the trenches, soldiers could hide their body. However, their head and face were exposed

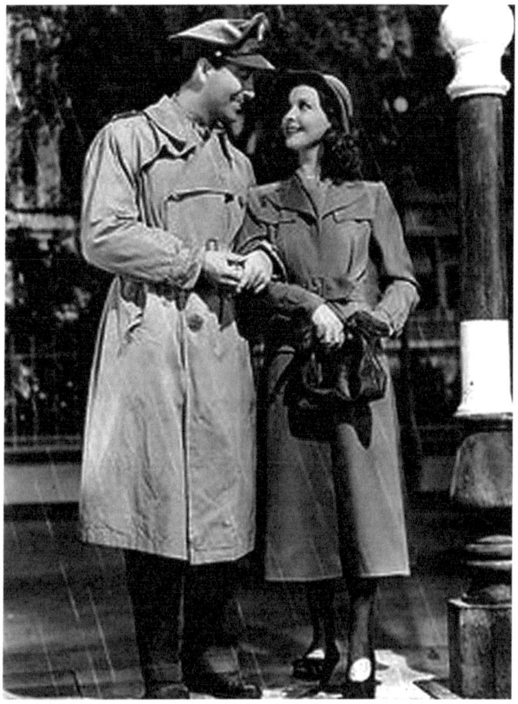

Fig. 9.4 Robert Taylor and Vivien Leigh are wearing stylish trench coats in "Waterloo Bridge (1940)"

to the enemy's fire, and therefore, head and facial trauma occurred frequently.

Harvey Cushing (1869–1939) made major contributions to the treatment of head injuries. When he was at a French military hospital in 1917, he extracted fragments of metallic missile shrapnel that were lodged deeply within the brain using electromagnets. During 4 months in 1917, he treated 219 wounded soldiers, including 133 gunshot wounds that penetrated the dura mater. He developed debridement, using negative pressure, and dura repair, using the fascia lata. He also systematized the treatment of head injuries, reducing mortality among head injury patients.

When WWI began, Gillies joined the Royal Army Medical Corps and met many soldiers who had facial trauma. After his returned to England, he devoted himself to facial repairs at the Queen's Hospital. He developed many plastic surgery techniques. From 1917 to 1925, he performed more than 11,000 operations on 5000 soldiers with facial injuries. His experiences with head and facial injury became the basis of craniofacial surgery, and his advances were also applied to congenital craniofacial malformations. He wrote "A new principle in the surgical treatment of 'congenital cleft palate' and its mechanical counterpart" in 1921. His technique for the treatment of cleft hard and soft palate was based on a combined surgical and dental treatment strategy.

Through treating severely injured faces, he accumulated surgical experiences with the face that led to the development of aesthetic surgery. Most of the principles of modern facial plastic surgery were developed during the 20 years between WWI and WWII. As such, plastic surgery aims for humanity before beauty.

9.3 Portraits of Two Innovative Plastic Surgeons in the National Portrait Gallery

It must at all times be kept in mind that the most important person is first, last, and all the time the patient [4].—*Archibald McIndoe*

As a medical doctor, when I visit a gallery or museum, I look for portraits of medical doctors. During my stay in London, I visited the National Portrait Gallery, where I happened to see the portraits of two famous plastic surgeons: Sir Harold Delf Gillies (1882–1960, Fig. 9.5) and Sir Archibald Hector McIndoe (1900–1960, Fig. 9.6). The name "Gillies" caught my eye because the approach named after him is one of the indirect approaches for the reduction of the zygomatic arch (Gillies, temporal; Keen, transoral; and Dingman, lateral brow). The name "McIndoe" was also familiar because of the "McIndoe operation" for reconstruction of the vagina in the congenital absence of the vagina, using an indwelling skin graft [5].

World War I (WWI, 1914–1918) was characterized by trench warfare, during which Combatant's head and neck were exposed to high-energy weapons, resulting in severe facial wounds [6].

Gillies was born in New Zealand and studied medicine at Cambridge University. When WWI began, he joined the Royal Army Medical Corps.

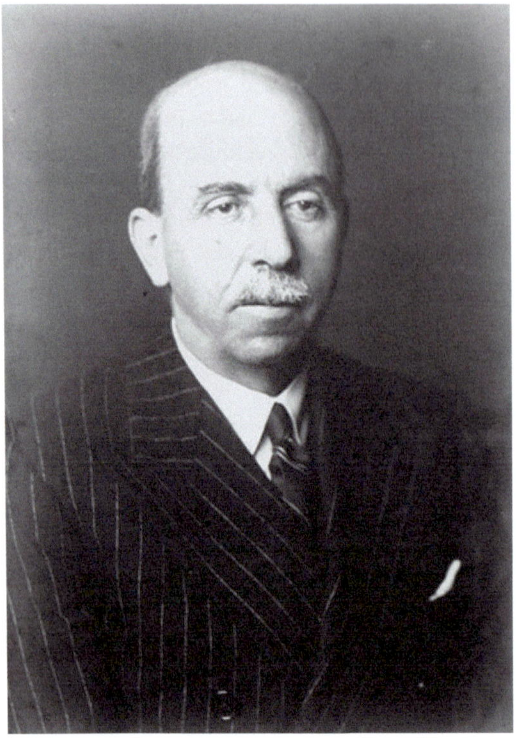

Fig. 9.5 Sir Harold Delf Gillies (1882–1960), plastic surgeon

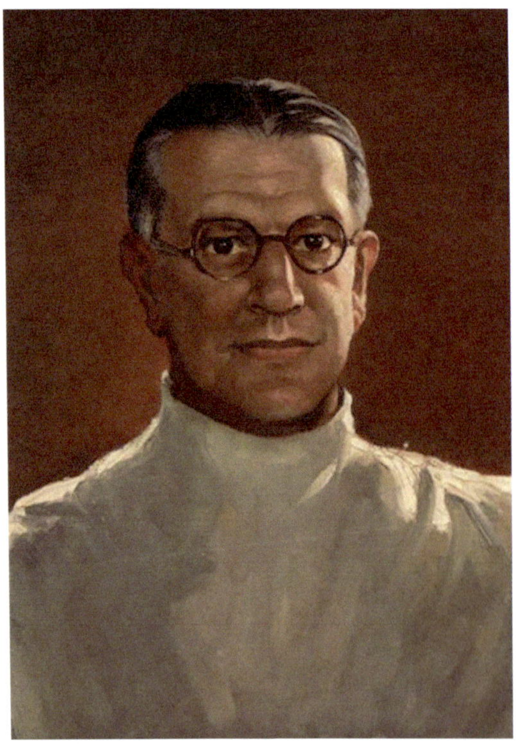

Fig. 9.6 Sir Archibald Hector McIndoe (1900–1960), plastic surgeon

While working in France, Gilllies met French-American dentist, Charles Valadier, and learned the basics of repairing jaw injuries, including how to do bone grafting. After his return to England, he worked at the Queen's Hospital, which was devoted to facial repairs. He developed many plastic surgery techniques. From 1917 to 1925, he performed more than 11,000 operations for 5000 soldiers with facial injuries [7]. His pre- and postoperative results were drawn by artist Henry Tonks, with pastels, and by Daryl Lindsay, with watercolors.

McIndoe was born in New Zealand and studied medicine at the University of Ontago and moved to London at the age of 30. When McIndoe arrived in the United Kingdom, his cousin Gillies got McIndoe a temporary position at St Bartholomew's Hospital in London. McIndoe worked here for less than a year and obtained his British qualifications. Gillies put McIndoe forward for a lecturer position at the Hospital for Tropical Diseases. McIndoe was successful but he soon became bored of this position, so Gillies invited him to join his private practice. From 1931 to 1939, they performed hundreds of operations together and devised new techniques.

In World War II (1939–1945), the survival rates from the combat wounds increased due to the development of blood transfusion, endotracheal intubation, and rapid evacuation by aircraft [8]. Severe burn cases appeared due to massive air strike from bombers. Thereafter, burn care significantly advanced during World War II.

Following the outbreak of World War II, McIndoe moved to the newly built Queen's Hospital and treated deep burn injuries and serious facial deformities, like the loss of eyelids.

At that time, the standard treatment for burns was coagulation with tannic acid, which is very painful. He observed different healing rates in extensively burned pilots who had come down on land and in the sea. From this, he discovered that immersion in saline promoted healing as well as improving survival rates and thus began saline baths and early grafting instead of tannic acid. He recognized the importance of rehabilitation and social reintegration back into normal life [4]. In fact, over 80% of his aircrew patients returned to duty [9].

On arriving home from the museum, I searched for the number of papers they wrote and their titles. Gillies and McIndoe published 12 and 17 papers, respectively. Among them were two articles they coauthored [10, 11].

Gillies wrote "A new principle in the surgical treatment of "congenital cleft palate" and its mechanical counterpart" (1921, cited 113 times) [12] and "The design of direct pedicle flaps" (1932, cited 29 times) [13], among others.

His technique for the treatment of cleft of hard and soft palate was based on a combined surgical and dental treatment. Soft palate was paired and lengthened surgically by separating the soft palate from the hard palate. A dental apparatus was applied on the hard palate, and skin graft was applied to the raw anterior edge of palate. After healing, Fry's apparatus was applied for stretching the soft palate [12].

McIndoe developed many new techniques, reflected in his publications which included "Total reconstruction of the burned face. The Bradshaw Lecture" (1958, cited 41 times) [14], "Symposium: radiation necrosis" (1947, cited 32 times) [15], "Operation for the cure of adult hypospadias" (1937, cited 23 times) [16], "Surgical and dental treatment of fractures of the upper and lower jaws in war time" (1941, cited 15 times) [17], "The burned hand" (1945, cited 12 times) [18], and "Congenital absence of the vagina, treated by means of an indwelling skin-graft" (1938, cited 9 times) [5].

His methods were very innovative and the first successful reconstruction for congenital absence of the vagina. A hollow vulcanite mold was used, which was completely closed at both ends, with the size and shape of a distended virgin vagina. A split thickness skin graft (9.5 inch long by 2.5 inch wide) was harvested from the inner thigh. An incision was made from a point half an inch posterior to the urethral meatus and carried vertically backwards to a point 3/4 inch in front of the anus. Blunt dissection was carried between the rectum and the bladder, and a cavity was made for the mold. The mold was covered with the skin graft, raw surface outwards. The skin-covered mold was inserted into the cavity, and the labia minora were sutured across its lower end, leaving a small hole anteriorly just behind the meatus for drainage. The skin-covered mold was maintained for 5 months after operation [4].

It goes without saying that these two New Zealand born cousins were innovative plastic surgeons. Where did their innovative thinking come from? As in Gillies' case, innovation can come from being informed by other subjects of study or specialties. Innovation comes also from close observation, as in McIndoe's case. However, innovation mostly arises out of necessity, as when Gillies and McIndoe pursued their field practice.

9.4 Meet Dr. Kilner at the Hunterian Museum

> Why do we operate? To make patients look, speak, and eat well.
> Your slogan should be 'The simplest possible repair with minimum sacrifice of material.'—*Thomas Pomfret Kilner (1890–1964, at the lecture for a course of Postgraduate Education of Plastic Surgery at Royal College of Surgeons, February 23, 1948)*

The V-Y pushback palatoplasty is one of the most frequently performed procedures in cleft palate repair. From my training period until now, I am using this technique since I believe it is the best method.

My first exposure to the literature of palatoplasty procedures was *Cleft Craft: The Evolution of its Surgery* written by Dr. Ralph Millard at the beginning of my residency training (1987) [19]. This book provided me a history and evolution of the techniques. A year later, I encountered the detailed procedures by reading Chapter 29 (V-Y Pushback Palatoplasty) written by Dr. James Calnan in the *Cleft Lip and Palate Surgical, Dental, and Speech Aspect by 71 Authors*, edited by Dr. Grabb et al. Dr. Calnan described each step of the Kilner's palate operation in meticulous detail [20].

It was very easy to read because it gave precise explanation and fine illustration of each step, including detaching the nasal mucosa from the posterior border of the hard palate, by passing the instrument behind the palatine vessels, or from posterior nasal spine, using curved hook.

I photocopied that chapter and read it again and again and made underlines, marks, and numbers until it was worn out. I still memorize the sequence of all the procedures that includes freeing of lateral pharyngeal mucosa from the medial pterygoid plate.

It is well-known that Dr. Hugo Ganzer was the first surgeon who stated that von Langenbeck palatoplasty results in short velum. He introduced V-Y type of retropositioning of the palate, which resulted in about 1 cm length gain. Dr. Franz Ernst proposed that circular narrowing of the pharynx can facilitate the velar approximation to the pharyngeal wall [19].

The V-Y pushback palatoplasty is also known as Wardill–Kilner–Veau method. Dr. Victor Veau discarded the closure under tension of the Langenbeck procedure, and his two major contributions are nasal mucoperiosteal closure of the hard palate cleft, including vomer flap and his muscle sutures [21]. In 1937, Dr. Kilner in London and Dr. Wardill in Newcastle independently published a technique, the "V-Y retroposition" operation. The major difference between the two surgeons is posterior palatine artery. Dr. Wardill divided posterior palatine artery; however, Dr. Kilner saved it [22, 23].

Since the palatoplasty method I have been using for almost 30 years was derived from Dr. Kilner via Dr. Calnan, I did want to see some relics belonging to Dr. Kilner. Thereafter, I contacted the Hunterian Museum, London, and could see three boxes of Dr. Kilner's relics: draft of papers, pictures of his patients operated, and schemas submitted to journals and his handwritten notes.

Among them, I impressively read the draft for a course of lectures in plastic surgery, arranged by the Postgraduate Education Committee of the Royal College of Surgeons (Cleft Lip and Palate Repair, February 23, 1948). He wrote "The operation we perform and have performed for many years is a composite one but owes most to Victor Veau who discarded the closure under tension of the Langenbeck procedure and developed the use of rotation flaps. To this we added the resuscitative procedure of hamular process fracture to put out of court (temporarily at any rate) the action of the tensor palate muscles and the lateral freeing used by Ernst and Axhausen of Berlin."

Several hours passed very swiftly in the BAPRAS archive room of the Royal College of Surgeons. In the room, globes were on my hands to protect the papers. While I was reading his lecture draft written 68 years ago, I felt as if I was listing his lecture in the lecture room downstairs.

Most of the drawings were printed ones; however, only one drawing of palatoplasty was drawn by pencil (Fig. 9.7). Interestingly, it was not made on the ordinary paper or card. It was drawn on the reverse side of a letter envelope of "Queen's Hotel, Birmingham" (Fig. 9.8). I think that the human brain is like a molten bronze that should be poured into a mold. When inspired, it should be written or drawn before it disappears. It is thought that Dr. Kilner got an idea when he stayed at that hotel. Before the vivid idea went

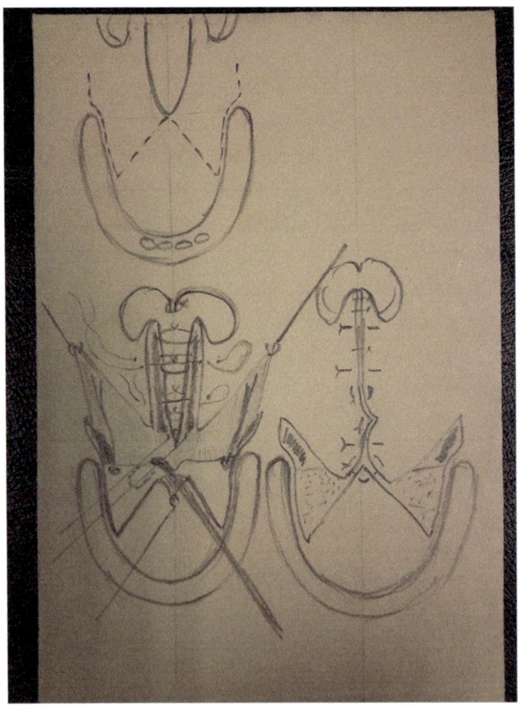

Fig. 9.7 Dr. Kilner's pencil drawing of V-Y pushback palatoplasty. (Upper) Design of V-Y flaps. (Lower left) Nasal mucosae are detached from the posterior border of the hard palate and posterior nasal spine using periosteal elevator. Palatine vessels are preserved. Palatal muscles of each side are sutured together. (Lower right) Closure of buccal layer with simple interrupted suture and vertical mattress sutures alternatively. Two posterior flaps are joined to anterior flap

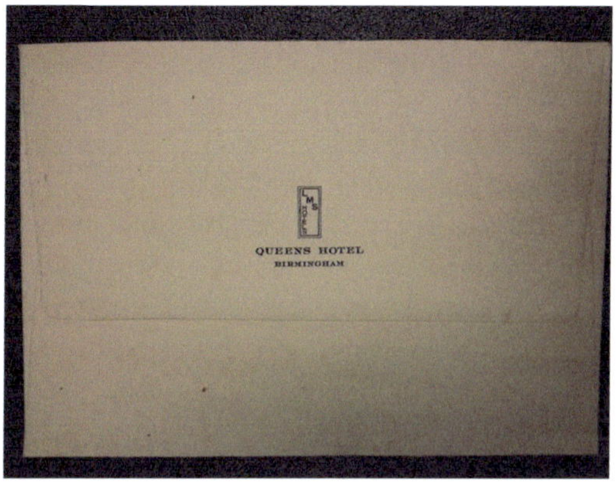

Fig. 9.8 Reverse side of the pencil drawing: a letter envelope of "Queen's Hotel, Birmingham"

away, he made the schema with his nearest paper, the letter envelope, I believe.

There is an oriental saying, "Tigers leave fine hides when they die, and people leave their name on their departure." Dr. Kilner has surely left his good name on the famous operation that will be continued for generations to come.

9.5 Origin of Lee Quedae's Knowledge of Artistic Anatomy

9.5.1 Art and Medicine

The purpose of medicine is to heal the sick and relieve suffering. Empathy, which refers to the ability to be aware of the feelings and emotions of other people, is needed to be a good doctor. Teaching art to medical students helps them sharpen their observational skills and makes them more empathetic. Art helps make medical students become more thoughtful and listen carefully to a patient's narrative of his/her symptoms, and this allows doctors to make a more informed diagnosis [24].

Art is a creative human endeavor that appeals to the senses. Art in medicine, especially in anatomy, is the creative expression of the structural form of life, specifically life as manifested in human anatomy. For example, Gustav Klimt (1862–1918) made *Liebespaar* (*The Lovers*) based on anatomical knowledge and communication with an anatomist [25].

9.5.2 Art and Anatomy in the Renaissance

In the Renaissance, anatomical science was a major source of inspiration for artists. By the fifteenth century, interest had emerged in anatomy as an area of research, and the artists of the period dissected cadavers. Artists performed dissections in order to pursue divine beauty, in the belief that God created humankind in his image, whereas anatomists' goal was to gain scientific knowledge [26].

Artists witnessed or participated in dissections to gain a better understanding of the relationships among bones, tendons, muscles, and the overlying skin in particular postures. Renaissance artists sought to accurately portray facial expressions, positions, reflexive motions, and draped clothing. Observations of living subjects constituted the primary source of artists' expertise. Some artists thought that anatomy was a tool to be used in their drawings and paintings; however, other artists, such as Leonardo, approached anatomy as an academic field. Dissection provides a fixed model without flowing blood, which cannot be used as an animated model. It is thought that these artists learned about the origins of vivid expressions from the anatomy of the muscles lying beneath the skin. Artists and anatomists together produced images of the body that combined medical knowledge and an artistic vision [27, 28]. Artists' general enthusiasm for studying cadavers decreased in the seventeenth century, when art academies became amply stocked with skeletons and skinned specimens and illustrated anatomical texts became readily available [29].

9.5.3 Pioneer of Artistic Anatomy in Korea

Lee Quede (1913–1965) was a master artist of the early 2twentieth century of Korea. After graduating from Whimoon High School, he went to Japan to attend the Teikoku Art School (Imperial Art School, 帝國美術學校). During the Korean War (1950–1953), he suffered a tragic fate. He could not escape from the North Korean army due to his elderly mother and pregnant wife. He had no choice but to help produce North Korean propaganda paintings. He was later kept in a prisoner of war camp run by the South Korean army.

In the Geoje prisoner of war camp (PWC), Lee Quede produced anatomical drawings and notes about the human body to teach artistic anatomy to his fellow refugee Lee Ju-yeong. Human anatomy, physiognomic differences among races, and phrenology are explained in those drawings (Fig. 9.9). Since no references were available in the PWC, Lee Quede's drawing notes solely relied upon his own memories of what he had learned at Teikoku Art School in Japan, where he obtained knowledge on artistic anatomy from Professor Nishida Masaaki (西田正秋, 1894–1961) [30, 31].

His drawings and notes comprised two textbook-format books that spanned over 48 pages. Seventy-four drawings and their explanations were produced. The table of contents was ordered starting from body proportions, followed by the skeleton, the muscles, and the head. There were four drawings of the trunk, 51 of the head, seven of the arms, nine of the legs, and three of the full body. The drawings of the head and face were detailed. The essential forms, proportions, and movement were included [32].

Later, he produced some of his masterpieces amid political turmoil arising from tension between the left wings and the right wings of society after independence. He described the hope and confusion that existed across Korean society after independence in his painting "Group of People 1" (群像), in which many masculine male nudes are expressed.

9.5.4 Origin of Artistic Anatomy in Japan and Korea

In 1887, artistic anatomy lessons (2 h per week) were launched at Teikoku Art School in Japan.

From 1891 to 1895, Mori Ogai (森林太郎, 1862–1922) taught artistic anatomy. He received

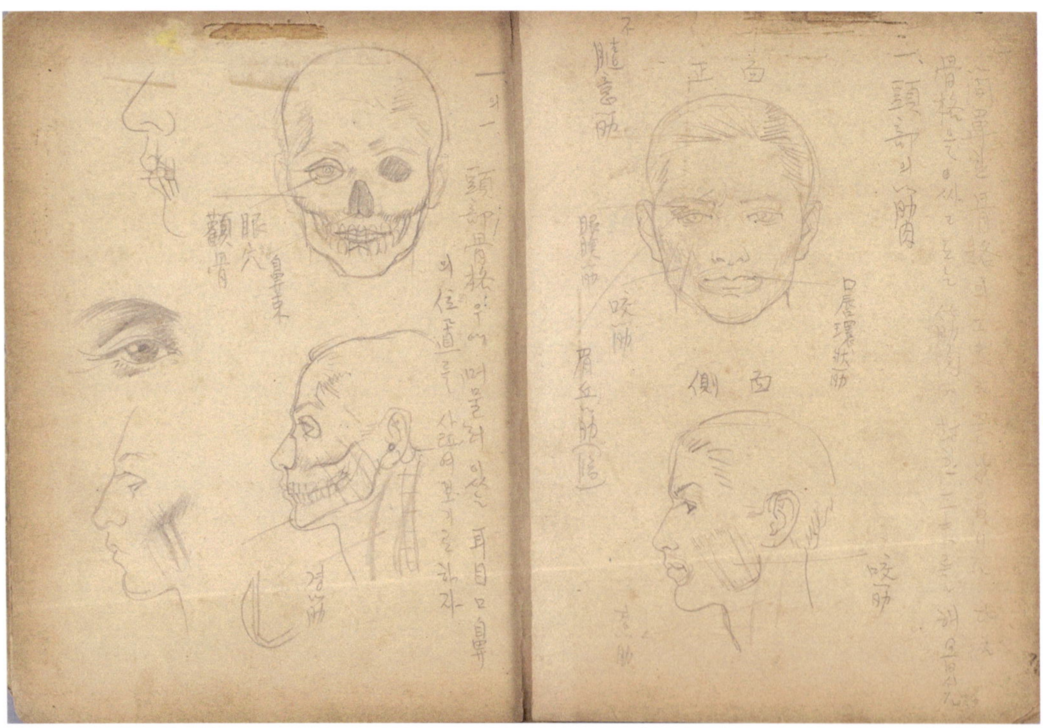

Fig. 9.9 Lee Quede's drawing notes. Available at: https://www.chosun.com/national/weekend/2022/02/19/K4JBOKM3ZNBDPBUM35OF4DN63M/. Assessed March 22, 2022

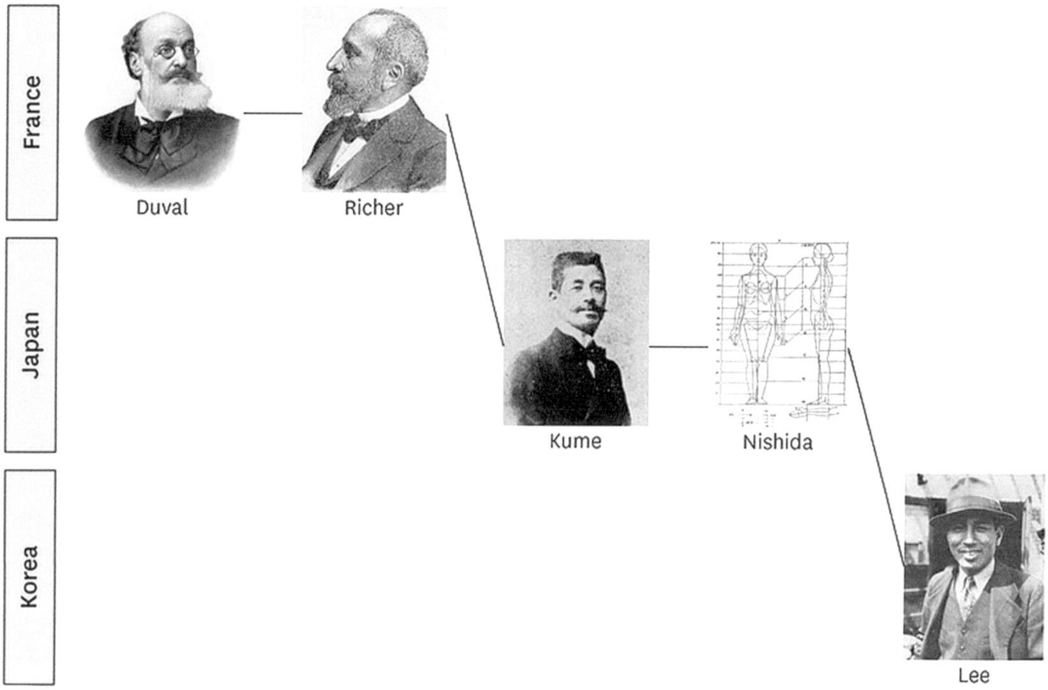

Fig. 9.10 Pedigree of artistic anatomy from nineteenth century French art school to Korean artist Lee Quede through Japanese Kume and Nishida

specialized training in hygiene in Germany and referenced Kollmann's anatomy textbook (*Plastische Anatomies des menschlichen Körpers,* 1866) [33].

Starting in 1896, Kume Geichiro (久米桂一郎, 1866–1934) took over these lectures. When he was a student at the École Supérieur des Beaux Arts in France, Kume was a pupil of Mathias Duval (1844–1907). After Duval's retirement, Paul Richer (1849–1933) served as an instructor at that school. In Japan, Kume taught using the books written by Duval and Richer [34–36].

On retirement, Kume handed over his lectures to Nishida Masaaki, his beloved pupil. Nishida's knowledge was based on French artistic anatomy of the nineteenth century, succeeded by Kume [37].

The Korean artist Lee Quede learned artistic anatomy from Nishida during his stay at Teikoku Art School. Therefore, Lee Quede's anatomical knowledge was based on the French artistic anatomy of the nineteenth century, succeeded by Kume and Nishida (Fig. 9.10).

Until now, learning human anatomy is needed in human figure paintings education in art schools in Korea [38].

9.5.5 Conclusion

Lee Quede's anatomical knowledge was based on the French artistic anatomy of the nineteenth century, succeeded by Kume and Nishida. Lee Quede's drawing notes are valuable documents for assessing the influence of Japanese artistic anatomy on Korean artistic anatomy. The human anatomy adds reality to portraits as a branch of contemporary art; therefore, it can work as a contemporary logic to express spirituality.

9.6 Textbooks in Plastic Surgery: Paper or Digital?

> A computer does not smell … if a book is new, it smells great. If a book is old, it smells even better… And it stays with you forever. But the computer doesn't do that for you. I'm sorry. —*Ray Bradbury*

Being a faculty member at a training hospital, I usually purchase new textbooks when they come out. The trainees have to buy the newest version to prepare for their board certification. CD versions are available, but nonetheless, I purchase the printed books. They come in six volumes, which are bulky, so that I either need to put them on a new shelf or get rid of the old versions. In fact, my shelves are crowded with textbooks.

Recently, I found the fourth edition of *Plastic Surgery* in the residents' lounge and realized that time flies. Five years have passed since I bought the previous third edition. When I was a trainee, we studied with teo books: Grabb and Smith and Converse. In my last year of training, McCarthy appeared. Remembering my young days, I created a list of plastic surgery textbooks for young plastic surgeons who need to know their roots.

About 100 years ago, two landmark books appeared. *Plastic Surgery: Its Principles and Practice* (1919) by John Staige Davis contained comprehensive information on reconstructive plastic surgery from head to toe with over 2000 references. This book has been cited 132 times. One year later (in 1920), Harold Gillies published *Plastic Surgery of the Face*, which focused on the face and has been cited 88 times as of 2017.

Thirty years later, Varaztad Kazanjian and John Converse published *Surgical Treatment of Facial Injuries* (1949), and the second edition was published in 1959. In 1974, Converse revised the book and renamed it *Kazanjian and Converse's Surgical Treatment of Facial Injuries*, and this book has been cited 635 times. These editions were focused on facial injuries.

For a comprehensive review, Grabb's *Plastic Surgery* first appeared in 1968. New editions appeared in 1973 (2nd), 1979 (3rd), 1991 (4th), 1997 (5th), 2007 (6th), and 2014 (7th). The third edition has been cited 364 times and the seventh edition 239 times.

In 1977, Converse published *Reconstructive Plastic Surgery*, and this book has been cited the most often (744 times) of all plastic surgery textbooks. After his death, Joseph McCarthy, one of his pupils, revised it, giving it a new title (*Plastic Surgery*; 1990, Saunders), and this book has been cited 369 times.

Sixteen years later, Saunders published another version of *Plastic Surgery* (2006), edited by Stephan Mathes, and this book has been cited 275 times. Six years after Mathes's edition, the third edition of *Plastic Surgery* edited by Neligan appeared and has been cited 62 times. Finally, the fourth edition by Neligan came out in 2017 (Fig. 9.11).

Citations of the textbook are far less than I expected (least 6, most 744 hits). The reason for this low citation is thought to be the transformation of the art to digital world.

We training staffs should not urge our resident just to memorize the old achieved books. For what is new and getting for a solution, we ought to touch the searching engines. However, these textbooks are historical encounter I want my residents to read.

Recently, in one of my editorials ("Rob Peter to pay Paul"), I cited the "Barter principle" in McCarthy's textbook. My most regretful memory is giving Converse's 1977 textbook to a friend when I received my board certification. I still miss the books I marked with pen and highlighted many times. Fortunately, I downloaded two books for free: Davis's textbook (1919) and Gillies's textbook (1920). Although I cannot the smell the old paper, I can read the preface, between the lines and the text, and it seems as if the old authors are still living and are teaching me, as a young surgeon.

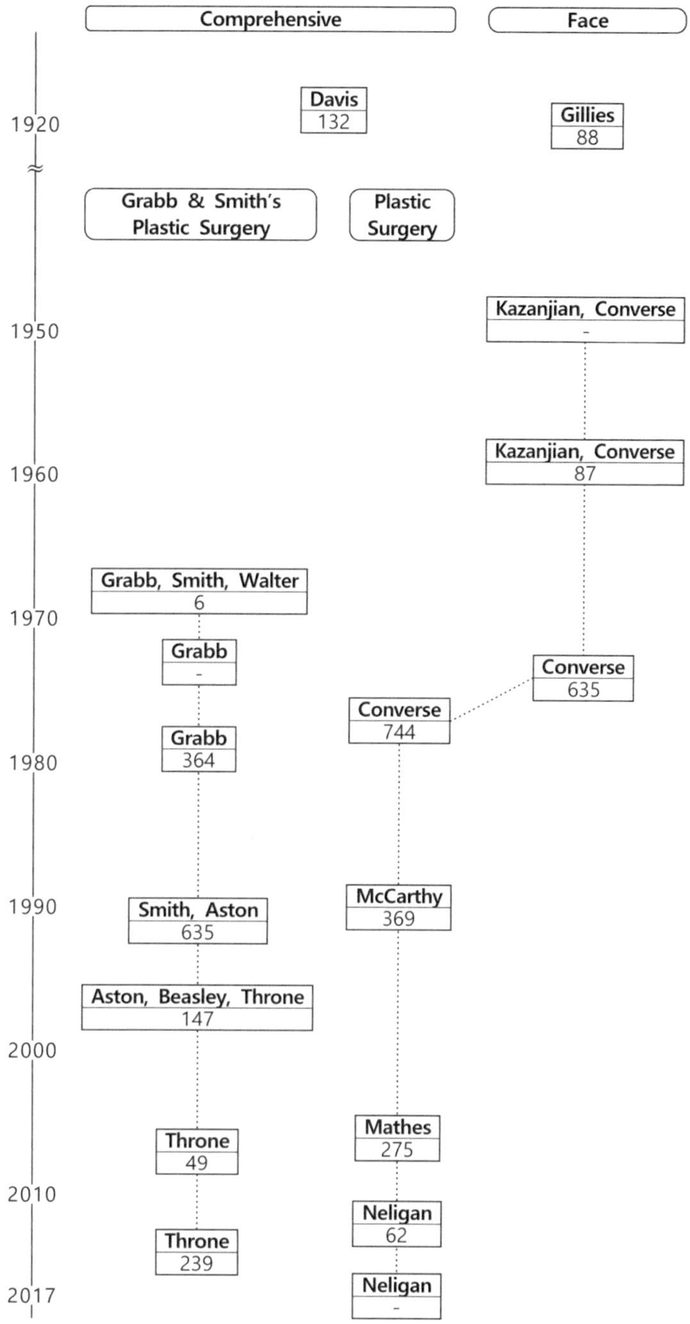

Fig. 9.11 Genealogy of textbooks in plastic surgery

9.7 My Lawful Wife and my Mistress

How would you feel if you received the following letter from a fellow surgeon confessing infidelity? "I feel more confident and more satisfied with myself when I reflect that I have two women and not one; my lawful wife and my mistress. When I get tired of one, I spend the night with the other. Though it is irregular, it is less boring this way, and besides, neither of them loses anything through my infidelity."

I would be very envious of him, but I would suggest that he either focus on his "lawful wife" or divorce her and unite with his "mistress."

By adding "medicine is my lawful wife" and "literature is my mistress," the letter can be completed. This letter was sent from Anton Chekhov (1860 to 1904) (Fig. 9.12, *left*) to his friend Alexei Suvorin. Unlike other successful writers with a background of medical training, Chekhov practiced as a medical doctor throughout most of his literary career.

Many doctors enjoy music or literature as hobbies; very few doctors (1.4–2%) leave medicine [39]. Participation in music appears to be higher among doctors than other professions, and some doctors hold regular concerts. Writing is also a popular pursuit among doctors who prefer activities outside medicine. However, it is rare that medical doctors have two professions, like Chekhov had. To have literature as a "mistress," one must at least write something and publish it.

Who can bear comparison with Chekhov among plastic surgeons?

In my training period in 1989, I was sent to Asan Medical Center, Seoul, South Korea, for a month under the direction of Dr. Robert S. Chung. We had daily meetings, and we read and discussed the editorials in plastic surgery journals. The first editorial we read was titled "Overobliging and Underappreciated" [40]. Dr. Chung interpreted the meaning between the lines written by Dr. Robert Goldwyn (1930 to 2010) (Fig. 9.12, *right*). After completing my training, I came across the book *The Operative Note [41]*. I expected it to contain detailed descriptions of operations, helping to make operative records. However, the book was a collection of Dr. Goldwyn's editorials.

As a professor of plastic surgery, Dr. Goldwyn operated on patients from 1961 to 1996. As a writer, he authored or coauthored more than 350 articles, including impressive editorials and more than 50 chapters. He surely deserves recognition as a "plastic surgeon–writer" who had a "lawful wife and mistress" in the sense of Chekhov.

I saw him only once in Yokohama. At the 1995 Congress of the International Confederation for Plastic, Reconstructive, and Aesthetic Surgery, he gave an eye-opening lecture ("The young plastic surgeon: Threat or necessity or both?"). I, a young surgeon, was in the audience but did not have a chance to talk with him. After that conference, I started to write papers; some of them were accepted, others rejected.

It has been more than a decade since Dr. Goldwyn passed away. Several years ago, I started writing editorials and submitting them to journals.

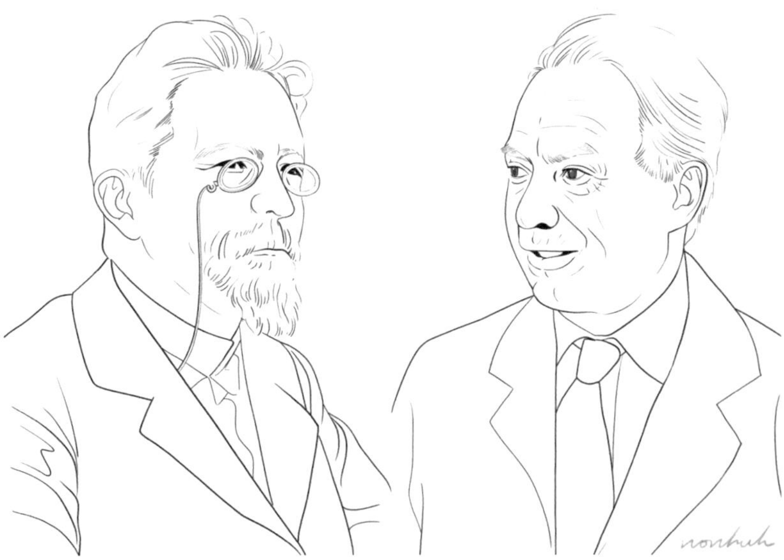

Fig. 9.12 Anton Chekhov (left) and Robert Goldwyn (right). Drawing by Hye Won Hu, M.F.A

I hope that my editorials will be as enjoyable and interesting to read as Dr. Goldwyn's were.

9.8 Harold Ellis: A Surgeon's Contribution to Anatomy Education

It is safe to say that the majority of Korean anatomists possess either "Gray's Anatomy" [42] or "Clinical Anatomy: Applied Anatomy for Students and Junior Doctors" [43]. However, it is likely that their knowledge of Professor Ellis, who has been the author of "Clinical Anatomy" since 1960 and the leading editor of the 39th edition of Gray's Anatomy [42], is scanty. This paper is not aimed to be a bibliography of Professor Ellis; it is an introduction to this man and his work and discusses how he contributed to the field of anatomy education.

In 1986, while I worked as an intern in a hospital, my teacher Professor Key June Seoung, an anatomist at Seoul National University, Korea, gave me a book titled "Clinical anatomy: a revision and applied anatomy for clinical students," the First P. G. Asian Economy edition [44]. During my internship and plastic surgery residency training, I referred to that book frequently, because it was very easy to find information in it and it contained simple drawings that were easy to understand. For example, one figure in that book shows a clear illustration of how the sixth cervical vertebra corresponds to the lower border of the cricoid cartilage, how the junction of the larynx relates to the trachea, how the junction of pharynx relates to the esophagus, and the level at which the inferior thyroid artery and the middle thyroid vein enter the thyroid gland. After 22 years of owning that book, I gave the book to my first son who just entered medical school in the United Kingdom, and subsequently the book became one of his favorite books.

Professor Ellis qualified as a doctor at the University of Oxford in 1948. From 1950 to 1951, he undertook national service as a Captain in the Royal Army Medical Corps; afterwards he continued his training as a surgical registrar in London, Sheffield and Oxford before taking up a post as a senior lecturer in the University of London. In 1960, he was the foundation chair of surgery at Westminster Hospital, a post which he held until his retirement from practice in 1989. He was also a professor in the Department of Anatomy and Human Sciences at King's College London School of Medicine. After a stint teaching anatomy at the University of Cambridge, he took up his present position as a professor in the Department of Anatomy and Human Sciences at King's College London School of Medicine in 1993.

The first edition of "Clinical Anatomy" was written in 1960 when he had just become the foundation chair of surgery at Westminster Hospital. In 2010, the tenth edition was published as a 50th anniversary edition [43].

In December 2010, I was writing a paper about a British anatomist, and I visited the Anatomical Society in Guy's cam pus to find some of his relics, such as the books or the instruments he had used, but met without success. In the Hodgkin's building I met the author of "Clinical Anatomy," Professor Harold Ellis. He was 84 years old at the time. Wearing a green lab jacket, he was teaching medical students in the dissecting room.

In December 2011, I met him again at the winter meeting of the Anatomical Society, which was held at Cardiff University. His lecture entitled "Learning, using and teaching anatomy" was a history of the teaching of anatomy in the United Kingdom. His words were like a breath of fresh air and they were a real inspiration. After his lectures, the whole audience gave this living legend in the field of clinical anatomy a huge round of applause.

Professor Ellis should be remembered as a pioneering clinical anatomist as well as a proficient surgeon. He left a very fine user-friendly book titled "Clinical Anatomy." I believe more new editions of this book are forthcoming. There is an oriental saying which states that "Tigers leave fine hides when they die, and people leave their names on their departure." Professor Ellis will leave his good name—a name that will be remembered for generations to come.

9.9 On Entering a New Decade: Foolish Old Surgeons Removing the Mountains

The Korean Cleft Palate-Craniofacial Association (KCPCA), with its 28-year history, has developed into a well-regarded professional society with 1228 members. In 2021, we are starting a new decade and we hope to make a new leap forward.

I am grateful to the members of the KCPCA for electing me as the 16th president of our association. It will be my last opportunity to serve the KCPCA since I have only 2 years before my retirement.

In my role as president, I would like to enhance knowledge sharing among our members by providing more opportunities for academic communication. I also hope to raise our association's status to a higher level in the global academic community. To achieve this goal, we will need active participation from all of our members.

Of particular note, our official journal, *Archives of Craniofacial Surgery (ACFS)*, which was registered in PubMed Central (PMC) since 2014, was indexed in Scopus in 2019. As the president of the KCPCA and the ethics editor of *ACFS*, I will help the chief editor of *ACFS* for indexing *ACFS* in more databases. To echo the words of President John F. Kennedy, please do not ask what KCPCA can do for you but ask what we can do for our KCPCA together. I eagerly hope that our members will submit valuable manuscripts to *ACFS*.

I know that being registered in MEDLINE or SCIE (Science Citation Index Expanded) may seem like a distant goal. However, it is not so far off that it cannot be reached eventually. A well-known fable that emphasizes the virtues of perseverance and willpower comes to mind.

A 90-year-old foolish man (愚公) lived near a pair of mountains. He was annoyed by the obstruction caused by the two mountains and sought to dig through them with hoes and baskets. When questioned by his clever neighbor as to the seemingly impossible nature of his task, this foolish man replied that while he may not finish the task in his lifetime, through the hard work of himself, his children, and their children, and so on through many generations, someday the mountains would be removed if he persevered (Fig. 9.13). The gods in Heaven, impressed with his hard work and perseverance, ordered the mountains to be separated ("Foolish old man removes the mountains," 愚公穆山).

Perhaps the goals of achieving a higher level in the global academic community or attaining a glorious future will not be reached while I am the president of the KCPCA, or even before my retirement. However, I do believe that if we foolish old surgeons start building a stone bridge, one by one, to cross the stream, and if our junior surgeons continue the task, it will be completed someday in the future.

Indeed, "foolish old surgeons remove the mountains (愚公穆山)."

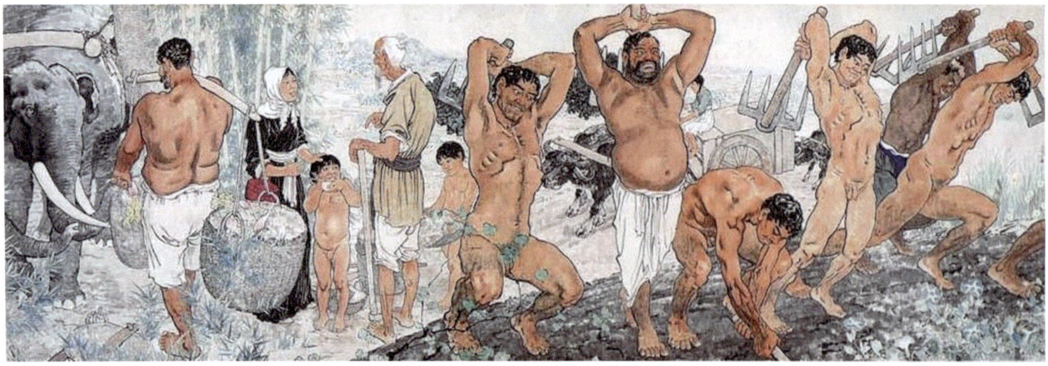

Fig. 9.13 A foolish old man removes the mountains (愚公移山) drawn by Xu Beihong (餘悲鸿) (1895-1953). Source: Wikimedia Commons

9.10 Learning from the Masters: The Pilgrimage of a Plastic Surgeon

During residency training, trainees learn basic principles and skills from their program director and supervisors. However, not every institution can afford a sufficient education in every field of plastic surgery because each institution has its pros and cons. Therefore, we learn from textbooks, journal articles, and books. Although we are familiar with famous books themselves, knowledge about the philosophy or motto of the author might be rather superficial.

Recently, I attended a valuable lecture entitled "Learning from the Masters" at the Twentieth Anniversary Symposium of the Department of Plastic Surgery at Ajou University, Suwon, Republic of Korea. The speaker, Henry Kawamoto, introduced us to the mottos and principles of the masters of plastic surgery that he had met and learned from.

At the end of his lecture, I recalled a Buddhist scripture I read several years ago, *Flower Ornament Scripture* (*Avatamsaka Sutra,* 華嚴經) [45]. It describes a cosmos of infinite realms upon realms, mutually containing one another. It consists of 10 stages, and the last chapter of it is known as the "Gandavyūha Sutra" (入法界品, "Entering the Dharma Realm"). This section details the pilgrimage of the youth Sudhana to various lands at the behest of the bodhisattva Mañjuśrī (文殊菩薩). In his quest for enlightenment, Sudhana would converse with a diverse array of 52 wise advisors. The final master that Sudhana visits is bodhisattva Samantabhadra (普賢菩薩), who teaches him that wisdom only exists for the sake of putting it into practice; that it is only good insofar as it benefits all living beings [46].

As Sudhana's pilgrimage for enlightenment started from bodhisattva Mañjuśrī, Kawamoto's lecture began with Varaztad Kazanjian (1879 to 1974), who pioneered techniques for plastic surgery and is considered to be the founder of the modern practice of plastic surgery [47]. At the beginning of his book *Surgical Treatment of Facial Fractures*, Kazanjian's pupil John Converse wrote that it is "imaginative and resourceful, he taught to improve new methods rather than follow the conventional. 'Do it just right' he would say, meaning in his laconic way that each patient's problem required an individual solution." He never denigrated a colleague's work [48].

Kawamoto's boss was John Converse (1909 to 1981). He was a man of curiosity and energy, was full of ideas, and had a great sense of humor. He kept an open mind and never swore. He preferred autogenous materials in reconstruction. He appreciated history and photographic documentation and team competition.

After completion of his plastic surgery residency, he met many great plastic surgeons and learned a lot from them: Gillies, Harrison, Robinson, Mulkey, Obwegeser, Ortiz-Monasterio, del Capmo, and Ricketts. Ralph Millard (1919 to 2011) said to him, "If you don't know how to assist, you will never be a good surgeon." In the operating room, he himself set the position of assistant and the direction of light. To reduce glare, he preferred black instruments. He emphasized purposeful economic movement and precision.

The final master that Kawamoto visited was Paul Tessier (1917 to 2008). He never examined a radiograph before seeing a patient. Kawamoto had a special relationship with his best mentor, Tessier, who passed away on June 6, 2008, and Kawamoto participated in Tessier's funeral in Héric, France. At the end of the lecture, I asked Kawamoto who he thought was the greatest contributor. The answer was of course Tessier.

As Sudhana was enlightened when Samantabhadra concludes with a prayer of aspiration to Buddhahood, I am sure that Kawamoto became a real master when he lowered the rope holding Tessier's coffin at his funeral.

Finally, I have to say something about the invaluable lesson at the International Confederation of Plastic, Reconstructive, and Aesthetic Surgery meeting that was held in Yokohama, Japan, in 1995. At the opening ceremony, Joseph Murray (1919 to 2012), who wrote the preface of Deranian's book about Kazanjian, had the keynote lecture [49]. The elder retired plastic surgeon emphasized that scientists should remember three important words: curiosity, imagination, and persistence [50]. After listening to his lecture, those three tips have been the source of much research.

9.11 Let's Salute Our Deceased Predecessors: Academic Obituaries in the Journal of Craniofacial Surgery

> Let me not then die ingloriously and without a struggle, but let me first do some great thing that shall be told among men hereafter.—*Hector's last word in Iliad*

Recently I enjoyed a movie, "The Last Word" (2017; director: Mark Pellington) (Fig. 9.14a).

Harriet, played by Shirley MacLaine, is a successful businesswoman with the goal of completely controlling her surroundings in retirement. She even pays the local newspaper to write her obituary in advance, under her supervision, to make sure that the story of her life is told in the way that she wants. Harriet says to Anne (Amanda Seyfried), the young journalist assigned to the task, that there are "four essential elements to a really great obituary": for the deceased to be loved by his or her family, for the deceased to be admired by coworkers, for the deceased to change someone's life unexpectedly, and the "wild card." However, Anne does not agree to follow Harriet's script and instead insists on discovering the truth about Harriet's life, and their relationship develops into a life-altering friendship.

Because two of my teachers who trained me passed away recently (Yoon-Ho Lee in 2019, Chull-Gyoo Park in 2020), I searched for the definition of "obituary" and how many obituaries

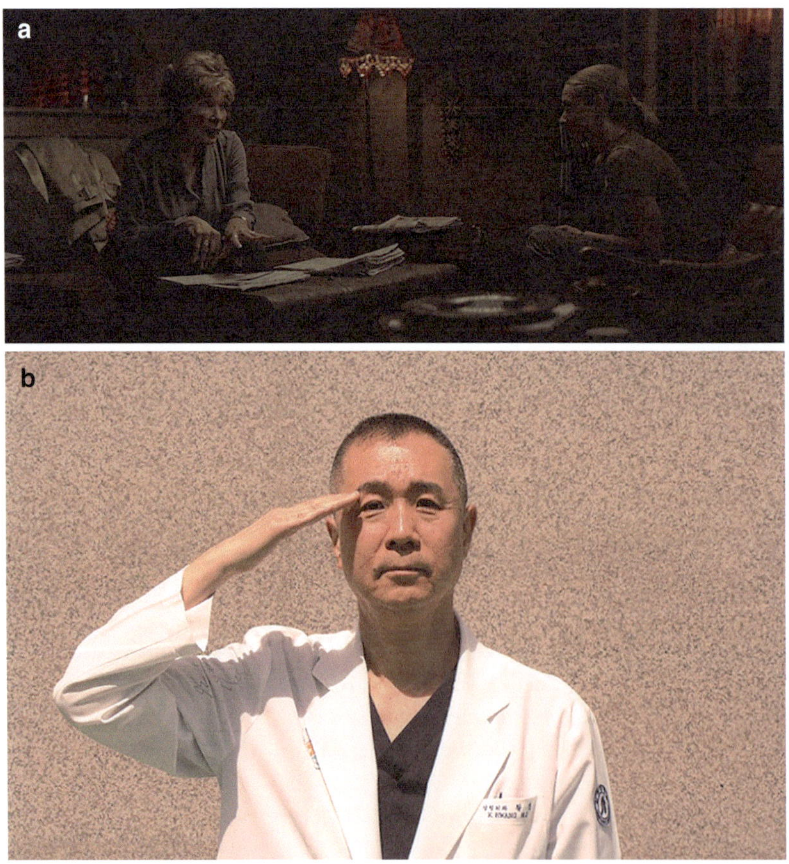

Fig. 9.14 (**a**) Shirley MacLaine explains "four essential elements to a really great obituary" to Amanda Seyfried. From https://youtu.be/kx-B4SYbglE. (**b**) Salute to predecessors

have been published in the *Journal of Craniofacial Surgery* (JCFS).

An obituary is defined as a report, especially in a newspaper, that gives the news of someone's death and details about their life. Since 1990, when the journal started publication, only 10 obituaries (in memory of, in memoriam) have been published as special editorials rather than obituaries.

The first volume of JCFS appeared in 1990. As time goes by, the pioneers of the JCFS are getting very old; some of them have even passed away.

As an editorial board of the JCFS, I have been thinking how to express our respect to our predecessors, especially the pioneers of craniofacial surgery. One of the ways to show respect would be academic obituaries saluting our deceased predecessors. However, I think that academic obituaries should be different from those published in newspapers or for funerals.

Biographical narratives connect a series of positions by the notion of a "subject," thereby making sequences understandable [51]. Once evoked, the academic subject is endowed with personal agency and internal motives through descriptors such as "talent" or "diligence," whereas external determinants, such as class, sex, and biographical hurdles, receive little attention or are ignored altogether. Through this process, obituaries act as a narrative vehicle through which information is transmitted about the researchers regarded as important or noteworthy across generations of scholars. Specific portrayals of events in a deceased researcher's life are thereby transferred into the collective memory, whereas negative aspects, such as biographical constraints and hurdles, are subjected to collective forgetting. The memorial function of academic obituaries relies on the existence of colleagues, pupils, or even a school or community with a stake in perpetuating the reputation of the decedent [52].

The author of an obituary must act as a spokesperson for a community that, in turn, serves as a supervisory authority with responsibility for the evaluation. If an obituary makes a judgment that appears unjust, the author is held to account, and her or his reputation may suffer [53].

In summary, obituaries should not merely be a space for parading details about brilliant personal careers. Instead, an obituary should contain true facts about the surgeon's life. The writer should find out the "wild card" that is meaningful and should convey who the decedent was.

There is an Asian saying that "tigers die and leave their skins; people die and leave their names." We should salute to our predecessors' and preserve their spirits (Fig. 9.14b).

References

1. Oxford dictionaries. Oxford Dictionaries English. Oxford: Oxford University Press; 2013. http://oxforddictionaries.com/definition/english/Colles-fracture
2. Colles A. On the fracture of the carpal extremity of the radius. Edinb Med Surg J. 1814;10:181.
3. Wikipedia. Abraham Colles. Wikipedia; 2013. http://en.wikipedia.org/wiki/Abraham_Colles#cite_note-boy-3.
4. McIndoe AH. Surgical responsibility in relation to injury. J R Inst Public Health. 1946;9:335–42.
5. Banister JB, McIndoe AH. Congenital absence of the vagina, treated by means of an indwelling skin-graft. Proc R Soc Med. 1938;31:1055–6.
6. Backstein R, Hinek A. War and medicine: the origins of plastic surgery. Univ Tor Med J. 2005;82:217–9.
7. Wikipedia. Harold Gillies. 2017. https://en.wikipedia.org/wiki/Harold_Gillies.
8. Chambers JA, Ray PD. Achieving growth and excellence in medicine: the case history of armed conflict and modern reconstructive surgery. Ann Plast Surg. 2009;63:473–8.
9. Wikipedia. Archibald McIndoe. 2017. https://en.wikipedia.org/wiki/Archibald_McIndoe.
10. Gillies HD, McIndoe AH. The role of plastic surgery in burns due to roentgen rays and radium. Ann Surg. 1935;101:979–96.
11. Gillies H, McIndoe AH. The late surgical complications of fracture of the mandible. Br Med J. 1933;2:1060–3.
12. Gillies HD, Fry WK. A new principle in the surgical treatment of "congenital cleft palate" and its mechanical counterpart. Br Med J. 1921;1:335–8.
13. Gillies HD. The design of direct pedicle flaps. Br Med J. 1932;2:1008.
14. McIndoe AH. Total reconstruction of the burned face. The Bradshaw lecture 1958. Br J Plast Surg. 1983;36:410–20.
15. McIndoe AH, Forbes R, Windeyer BW. Symposium: radiation necrosis. Br J Radiol. 1947;20:269–78.
16. McIndoe AH. Operation for the cure of adult hypospadias. Br Med J. 1937;1:385–404.
17. McIndoe AH. Surgical and dental treatment of fractures of the upper and lower jaws in war time a review

of 119 cases: (section of odontology). Proc R Soc Med. 1941;34:267–88.
18. McIndoe AH. The burned hand. Mod Treat Yearb. 1945:221–31.
19. Millard DR Jr. Cleft craft: the evolution of its surgery, vol. 3. Boston, MA: Little Brown; 1976.
20. Calnan JS, Grabb WC, Rosenstein SW, Bzoch KR. Chap 29: V-Y pushback palatoplasty. In: Cleft lip and palate surgical, dental, and speech aspect by 71 authors. Boston, MA: Little Brown; 1971. p. 422–31.
21. Veau V. Division Palatine. Paris, France: Masson; 1931.
22. Kilner TP. Cleft lip and palate repair technique. St Thomas Hosp Rep. 1937;2:127–40.
23. Wardill WEM. The technique of operation for cleft palate. Br J Surg. 1937;25:117–30.
24. Hajar R. What has art to do with medicine? Heart Views. 2018;19(1):34–5.
25. Kim DH, Park H, Rhyu IJ. Gustav Klimt's the kiss-art and the biology of early human development. JAMA. 2021;326(18):1778–80.
26. Sellmer R. In: Whitelaw WA, editor. Anatomy and art in renaissance; Proceedings of the 10th Annual History of Medicine Days. Calgary, Canada: University of Calgary; 2001. p. 80–2.
27. Hwang K. Artists with anatomical knowledge after Anathomia (1316) and before Fabrica (1543). J Craniofac Surg. 2021;32(1):350–4.
28. Hwang K, Skinned S. Bartholomew before (1541) and after (1556, 1562) Fabrica (1543). Anat Rec (Hoboken). 2022;305(1):5–7.
29. Wittkower R, Wittkower M. Born under Saturn: the character and conduct of artists: a documented history from antiquity to the French revolution. New York, NY, USA: WW Norton; 1963.
30. Kwon H. Modern male's body and the artistic anatomy: the anatomical drawing note of lee Quede. J Kor Modern Contemporary Art History. 2020;40:169–206.
31. Nishida M. Review of artistic anatomy. Tokyo, Japan: Seikishobou (聖紀書房); 1944.
32. Youn KH. The significance and limits of lee Quede's anatomical drawings. Korean J Phys Anthropol. 2018;31(3):71–6.
33. Shimada K, Michiyo M. Foreign artistic anatomical textbooks at the beginning of artistic anatomy education in early modern Japan. J Art Anat. 2007;11(1):76–84.
34. Ito S. Kume Keiichiro and artistic anatomy: the review of the special exhibition "bi no Naikei". J Art Anat. 2012;16(1):91–7.
35. Richer P. Artistic anatomy: description of the external forms of the human body at rest and in the main movements: with 110 plates containing more than 300 drawn figures (Anatomie artistique: description des formes extérieures du corps humain au repos et dans les principaux mouvements: avec 110 planches renfermant plus de 300 figures dessinées) Paris, France: Plon Nourrit et Cie; 1890.
36. Richer P. Artistic anatomy. Pitman, New York, London: Watson-Guptill Publications; 1986.
37. Kato K, Sakai T. History of Western artistic anatomy in the 19th century: prehistory of artistic anatomy in Japan. J Japanese Soc Hist Med. 2017;63(1):23–42.
38. Kim KH. A study on the necessity of human anatomy in human figure paintings education in Korean art departments of Korean art universities: with a focus on portraits and human anatomy. Art Education Research Review. 2013;27(2):139–70.
39. Koh C. A is for aphorism: "Medicine is my lawful wife, and literature is my mistress. When I get [fed up with] one, I spend the night with the other". Aust Fam Physician. 2013;42:663–4.
40. Goldwyn RM. Overobliging and underappreciated. Plast Reconstr Surg. 1989;83:326–7.
41. Goldwyn RM. The operative note: collected editorials. New York: Thieme; 1992.
42. Standring S. Gray's anatomy: the anatomical basis of clinical practice. 39th ed. Edinburgh: Churchill Livingstone; 2005.
43. Ellis H, Mahadevan V. Clinical anatomy: applied anatomy for students and junior doctors. 10th ed. London: Wiley-Blackwell; 2010.
44. Ellis H, First P.G. Asian Economy. Clinical anatomy: a revision and applied anatomy for clinical student. 7th ed. Singapore: P. G. Publishing; 1983.
45. Cleary TF. Entry into the realm of reality. In: The flower ornament scripture. Boulder Shambhala; 1987. p. 369–404.
46. Hua H. Entering the Dharma realm. In: Flower Adornment Sutra. Ukiah, California: Dharma Realm Buddhist Association; 1980. p. 1–245.
47. Wolfe A. A man from Héric: the life and work of Paul Tessier, MD, father of craniofacial surgery: Volume I and II. Raleigh: NC Lulu Enterprises; 2012.
48. Converse JM. Kazanjian & Converse's surgical treatment of facial fracture. 3rd ed. Baltimore Williams & Wilkins; 1974.
49. Deranian HM. Miracle Man of the Western Front: Dr. Varaztad H. Kazanjian: Pioneer plastic surgeon. Worcester: Mass Chandler House Press; 2007.
50. Hwang K. How to write a scientific paper: three tips to remember. Arch Plast Surg. 2012;39:77.
51. Foucault M, Foucault M. What is an author? In: Language, counter-memory, practice: selected essays and interviews. New York, NY: Cornell University Press; 1977. p. 113–38.
52. Fowler B. Collective memory and forgetting: components for a study of obituaries. Theory Culture & Society. 2005;22:53–72.
53. Hamann J. Let us salute one of our kind. How academic obituaries consecrate research biographies. Poetics. 2016;56:1–4.

10 Plastic Surgeon as a Spiritual Healer

10.1 Hallucinations in Children with Plague: A Point of View from 400 Years Ago

Fever is one of the symptoms of coronavirus disease 2019 (COVID-19), which is prevalent both in Korea and in other countries throughout the world. Fever is defined as an oral temperature of 37.8 °C or higher or a rectal temperature of 38.2 °C or higher. There are many causes of fever, including infections such as bacteria and viruses. When the body heat rises, blood vessels dilate to lower the core body temperature, increasing sweat secretion.

In children, a high fever can cause febrile convulsions. Due to a high fever, one becomes mentally confused and unable to understand the surrounding environment, with very unstable emotions, causing conscious and cognitive disturbances such as illusions or hallucinations—that is, delirium.

How did Koreans interpret these symptoms before it was discovered that pathogens are the cause of infectious diseases that result in high fever? In the late Joseon Dynasty, many infectious diseases, such as smallpox, measles, and cholera, occurred. These "plagues" would spread suddenly and frighten the populace, but they would disappear after a while. The people's awareness and perceptions of plagues can be seen vividly in the tales of that time.

This paper introduces an example of "child fever" from the examples of plagues described in the book *Eoyuyadam,* published in 1622 by Mongin Yu (1559–1623) [1]. Relevant materials were found and verified by searching the Research Information Service System provided by the Korea Education and Research Information Service [2].

In section 159 of *Eoyuyadam*, related to religion, the following is recorded:

In this era, if a child was afflicted with a plague and had hallucinations, people believed that the child became numinous. Since their parents only responded through prayer, due to ignorance regarding effective treatments for the disease, most children affected by this condition died (Fig. 10.1). It is truly a pity for clever children to die and disappear from a single illness. People say, "People afflicted with this disease sometimes show magical powers and in other cases engage in strange behaviors. What can they be other than ghosts?"

My thoughts are as follows: Plague causes fever, and heat is fire. The nature of fire is bright, and fire controls the heart. Since the heart is inherently futile, when it has a fever, it becomes as powerful as a ghost and as bright as fire, hearing without hearing and seeing without seeing. That is why an afflicted child is able to respond to external events even in a dark, quiet room and sometimes can surprise and deceive people by

K. Hwang, *Good Physician, Good Plastic Surgeon*, https://doi.org/10.1007/978-981-97-1864-1_10

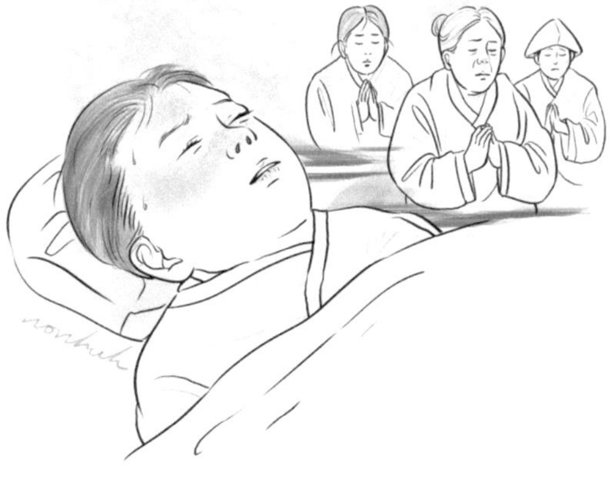

Fig. 10.1 A child with halluciations. If a child was afflicted with a plague and had hallucinations, people believed that the child became numinous. Parents responded through prayer. Illustration by Hye Won Hu, MA

revealing things they had no way of knowing about in casual talk like sleep talk.

In my opinion, both plague and measles are febrile diseases. This is because heat and fire are so bright that they can see even things that have no form. When women see such things, they put their hands together and pray to God, which is ridiculous.

People said that children affected by plagues were unusually smart and could understand things they had not seen and heard, but Mongin Yu said that even if something like this happens, it is not because the child is smart but because of the fever, which makes that mind temporarily weak. He criticized others' viewpoints based on the theory of the five elements as the principle of yin and yang.

In fact, children with high fever and delirium can progress to encephalitis or encephalopathy, especially in cases of influenza infection. Delirium due to hyperthermia requires differentiation from benign parasomnia, which is characterized by fearful expressions, a positive past history, and autonomic nerve symptoms. Instead, in delirium, visual hallucinations occur in association with sleep. Meningeal signs and disturbed consciousness also appear. Marked slowing of the background activity of electroencephalography is a warning sign of delirium [3, 4].

When a fever above 38.5 °C persists in children, it is best to first take off all clothes and continue to wipe their head, chest, stomach, armpits, and groin, which generate abundant heat, with tepid water at about 30 °C so that the heat can gradually go down. When the body temperature rises, the basal metabolic rate increases, the heart rate increases, and water loss occurs. When the body temperature rises by 1 °C, the basal metabolic rate increases by 10–12%, the oxygen consumption rate by 13%, the heart rate by 15 beats per minute, and daily insensible water loss increases by 300–500 mL per square meter of body surface area. Therefore, it is important to drink plenty of water.

Mongin Yu was critical of the belief that children become spiritual when they are afflicted by a plague. He argued that although people said that children afflicted by a plague were unusually intelligent and could understand things they had not seen and heard, any such cases did not occur as a result of the child becoming intelligent. Instead, he said that this could be a temporary phenomenon. Although he understood the mechanism of fever differently from how it is understood in modern medicine, he recognized that fever causes "mental confusion" and hallucinations. He pointed out that the beliefs about plagues in that era were wrong and emphasized the necessity of treating sick children.

In Korea, scientific prevention and treatment measures are being implemented in response to COVID-19. However, some people vocalize unscientific and religious opinions and recommend traditional prescriptions. It is worth remembering that a Joseon dynasty scholar, although he worked within a framework based on yin and yang, argued for a relatively empirical and scientific approach to prevention and treatment 400 years ago.

10.2 A Safe Distance Between Doctor and Patient

If the distance is great, then the degree of love is great; if the distance is small, the degree of love is small. From "Measurement of Love" by *Han, Yong-un (1879–1944)*

When I visited Edinburgh last year, I enjoyed exploring the Surgeons' Hall Museums. Among the many famous surgeons from that city, a surgeon with a special costume caught my eye. The costume comprised an ankle-length overcoat and a birdlike beak mask, and the surgeon was also wearing gloves, boots, a wide-brimmed hat, and an outer garment.

When the worst outbreak of the plague was ravaging Edinburgh in 1645, Dr. George Rae was appointed as the "Plague Doctor" of that city. Although the available treatments at that time were limited, he did his utmost. He lanced patients' boils to allow the poison to drain. After the wound was cleaned, he cauterized it, thereby disinfecting and sealing the wound site. To protect himself against airborne miasmas, which were then thought to be the causative agent of the plague, Dr. Rae wore a special outfit. In addition to a long cloak, which protected his skin from the infectious air, he also wore a beak-like mask that was filled with spices and rose petals, which would prevent entry of the miasmas through his nose. The length of the beak-like mask secured a safe distance from the patient (Fig. 10.2). Although miasmas do not cause the plague, as we now know, it is remarkable to note that Dr. Rae's outfit still did its job—by protecting him from fleabites, it enabled him to survive the plague.

In recent months, severe acute respiratory syndrome coronavirus 2 (SARS-CoV-2) has spread throughout the world. When patients visit my outpatient clinic, both plastic surgeons and patients are recommended to wear facial masks. However, when patients with facial trauma are being examined, they must take off their masks. When a patient is sitting too close to me, a feeling of uneasiness sometimes arises.

This leads to an important question: how much distance is needed between doctor and patient?

Maintaining a certain distance from others can convey a nonverbal message. According to Hall [5], an anthropologist, doctors and patients should use a wider personal distance (90 to 150 cm) for discussions with one another. This distance is also highly convenient for discussions while sitting down. This guideline applies to situations where a doctor has a discussion with a patient who is in bed. During ward rounds, in which conversations take place at the foot of the bed, the doctor is already out of the patient's personal distance and has entered the so-called business distance, which is no longer suitable for confidential conversations.

In airborne infections, large droplets can travel approximately 101 cm (39.9 inches). Surgical masks provide highly effective protection against large airborne droplets. For small droplets, which can travel longer distances along unpredictable paths affected by wind gusts and other factors, traditional masks are less effective, as it is possible to inhale droplets around the sides of the masks.

Compared to other physicians, plastic surgeons are especially prone to shortening the clinical distance to examine the patient's face. As a result, we are vulnerable to small droplet infections under the current circumstances. Therefore, the patient's history and temperature should be checked before we meet them.

Remember, doctors are no exception to sickness!

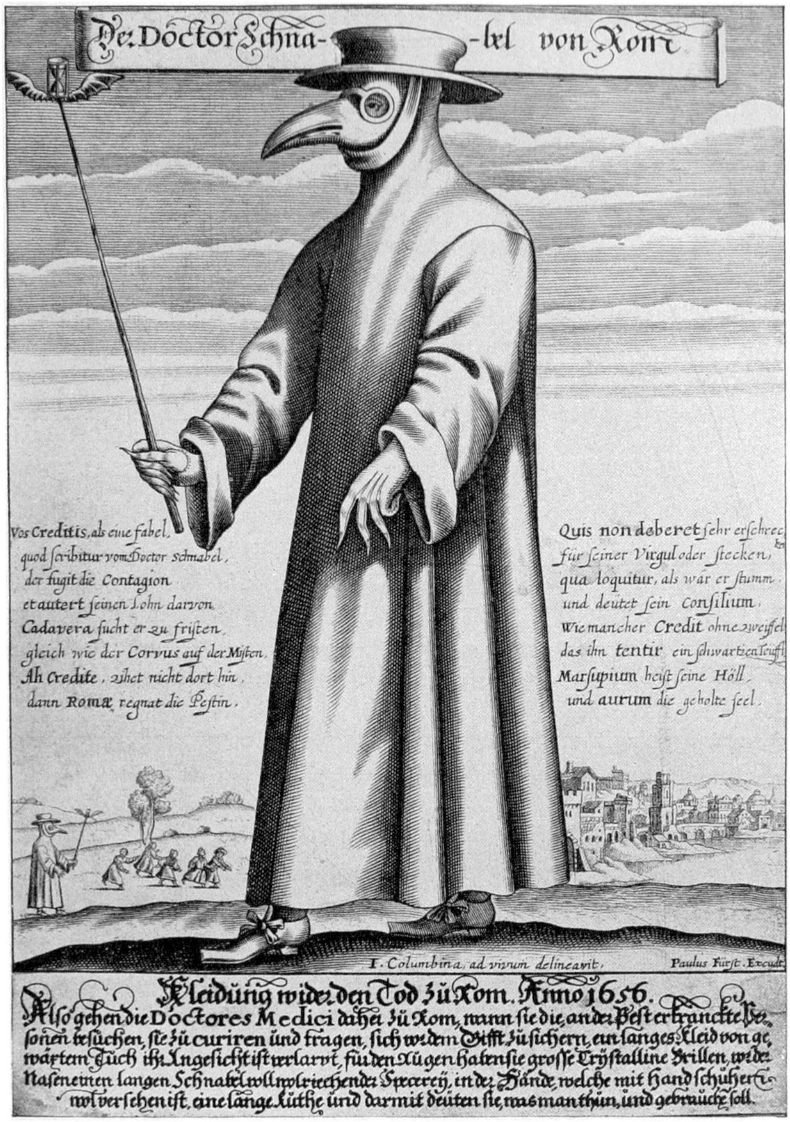
Der Doctor Schna-
-bel von Rom
I. Columbina ad vivum delineavit.
Paulus Fürst Excudit
Kleidung wider den Tod zu Rom. Anno 1656.

Fig. 10.2 Plague doctor of Marseilles Paul Fürst, engraving, c1721

10.3 Trauma Surgeons: Heroes of a Moment

Because of COVID-19, it has not been possible for me to attend mass recently. Instead, I listen to sermons and hymns online. My favorite hymn is "The Lily of the Valley": "He's the 'Lily of the Valley', the Bright and Morning Star/He's the fairest of ten thousand to my soul".

This hymn was written by William Charles Fry (1837–1882) for the Salvation Army and first published in 1881. The words were arranged to the music of "The Little Old Log Cabin in the Lane." It became a gospel standard and appears in almost all Protestant hymnals. It is generally understood that Fry took the term "Lily of the Valley" from the book of Song of Solomon 2:1 ("I am the rose of Sharon, the lily of the valley").

However, the French novelist and playwright Honoré de Balzac (1799–1850) wrote a novel of same name about a half century before Fry (1835). Balzac wrote this novel, dealing with themes of emotionally vibrant but never consummated affection, and titled it Lily of the Valley, representing the character of Henriette de Mortsauf.

Touched by this novel portraying the theme of affection, I read Balzac's other short stories and found a very interesting story about a great surgeon: "The Atheist's Mass" (Fig. 10.3). The protagonist, Desplein, is a successful surgeon and an atheist. One day his former assistant Bianchon sees Desplein going into a church and alone attending a mass. Bianchon questions the priest and finds that Desplein attends a mass at the church four times a year, which he himself pays for. Years later, Bianchon again sees Desplein going into the church and questions Desplein about it. Desplein explains that the mass is in memory of a water carrier named Bourgeat, who was his friend and father figure. When Desplein was a poor medical student, Bourgeat helped to pay for Desplein's education and did menial tasks like cutting wood. After Desplein became successful, he bought Bourgeat a horse and cart for his water-carrying work. After Bourgeat's death, knowing that Bourgeat was a devout Catholic, Desplein decided to have four masses a year for him at church.

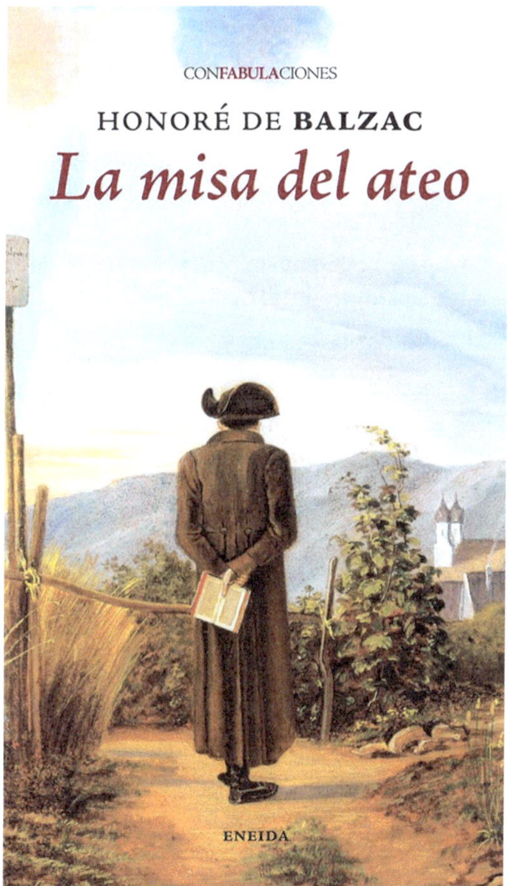

Fig. 10.3 The atheist's mass and other stories (La Misa del ateo, 2013, Spanish Edition) written by Honoré de Balzac (1799–1850). Madrid: Edtorial Eneida

In this novel, Balzac defines the glory of a surgeon as follows: "The glory of a surgeon is like that of an actor: they live only so long as they are alive, and their talent leaves no trace when they are gone. Actors and surgeons, like great singers too, like the executants who by their performance increase the power of music tenfold, are all the heroes of a moment."

When trauma patients arrive at a trauma center, we make decisions and move fast like actors. When a trauma victim's life is saved and stabilized, our performance is over. We are the heroes of a moment like actors. As a trauma surgeon, I completely agree with Balzac that surgeons live only so long as they are alive and their talent leaves no trace when they are gone. Like a "Lily of the Valley" and the "Bright and Morning Star," we trauma surgeons give "every care on them to roll."

10.3.1 Keep Playing Tug-of-War Against Grim Reaper

As you all know well, the aim of the Korean Society of Traumatology (KST) is to reduce the death and disability rates of trauma victims through academic progress in the treatment of trauma patients. The KST held its first annual conference in 1986 and its 27th conference in 2012. Starting in 2013, the KST collaborated with the Armed Forces Medical Command (AFMC) to host the Pan-Pacific Trauma Congress (PPTC) annually; this continued until the seventh congress in 2019. In 2020, an online congress was held because of coronavirus disease-19; however, we will continue to host the PPTC as soon as the pandemic subsides. The KST is participating in major national projects, such as a consultation guideline for trauma patients in Korea and a quality control guideline.

The Korean government implemented a regional trauma center (RTC) project in 2012, with the goal of reducing the preventable trauma death rate (PTDR) to the level of developed countries. RTCs should organically cooperate with the Korean government and the KST to ensure that seriously injured patients are treated at regional level 1 trauma centers [6]. Owing to the efforts of our KST members, the PTDR decreased from 50.4% in 1990s to 19.9% in 2017 [7, 8].

I am honored to become the president of the KST this year. This will be my last opportunity to serve the KST, because only 2 years are left before my retirement.

In my role as president, I would like to enhance knowledge-sharing among our members by providing more opportunities for academic communication. I also hope to raise KST's status to a higher level in the global academic community.

Of particular note, our official journal, *Journal of Trauma and Injury* (JTI), which published its first issue in 1988, was included in the Korean Citation Index (KCI) last year (2020). However, its impact factor is still not satisfactory (0.29). We have a long way to go to be registered in PubMed Central (PMC), Scopus, and SCIE. However, this goal is not so far off that it cannot be reached eventually. As the president of the KST and chairman of the ethics committee, I will help the editor of JTI (Gil-Jae Lee) work toward having JTI registered in more databases. I eagerly anticipate that our members will submit their valuable manuscripts to JTI and would be grateful for citations of papers published in JTI. To echo the words of President John F. Kennedy, please do not ask what KST can do for you, but ask what we can do for you and ask what we can do for our KST together.

A well-known movie entitled "Along with the Gods" (2017, starring Ha Jeong-Woo and Cha Tae-Hyun) comes to mind. This film tells the story of a firefighter (Kim Jahong) who dies while saving a girl in a fire in a skyscraper. He is led by three grim reapers who guide him through the seven trials in the afterlife. While watching the movie, I thought about the role of trauma doctors. As trauma doctors, we play tug-of-war against the grim reaper (Fig. 10.4). If we win, the trauma victim lives. If we lose, the patient dies. If we can decrease the PTDR, our winning rate increases—and to do so, we must share knowledge through academic communication. This is one of the roles of the KST.

The goal of a reaching higher level in the global academic community might not be reached while I am the president of the KST or before my retirement. However, I do believe that if we trauma doctors start building a stone bridge, one by one, to cross the stream, and if our junior trauma doctors continue the task, it will be completed someday in the future.

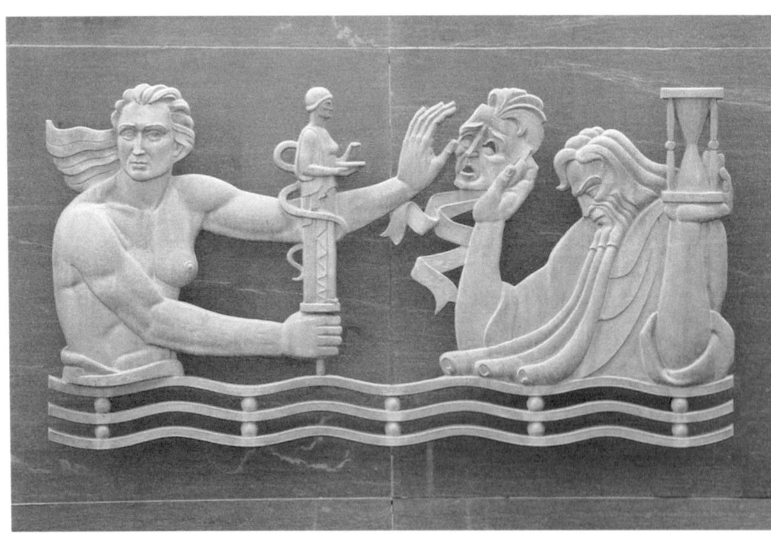

Fig. 10.4 Holding back the grim reaper. A sculpture on the side of the Fulton County Public Health Department in Atlanta, Georgia. Available from: https://playingintheworldgame.com/2015/09/10/holding-back-the-grim-reaper/

Here's to trauma doctors! Keep playing tug-of-war against the grim reaper!

10.4 Wrinkle the Skin, Wrinkle the Soul

> Years may wrinkle the skin, but to give up enthusiasm wrinkles the soul.—*Samuel Ullman*

In August of 2016, I enjoyed a movie titled *Operation Chromite*. Inspired by real events in Korean War, this movie focuses on a life-and-death mission of eight Korean operatives. Liam Neeson stars as General Douglas MacArthur and South Korea's Lee Jung-jae as his lieutenant (Fig. 10.5).

MacAuthur has been well-known worldwide since he officially accepted Japan's surrender after World War II and served as the effective ruler of Japan for 6 years. When the communists North Korea invaded South Korea in Jun 1950, he became supreme commander of the United Nations and defended South Korea.

In this movie, MacArthur (1880–1964) led the seemingly impossible marine landing at Incheon,

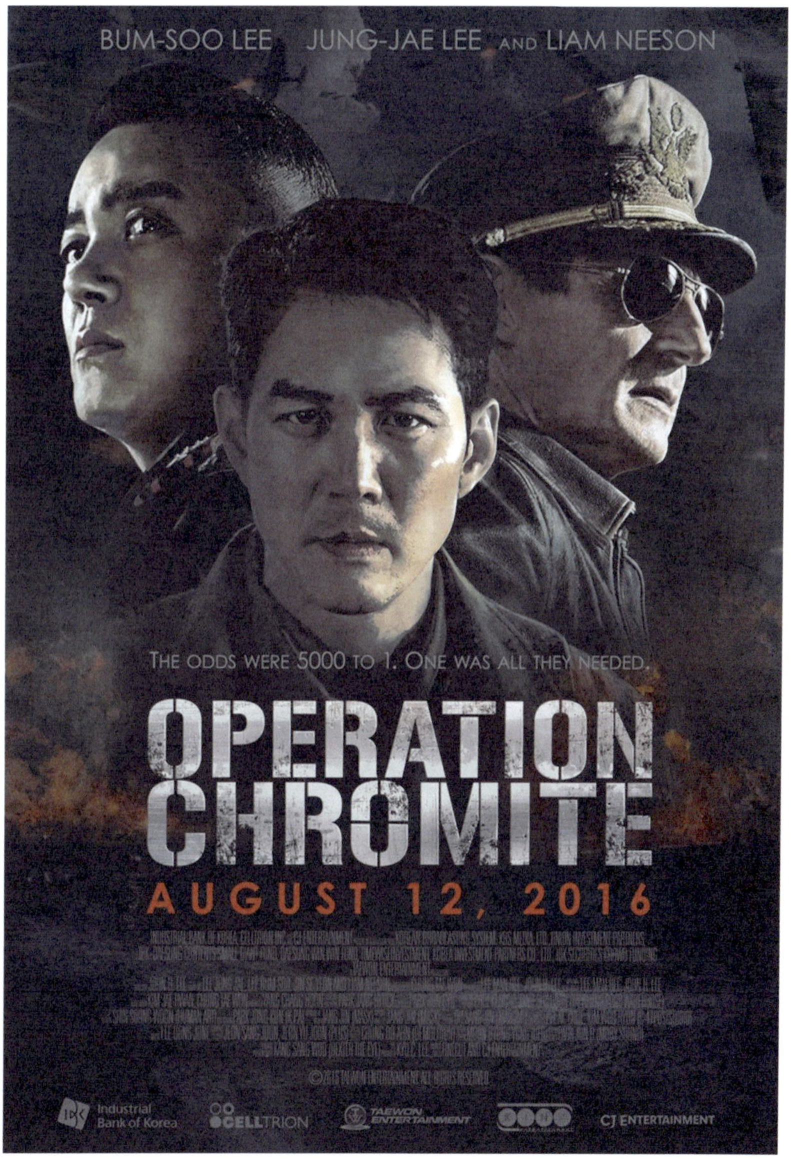

Fig. 10.5 Poster of Operation Chromite (2016)

which eventually succeeded (Fig. 10.6). When he was sailing to Incheon through the storm, he said to his officers: "People grow old only by deserting their ideals. Years may wrinkle the skin, but to give up interest wrinkles the soul."

This quote was from a poem of Samuel Ullman (1840–1924), *Youth*:

Nobody grows old merely by a number of years. We grow old by deserting our ideals. Years may wrinkle the skin, but to give up enthusiasm wrinkles the soul. Worry, fear, self-distrust bows the heart and turns the spirit back to dust.

In the center of your heart and my heart there is a wireless station; so long as it receives messages of beauty, hope, cheer, courage and power from men and from the Infinite, so long are you young.

MacArthur was so inspired that he even kept a framed copy of this poem in his office. He often quoted it in his speeches; thereafter, it became "MacArthur's Credo."

Wrinkles are caused by several factors: aging, ultraviolet light, smoking, and repeated facial expressions such as squinting or smiling. Plastic surgeons work to remove or at least reduce the wrinkles by "rejuvenation surgery."

Then, can the "operation rejuvenation" reduce the wrinkles of the soul as well as skin wrinkles?

If a young woman stops suffering from nervous hand sweating after successful aesthetic surgery of the face, the plastic surgeon could say he or she helped in getting her autonomic nervous system under control via an alternate route.

In order to be a good plastic surgeon, he or she should be a good physician first. Good physician is a doctor who can solve the patient's problems. For this, history taking and physical examination including the past medical history, social history, and systemic review are essential. When a preoperative patient has migraine headaches, instead of solely giving medications, we should take a look at all the potential factors that may be causing the person's headaches, such as other health problems, diet and sleep habits, stress, and personal problems.

To be able to help our patient reduce the wrinkle of soul, a plastic surgeon must have psychological and psychiatric knowledge as well as operating skills.

We should neither desert our ideals nor give up our enthusiasm. Instead, we should keep beauty, hope, cheer, and courage in our hearts. I

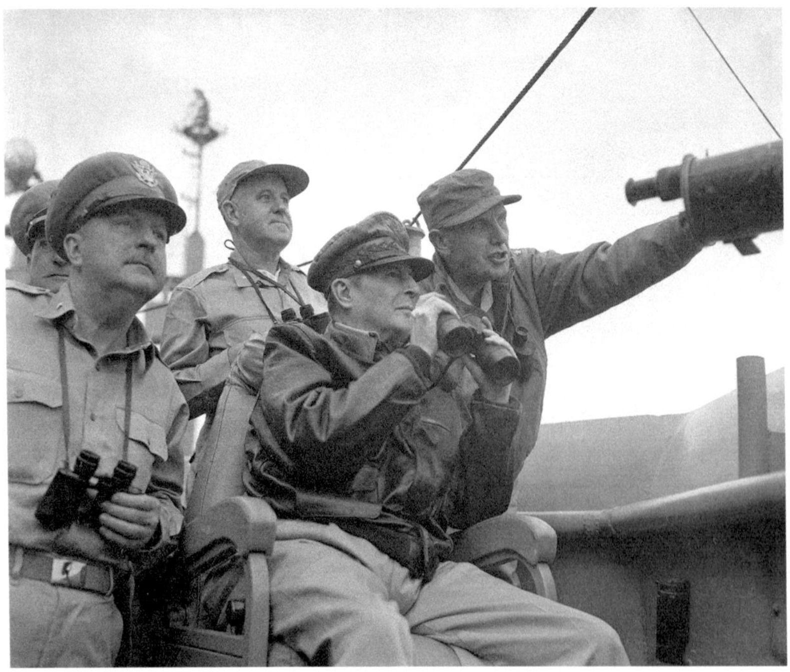

Fig. 10.6 MacArthur observes the naval shelling of Incheon from USS Mount McKinley, September 15, 1950, with Brigadier General Courtney Whitney (left) and Major General Edward M. Almond (right)

believe that there are wireless stations in my heart and heart of my patients as Ullman and MacArthur believed. As long as the hearts of our patients receive beautiful, hopeful, cheerful, and courageous message from our hearts, our patients will stay young.

Lastly, we should not forget that the plastic surgeon is a psychiatrist with a knife, and aesthetic surgery is a surgical psychotherapy [9, 10].

10.5 An Honorable Scar on the Face: A Scar Worthy of Satisfaction

> The scar had not pained Harry for nineteen years. All was well.—*J.K. Rowling*

As a plastic surgeon, I sometimes encounter patients who want to improve the appearance of a visible scar on their face or on an extremity. In contrast, some patients do not want to undergo scar revision, despite the presence of a visibly deformed scar.

In a well-known fictional example, Harry Potter's "lightning bolt" scar captured the wand movement required for the killing curse.

In the rhinoplasty set, we frequently use the Joseph knife and the Joseph elevator. These instruments were innovated to perform aesthetic rhinoplasty without leaving visible cutaneous scars. Jacques Joseph (1865–1934) innovated methods for aesthetic plastic surgery, especially cosmetic rhinoplasty.

In Jacques Joseph's picture, however, I immediately noticed a horizontal scar on his left cheek just above the nasolabial fold (Fig. 10.7). I wondered why he himself did not undergo scar revision on his cheek.

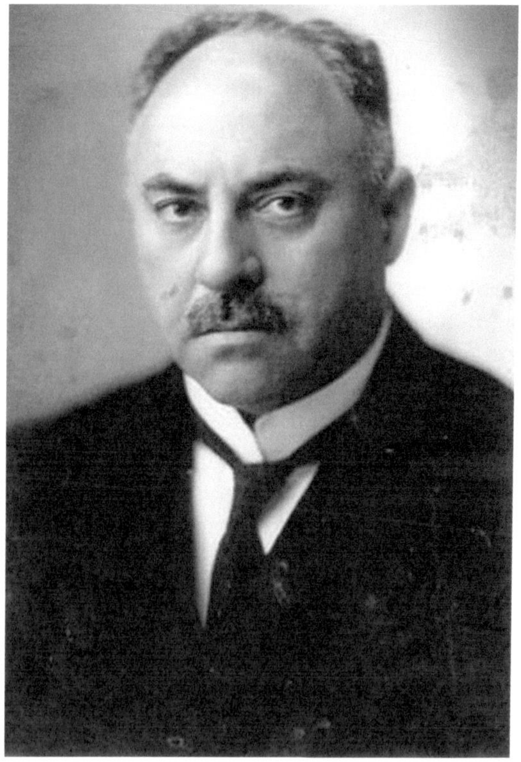

Fig. 10.7 Jacques Joseph (1865–1934). Note a horizontal scar on his left cheek just above the nasolabial fold

When he was studying medicine in Berlin and Leipzig, he understood the cultural marks of honor and dishonor in that social context. As a university student, he joined a conservative dueling fraternity and was proud to receive a scar from dueling with a saber. Joseph relished the test and the adventure of the duel, which was considered manly and edifying [11]. The scars from the duel were intentionally created. Students challenged each other to duels as a matter of course, without any real need for an insult to be exchanged. Being challenged was a process of social selection. The duelists had their eyes and throat protected, but their faces were purposely exposed to the blade of the saber. When a cut was made, it was treated in a way that maximized the resulting scar. The scar that Joseph carried with him throughout his life marked him as someone who was worthy of satisfaction, someone who had been seen as an honorable equal and thus had been challenged to a duel [11]. Marked on the duelist's face was his integration into German culture.

By the 1920s, such seemingly "false" scarring had become part of the German discourse on aesthetic surgery. An aesthetic surgeon named Levy-Lenz described the case of a young man who came to him after having won money in the lottery and wanted him to create artificial dueling scars through a "cosmetic procedure." In this way, he could "pass" as someone who was worthy of being challenged to a duel. Levy-Lenz refused to perform such an operation; the patient then went to a barber, who scarred the patient with a razor, severely damaging his salivary glands [12]. The visible scar enabled the young man to "pass" as a man of honor.

Can we differentiate an authentic mark of honor from a merely cosmetic mark?

Before persuading a patient to undergo scar revision, the plastic surgeon should become familiar with the cause and meaning of the patient's scar, in particular, whether it is an honorable or dishonorable scar.

10.6 Original Face for the Craniofacial Surgeons

In Zen Buddhism (禪佛教), original face (本來面目) is a term pointing to the non-duality of subject and object [13]. The term original face originates from Huangpo's *Chuanhsin fayao* (857) and the Hui-sin edition (967) of the *Platform Sutra of the Sixth Patriarch* (六祖壇經) [14]. A topic, "What is your original face before your parents were born?" tells us to let go of even more of our conditioning.

As Eastern Zen Buddhism seeks for the "my face before my parents were born," a similar concept of face can be found in Western literature: "The face I had before the world was made."

This other original face is the face of a person which she or he had before the world was made. In a poem titled "Before the World Was Made," Irish poet Yeats writes from the perspective of a beautiful woman responding to a jealous lover. She begins by acknowledging her efforts to make herself more attractive with cosmetics.

If I make the lashes dark.
And the eyes more bright.
And the lips more scarlet,
Or ask if all be right.
From mirror after mirror,
No vanity's displayed:
I'm looking for the face I had.
Before the world was made.

Then, what is original face of the craniofacial surgeons?

Congenital craniofacial abnormalities are a group of defects caused by abnormal growth and/or development of the head and facial soft-tissue structures and/or bones. Among them, cleft lip, cleft lip and palate, and isolated cleft palate are the most common congenital anomalies of the head and the neck, with a total prevalence of 2.1 per 1000 live births. The ultimate treatment for this malformation is surgical closure.

Dr. Millard (1919–2011), in the preface of his famous book *Cleft Craft: The Evolution of Its Surgery* (Fig. 10.8), emphasized surgeon should not ignore the first principle of plastic surgery; know the normal. He wrote "The plastic surgeon requires imagination for he must look into the puzzle of cleft. With this picture as transparency in his mind's eye superimposed over the cleft patient, the surgeon is abetted in the sorting out and fitting together of the pieces of the puzzle" [15].

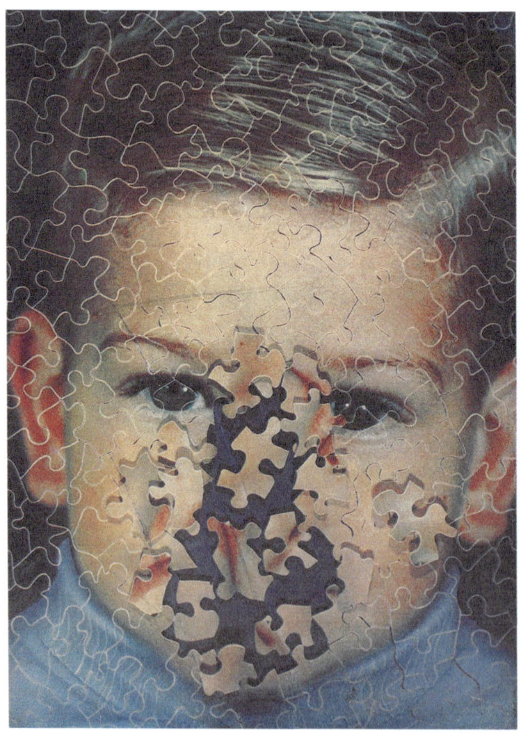

Fig. 10.8 Cover picture of Cleft Craft: The Evolution of Its Surgery

As Dr. Millard suggested, we craniofacial surgeons are trying repair the defect of the cleft lip patients similar to their original face using surgeon's imagination.

As written in the journal's homepage, the scope of *Archives of Craniofacial Surgery (ACFS)* is any aspect of craniofacial plastic and reconstructive surgery, operative procedures, clinical and laboratory research, and case reports. For seeking the normal or original face, I hope *ACFS* also welcomes anatomical studies of the head and neck and aesthetic procedures for the facial area.

10.7 What Would It be Like to Lose One's Nose? Gogol's the Nose and the Astronomer Tycho Brahe

> The nose looked at the Major and frowned a little.—*Nikolai Gogol, The Nose*

Last year at the Metropolitan Opera House, I enjoyed the opera *The Nose*, directed by William Kentridge. In the opera, a man named Major Kovalyov woke up one morning and found that his nose had gone missing in the night. The nose had developed a life of its own (Fig. 10.9). Although a police officer returned the nose to Kovalyov, a doctor was unable to reattach the nose. On 13th day after losing his nose, he woke up to find his nose reattached.

This satirical opera by Shostakovich was adapted from the classic short story by Nikolai Gogol (1809–1852). Kovalyov's nose acted as the source of his own pride; thereafter, the loss of his nose represented a loss of his identity. Since his identity was primarily defined by his outward appearance, the loss of that appearance devastated him.

Gogol wrote this story since he had an oddly shaped nose, which was often the subject of self-deprecating jokes in his letters [16]. Gogol opted for a comedy marked by the fantastic. However, parody is just a method of obscuring human suffering [17].

Today, an amputated nose can be reattached with microvascular anastomosis. If the stump is lost, the nose can be reconstructed with forehead flaps. In the Renaissance period, however, a nasal prosthesis was used instead.

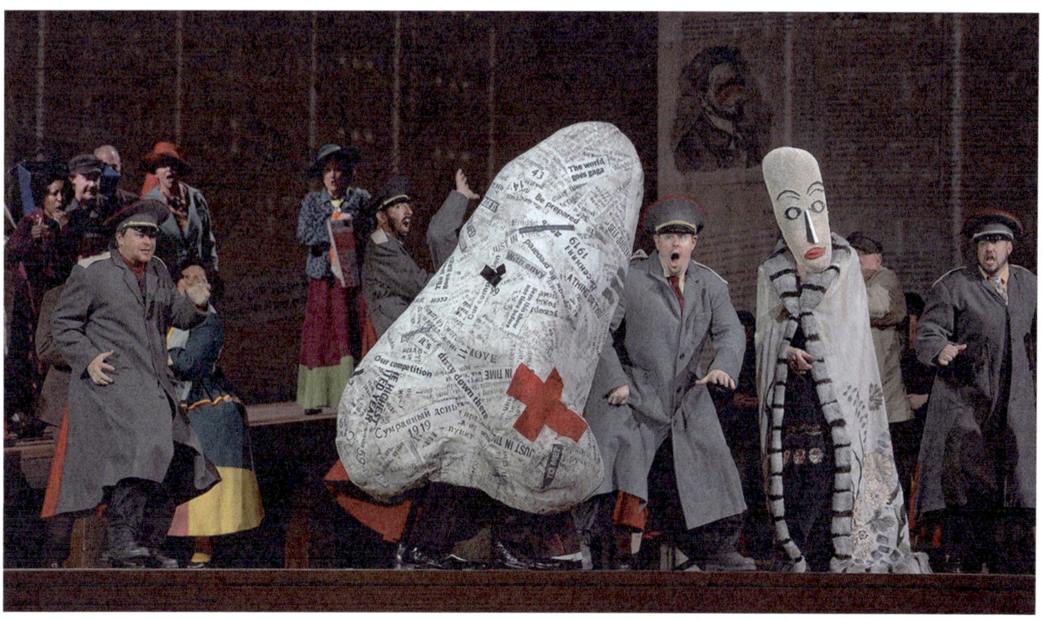

Fig. 10.9 The poster of the opera The Nose, as performed at the Metropolitan Opera House in New York City (reproduced with permission from "Courtesy of Metropolitan Opera")

Tycho Brahe (1546–1601) was a Danish astronomer. After his death, his assistant, Johannes Kepler (1571–1630), used Brahe's astronomical data and proposed the three laws of planetary motion: (1) the orbit of a planet is an ellipse with the sun at one of the two foci; (2) a line segment joining a planet and the sun sweeps out equal areas during equal intervals of time; and (3) the square of the orbital period of a planet is proportional to the cube of the semi-major axis of its orbit.

When he was 20, Brahe lost part of his nose in a sword duel with his third cousin, Manderup Parsberg. Manderup's blade cut away most of the nasal bridge, leaving the nasal cavity and septum exposed.

To hide his deformity, he constructed a prosthetic device made of wax, but it was unsatisfactory. Thus, he made a mold around the wax nose and fabricated a brass prosthesis. An artist matched the color of his skin. The prosthesis was held in place with glue. It is thought that this deformity altered his personality. He became defensive, depressive, and secretive [18].

Today, nasal prostheses made of polydimethylsiloxane are flexible and designed to move with the skin. They are retained by using an adhesive or osseointegrated implants.

A recent study found that the quality of life of patients with a facial prosthesis was reduced in comparison with a healthy group when the acquired defects were located at the eye or nose. The patients' body image and sense of their own sexual attractiveness were diminished. Some patients even believed they gave off an unpleasant odor [19].

Plastic surgeons should reflect on the examples of Major Kovalyov and Tycho Brahe as they consider the role of psychological care for patients who have lost a body part.

10.8 Use of the Theory of Reasoned Action in Plastic Surgery

In recent years, aesthetic plastic surgery has gained popularity worldwide. The American Society of Plastic Surgeons reported that 17.7 million cosmetic procedures were performed in 2017. Of these, 1.8 million were surgical procedures and 15.9 million were nonsurgical cosmetic procedures. Compared with 2016, the number of breast augmentation and liposuction procedures increased by 3% and 5%, respectively [20]. Thus, the popularity of aesthetic plastic surgery has attracted attention from the business sector.

Recently, I read an article regarding cosmetic surgery and services in Seoul from a journal in the field of management written by researchers in the fields of business and accounting from Malaysia and China [21, 22]. The researchers collected market data on women's willingness to undergo cosmetic surgery in Seoul. They interviewed 400 women aged 19 to 40 years using a self-administered questionnaire. Using the theory of reasoned action (TRA), they analyzed factors, such as attitudes, subjective norms (celebrities and the media), and psychological attributes (social status and self-esteem), that influence patients' intention to undergo cosmetic surgery.

The aim of the TRA is to explain the relationship between attitudes and behaviors within human action. This theory is most often used to predict how individuals will behave based on their preexisting attitudes and behavioral intentions. An individual's decision to engage in a particular behavior is based on the outcomes that the individual expects will come as a result of performing the behavior. In its simplest form, the TRA can be expressed as the following equation: $BI = (AB)W_1 + (SN)W_2$ (BI = behavioral intention, AB = one's attitude toward performing the behavior, W = empirically derived weights, and SN = one's subjective norm related to performing the behavior) (Fig. 10.10) [23].

This theory has been also used in medicine and behavioral science, such as in attempts to predict exercise in patients across stages of bariatric surgery [24].

In the cosmetic surgery field, three interesting studies in Iran, an Islamic country, used the TRA. In a paper from Islamic Azad University, Shahrekord Branch (Iran), 296 students were surveyed and analyzed using TRA. Intention to undergo cosmetic surgery showed significant relationships with attitudes toward one's body and subjective norms ($P = 0.013$). Higher body satis-

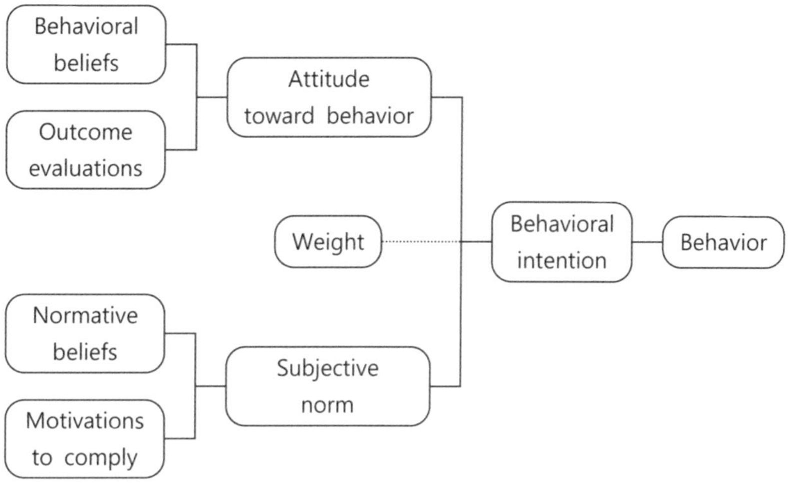

Fig. 10.10 Theory of reasoned action

faction was associated with less intention to use cosmetic surgery ($P = 0.01$). Surprisingly, the authors concluded that family status and feeling secure were the most important factors associated with intention to undergo cosmetic surgery. The authors argued that this intention is the result of psychological insecurity; therefore, community-oriented nurses with family support can improve these psychological traits [25].

Authors from a military medical school in Iran (AJA University of Medical Science) surveyed 233 female college students. Based on the TRA, they found a significant relationship between attitudes toward cosmetic surgery and participants' intentions ($P < 0.0001$). Because attitudes are an important predictor of cosmetic surgery, the authors drew the interesting conclusion that designing and conducting interventions are essential to reduce favorable attitudes toward elective cosmetic surgery among college students [26].

Authors from the Hamadan University of Medical Sciences, Iran, believed that cosmetic surgery is performed to change people's appearance and improve their self-esteem. They collected data from 340 female students at Hamadan University of Medical Sciences, to predict their intention to undergo cosmetic surgery, and analyzed the data using the TRA. They found a positive and significant correlation between the constructs of the TRA. Among the studied constructs, motivation for obedience, evaluations of behavioral outcomes, and behavioral beliefs played a significant role in explaining variance in behavioral intention [27].

The above three papers collected similar samples, used the TRA as a tool for the analysis, and drew similar conclusions. Although these papers appear to use TRA with the goal of finding ways to discourage people from cosmetic surgery, I still think that the TRA can be used in other parts of plastic surgery. We, as plastic surgeons, should conduct a prospective analysis of our market ourselves, instead of letting further surveys be done by marketing managers. In this analysis, TRA might play an important role.

10.9 Is Aesthetic Plastic Surgery a Form of Symbolic Consumption?

As a relatively rare example of a movie with a plastic surgeon as a major character, I love "A Woman's Face" (1938) directed by Gustaf Molander. The cast included Ingrid Bergman, as a woman criminal with a disfigured face, and Anders Henrikson, as a plastic surgeon who operates on her. Anna Holm, the character played by Ingmar Berman, is an embittered woman with a facial disfigurement involving distortion of her eye and mouth on one side and a scar on her cheek. In childhood, her face was burned in a house fire, and she was abandoned by her parents, who were also criminals. She became a criminal herself but is glad that her ugliness prevented her from an even worse fate. As an expression of her alienation from society, she became part of a criminal gang specializing in blackmail. Being a blackmailer, Anna threatens Mrs. Wegert, a plastic surgeon's wife. Dr. Wegert initially thinks that she is a burglar but becomes interested in the surgical problem of her disfigured face (Fig. 10.11). Therefore, he does not turn her in; instead, he hospitalizes her and operates on her face. After a successful operation, Anna becomes beautiful; her talks with Dr. Wegert also inspire her to become a different person.

This storyline of this movie reminds me of a psychological theory that I believe can help understand our patients' psychological perspective when they choose to undergo surgery.

A unique characteristic of humans, as distinct from other animals, is the ability to examine ourselves, to find ourselves lacking, and to attempt self-betterment. This sense of incompleteness leads us not only to create but also to self-create, and we consume goods and services in that process.

The psychological theory of symbolic self-completion holds that individuals seek to acquire and display symbols that are strongly related to what they perceive as the ideal self.[1] For example, relatively effeminate boys who want to appear macho may use products associated with manliness, such as a strong cologne or a silver watch, in hopes of symbolically fulfilling their self-definition of masculinity. Such cases of symbolic self-completion are seen in Internet communication, marketing and advertising, and consumer behavior.

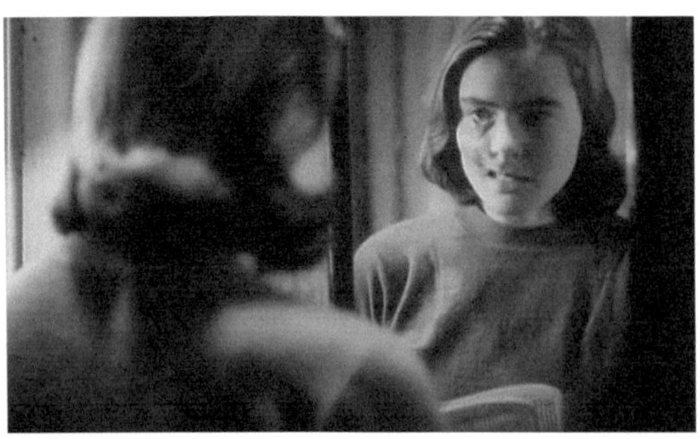

Fig. 10.11 Anna (Ingrid Bergman) is looking at her disfigured face in a mirror

Compared to other consumer goods and services, cosmetic surgery is irreversible, expensive, painful, and potentially dangerous. Symbolic self-completion theory provides insight into goal-striving and has been used to help explain patients' desire for cosmetic surgery [28].

A study collected data from customers who underwent cosmetic surgery in multiple, in-depth, ethnographic interviews regarding body image, impression management, and symbolic self-completion. Major changes in informants' roles or status often led to feelings of unconvincing role performance and then to behaviors interpretable in terms of self-completion theory. When particular physical attributes, such as a flat chest or a tired and wrinkled face, seemed incongruent with the roles they were attempting to cultivate, plastic surgery was seen to offer more appropriate bodily symbols and, consequently, greater self-confidence and self-acceptance in key role performance [29].

Of note, in "A Woman's Face," Anna forgets her past and starts a new life in Beijing.

The extent of a woman's conscious or unconscious concern about her outward appearance to others is predictive of the use of appropriate symbols for self-completion. Symbolic self-completion theory emphasizes seeking control over one's sense of self and social reality, in relation to the socially desirable female image. The extent to which a woman involves herself in this seeking is an important aspect of coping, as shown by Anna's trajectory.

As plastic surgeons, we are suppliers of a kind of service, that is, operations. Therefore, we would be well-served by understanding the dynamics of symbolic self-completion among our patients. Aesthetic plastic surgery is a form of symbolic consumption, and a plastic surgeon is a psychiatrist with a scalpel.

10.10 Breast Cancer, Planarians, and Plastic Surgeons

> ...This body's fenscape, manscaped, hills removed—the meaty joins

still livid, tight shut mouths

where distant territories were stitched in touch. Blood seeps in deltas over ribs…—*From Self-portrait without Breasts, by Clare Best*

It is generally accepted that the survival rate of breast cancer has dramatically improved, and the outcomes of breast reconstruction are also excellent. When we meet a patient who has breast cancer and is planning to undergo mastectomy, we can say, "Now it's a simple matter of cutting out the breast cancer and restoring the breast." However, surgical procedures intended to treat breast cancer or reduce the risk of developing the disease typically result in changes in appearance and scarring of the breast area and any donor sites [30]. Therefore, those who have not experienced these changes could never understand the indescribable pain.

Nonetheless, we might be able to sympathize with patients' pain and hurt through protagonists in literature. I introduce two examples.

In her project *Self-portrait without Breasts*, Clare Best, an English poet, reclaims the "flat simple scarred chest with no extras." In the title poem of the poem cycle she uses figurative expressions about the post-mastectomy body as a landscape (Fig. 10.12): "…This body's fenscape, /manscaped, hills removed—the meaty joins/still livid, tight shut mouths/where distant territories were stitched//in touch. Blood seeps in deltas over ribs… [31].".

A Japanese writer, Fumio Yamamoto (山本文緒, 1962–), wrote "Planaria," a collection of five stories about women without regular jobs, for which she won the Naoki literary prize in the second half of 2000 [32]. The title story is a vivid portrait of Haruka, a 26-year-old woman who is adrift in life, unable to reconnect to family and work after losing a breast to cancer 2 years earlier. A difficult person even before the operation, she sabotages her relationships with both her boyfriend and a slightly older woman who has given her part-time work at a confectionary store. In a memorable line, she says, while out drinking with friends, that she would like to be reborn as a "planaria," a small worm living in pure streams that can regenerate itself when a part of its body is cut off. In fact, a "planarian" is one of many flatworms of the traditional phylogenic class Turbellaria. Planarians exhibit an extraordinary ability to regenerate lost body parts. When split lengthwise or crosswise, a planarian will regenerate into two separate individuals. It can be cut into pieces, and each piece can regenerate into a complete organism. Cells at the location of the wound site proliferate to form a blastema, which differentiates into new tissues and regenerates the missing parts of the piece of the cut planarian. Thereafter, it is called "immortal under the edge of a knife" [33].

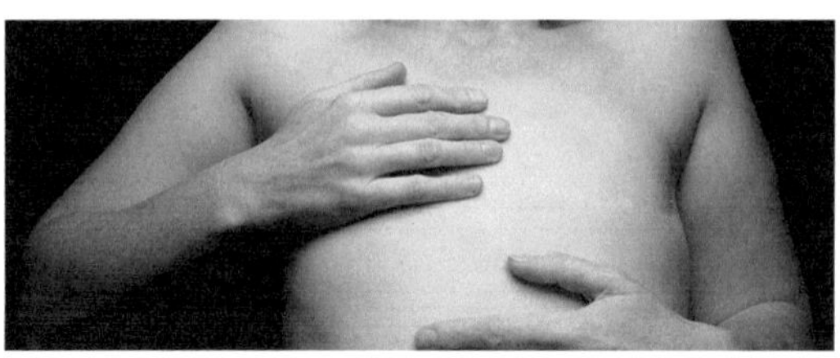

Fig. 10.12 Photography by Laura Stevens, collaborator of "Self-portrait without Breasts" written by Clare Best. Available at: https://clarebest.co.uk/projects/self-portrait/. Accessed on Aug 27, 2021. ©Laura Stevens. Used with permission

The reconstructive surgery following resection also bothered Haruka. "After I had breast reconstructive surgery, a place appeared where my skin was folded and sewn like the folds on my clothes. It itches terribly when I feel hot from time to time. I can't scratch it because it's under my clothes. Sometimes it really drives me crazy. Am I supposed to be okay with this?"

In a study, participants were asked open-ended questions about their experiences when seeing the postsurgical appearance of their breast/breast area (and donor site, if relevant) for the first time, and four key themes emerged: "preparedness and support," "first thoughts and emotions," "loss and grief," and "the reaction of others." Some felt prepared and emotionally supported at this time, whereas others felt this element of care was missing.[1] Another study explored the decision to undergo breast reconstruction surgery after mastectomy and found that the decision was made during stressful circumstances, and many women did not feel well prepared to make this decision. The most highly ranked reasons to choose breast reconstruction were the desire for the breasts to be equal in size, the desire to wake up from surgery with a breast in place, and the perceived bother of a scar with no breast. The most highly ranked reasons not to choose breast reconstruction were related to the surgical risks and complications [34]. A third study found that most women (76 of 93) made quick, "instant" decisions to undergo immediate breast reconstruction following mastectomy, whereas the remainder (14 of 93) sought further information before making their choice [35]. Women with complications were twice as likely to report feeling less feminine and dissatisfied with the appearance of their scar than those without problems [36].

Like Haruka in the novel, many breast cancer patients struggle with severe stress. What is needed to overcome these mental and physical sequelae is social rehabilitation. Therefore, the medical staff should encourage patients to return to daily life immediately after surgery and perform breast reconstruction or provide the patient an artificial breast. Thereafter, breast reconstruction restores both the resected breast itself and patients' communication with themselves, their family, and the society around them.

In this process, we plastic surgeons play the role of making patients who undergo mastectomy "immortal under the edge of a knife," much like planarians. I hope that both a poetic mind and anatomical knowledge will help surgeons achieve satisfactory results [37].

References

1. Yu M, Shin IC, Lee HD, Cho YH. In: Eoyuyadam. Paju: Dolbegae; 2006. p. 277–9.
2. Kwon HR. Disaster situation and the spirit of respect for humanity depicted in Eou-yadam as a disaster literature. The East Asian Ancient Studies. 2021;61:9–44.
3. Kashiwagi M, Tanabe T, Shichiri M, Tamai H. Differential diagnosis in children having delirium associated with high fever. No To Hattatsu. 2003;35:310–5.
4. Onoe S, Nishigaki T, Kosugi M. Usefulness of EEG recording for delirium in children with high fever. No To Hattatsu. 2003;35:29–35.
5. Hall ET. The hidden dimension. New York: Doubleday; 1966.
6. Park DJ, Park CY, Cho HM, Lee KH, Han HS. Current status and future prospects of trauma centers in Korea. J Korean Med Assoc. 2017;60:530–2.
7. Kim H, Jung KY, Kim SP, Kim SH, Noh H, Jang HY, et al. Changes in preventable death rates and traumatic care systems in Korea. J Korean Soc Emerg Med. 2012;23:189–97.
8. Jung K, Kim I, Park SK, Cho H, Park CY, Yun JH, et al. Preventable trauma death rate after establishing a national trauma system in Korea. J Korean Med Sci. 2019;34:e65.
9. Rozner L. Attitudes to cosmetic surgery. Med J Aust. 1973;2:513–6.
10. Hinderer UT. Dr. Vazquez Añón's last lesson. Aesth Plast Surg. 1978;2:375–82.
11. Gilman SL. Making the body beautiful: a cultural history of aesthetic surgery, Princeton. Princeton, NJ: Princeton University Press; 2001. p. 121–3.
12. Levy-Lenz L. Erinnerungen eines Sexual-Arztes: Aus den Memorien Sexologen. Baden-Baden, Germany: Wadi-Verlagsbuchhandlung; 1954. p. 460.
13. Hori VS. Koan and Kensho in the Rinzai Zen curriculum. In: Heine S, Wright DS, editors. The Koan: texts and contexts in Zen Buddhism. Oxford: Oxford University Press; 2000. p. 289.
14. Pine R. The platform sutra: the Zen teaching of huineng. Berkeley: Counterpoint Press; 2008.
15. Millard DR. Cleft craft: the evolution of its surgery. Boston: Little Brown; 1976.
16. Sicher E. Dialogization and laughter in the dark, or how Gogol's nose was made: parody and literary evolution in Bachtin's theory of the novel. Russ Lit. 1990;28:211–33.
17. Tainmont J. The ear and the nose in literary parodies. The "hymn of deafness" by Du Bellay and "the nose" by Gogol. B-ENT. 2011;7:309–17.
18. Greisman HC. Tycho Brahe: astronomer of renaissance Denmark. Clin Plast Surg. 1983;10:629–33.
19. Klein M, Menneking H, Spring A, et al. Analysis of quality of life in patients with a facial prosthesis. Mund Kiefer Gesichtschir. 2005;9:205–13.
20. American Society of Plastic Surgeons. Plastic surgery statistics report-2016 cosmetic plastic surgery statistics. Chicago, IL: American Society of Plastic Surgeons; 2016.
21. Hwang K. They are analyzing us: our own survey is needed. Arch Plast Surg. 2019;46:397–8.
22. Teng PK, Ling TJ, Seng KW. Propensity to undergo cosmetic surgery and services in Seoul. Int J Community Develop Manag Stud. 2019;3:1–16.
23. Hale JL, Householder BJ, Dillard JP GKL, Pfau M. Chapter. 14. The theory of reasoned action. In: The persuasion handbook: developments in theory and practice. Newbury Park, CA: Sage Publication; 2002. p. 259–86.
24. Hunt HR, Gross AM. Prediction of exercise in patients across various stages of bariatric surgery: a comparison of the merits of the theory of reasoned action versus the theory of planned behavior. Behav Modif. 2009;33:795–817.
25. Tahmasbi S, Tahmasbi Z, Yaghmaie F. Factors related to cosmetic surgery based on theory of rea-

soned action in shahrekord students. J Holist Nurs Midwifery. 2014;24:53–61.
26. Dehdari T, Khanipou A, Khazir Z, et al. Predict the intention to perform cosmetic surgery on female college students based on the theory of reasoned action. J Mil Caring Sci. 2015;1:109–15.
27. Barati M, Kazemi Kilehgolan F, Parsafar S, et al. Prediction of the intention to undergo cosmetic surgery among female students based on the theory of reasoned action. Am J Cosmetic Surg. 2020;37:75–80.
28. Wicklund RA, Gollwitzer PM. Symbolic self-completion theory. Hillsdale, NJ: Erlbaum; 1982.
29. Schouten JW. Selves in transition: symbolic consumption in personal rites of passage and identity reconstruction. J Consum Res. 1991;17:412–25.
30. Herring B, Paraskeva N, Tollow P, et al. Women's initial experiences of their appearance after mastectomy and/or breast reconstruction: a qualitative study. Psychooncology. 2019;28:2076–82.
31. Best C. Self-portrait without breasts. 2011. https://reframe.sussex.ac.uk/lifewritingprojects/body/breastless-encounters-with-risk-reducing-surgery-by-clare-best/. Accessed 21 Jan 2022.
32. Yamamoto F. Planaria (translated to Korean by Yang YO, ISBN 9788979198157). Seoul, Korea: Changhae Pub. Co.; 2008.
33. Dalyell JG. Observations on some interesting phenomena in animal physiology, exhibited by several species of Planariae. Edinburgh, Scotland: Archibald Constable; 1814.
34. Manne SL, Topham N, Kirstein L, et al. Attitudes and decisional conflict regarding breast reconstruction among breast cancer patients. Cancer Nurs. 2016;39:427–36.
35. Harcourt D, Rumsey N. Mastectomy patients' decision-making for or against immediate breast reconstruction. Psychooncology. 2004;13:106–15.
36. Potter S, Thomson HJ, Greenwood RJ, et al. Health-related quality of life assessment after breast reconstruction. Br J Surg. 2009;96:613–20.
37. Hwang K. Anatomical poems about the breast ("Le beau Tetin") and anatomical proportions. Plast Reconstr Surg Glob Open. 2021;9:e3652.

11 How to Become a "Good" Plastic Surgeon?

11.1 Goddess of Imagination

> At the left of Truth one sees Imagination, who positions herself to adorn and crown Truth.—*Denis Diderot (1751)*

Plastic surgeons are seen by those of other specialties as imaginative, original, inventive, and ingenious people. In the field of plastic surgery, many new ideas and skills are developed by surgeons and researchers. To develop new methods or improve surgical skill, creative activity is needed. Creativity is a phenomenon, whereby something new and somehow valuable is formed. Creative minds in plastic surgery have imagination that sparks the "brainstorming of ideas" [1].

To develop creativity, as Dr. Joseph Murray emphasized, scientists should remember three important words: curiosity, imagination, and persistence.

We can easily perceive what curiosity and persistence are. Curiosity is an emotion related to natural inquisitive behavior such as exploration, investigation, and learning. Persistence is the determination to do something even though it is difficult or other people oppose it.

For the concept of "imagination," however, the exact meaning is unclear from simply examining the definition: the creative ability to form images, ideas, and sensations in the mind without direct input from the senses, such as seeing or hearing.

Instead, I could find the "goddess of imagination" in a painting and a relief.

Denis Diderot (1713–1784) edited the *Encyclopédie* (1772) and devised a figurative system of three main branches of knowledge: "Memory"/History, "Reason"/Philosophy, and "Imagination"/Poetry. He put Anatomy, Physiology, and Medicine in the domain of "Particular Physics," a part of "Reason."

In the frontispiece of the *Encyclopédie* (first volume, 1751) drawn by Charles-Nicolas Cochin, many goddesses symbolizing each part of the book are depicted (Fig. 11.1). Diderot wrote, "Truth enveloped in a veil and radiating light which parts the clouds and disperses them. To the right, Reason and Philosophy are busy, one in raising the veil from Truth, the other in tearing it away. At the left of Truth one sees Imagination, who positions herself to adorn and crown Truth." It is thought that Diderot believed the imagination is essential to "adorn and crown" the truth, while reason and philosophy unveil the truth.

In the bronze door of the Library of Congress Thomas Jefferson Building, a "goddess of imagination" is carved in the relief panel by Olin Warner (1896). In the allegorical figure of the goddess with her head turned to proper right in three-quarters profile, her right arm is bent with hand pointing skyward and her left arm is holding a lute. She wears classical dress, and a pair of small wings is

K. Hwang, *Good Physician, Good Plastic Surgeon*, https://doi.org/10.1007/978-981-97-1864-1_11

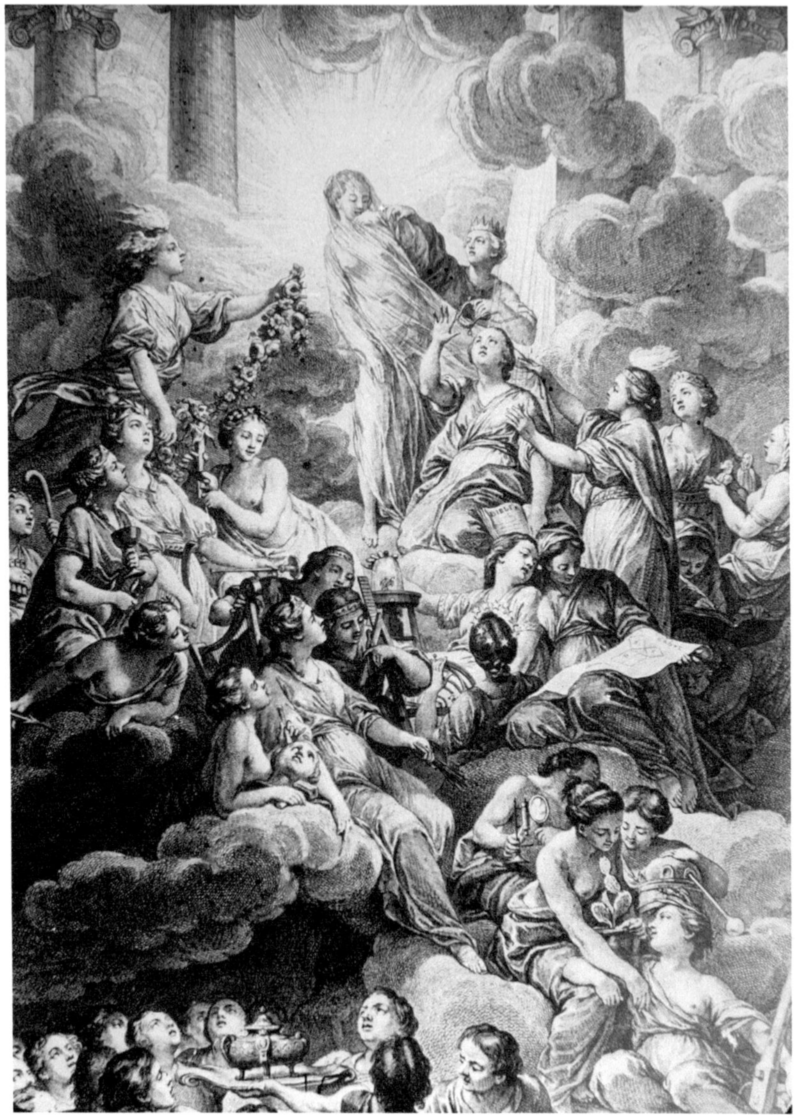

Fig. 11.1 The frontispiece of the Encyclopédie (Encyclopédie de Diderot et d'Alembert Tome I—A à E ou, Dictionnaire raisonné des sciences, des arts et des métiers Publication de 1751) drawn by Charles-Nicolas Cochin (1715–1790). Truth enveloped in a veil and radiating light which parts the clouds and disperses them. To the right, Reason and Philosophy are busy, one in raising the veil from Truth, the other in tearing it away. At the left of Truth one sees Imagination, who positions herself to adorn and crown Truth

attached to her head and a larger pair to her shoulders. The interpretation of the allegory of "imagination" is up to the imagination of the viewer.

Improvement in standards, modification of routine, and pioneering of new ideas in plastic surgery require innovation through creativity in which imagination sparks penetration beyond known boundaries [1].

Using Reason and Philosophy, we can unveil the truth. Using Imagination, we can adorn and crown the Truth, just as Diderot wrote.

11.2 Observational and Deductive Reasoning Ability for Plastic Surgeons

When you have eliminated all that is impossible, then whatever remains, however improbable, must be the truth.—*Sir Arthur Conan Doyle*

When I visited Edinburgh, I enjoyed looking around Surgeons' Hall Museums. Among the many famous surgeons from that city, Dr. Joseph Bell (1837–1911, Fig. 11.2a) caught my

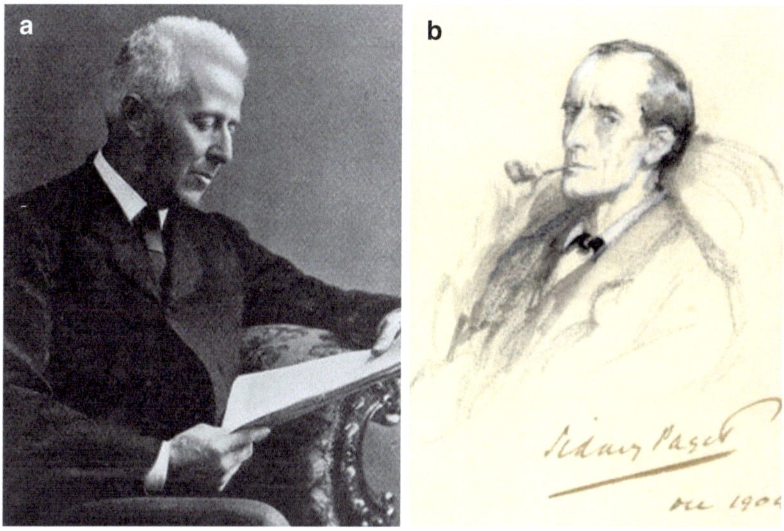

Fig. 11.2 Portraits of Dr. Joseph Bell (**a**) and Sherlock Holmes (**b**). Available at: https://uploads.disquscdn.com/images/8c5097f928af9024000cad554ace64793a4ff5bbf3a4669bec12fa6a46b8c0db.png. Accessed July 15, 2019

eye. He was the model for Sherlock Holmes (Fig. 11.2b), the protagonist of the famous detective stories written by Sir Arthur Conan Doyle (1859–1930).

A letter from Doyle, a doctor as well as writer, to his teacher Dr. Bell, was displayed there. Doyle wrote, "It is most certainly to you that I owe Sherlock Holmes … Round the centre of deduction and inference and observation which I have heard you inculcate I have tried to build up a man." In fact, Dr. Bell not only had the medical knowledge for diagnosis but also a great skill for being able to simply look at a person and tell their trade, their place of residence, their status in life, and many things about them. Reading the displays, I realized that observational and deductive ability is very important to detectives as well as physicians.

On my way home, I was reminded of my previous article and new idea about the reasoning which a good surgeon should have. I had written that a good doctor is the physician or surgeon who solves the patients' problem: correctly diagnoses their illness, cures them with safe evidence-based procedures, and is honest to them. A good surgeon should know how to operate, when to operate, and when not to operate [2].

In medicine, decision-making relies upon empirical knowledge as well as rational thinking to understand natural phenomena and determine causal inference [3].

In the sixteenth and seventeenth centuries, empiricism was developed by Francis Bacon and John Locke, where perceptions of natural phenomena were considered the ultimate source and judge of knowledge for assessing causality [4]. However, observations alone are not sufficient. Thereafter, inductive reasoning is needed to create causal inferences from observed instances to future instances.

Surgeons as well as physicians need to have an ability to see a problem and find out what steps are needed to solve that problem. When the scattered information is given to a surgeon, inductive reasoning—the ability to combine information to form conclusions—is needed.

For cardiovascular surgical training, Spencer found four activities very helpful in the development of deductive reasoning: (1) considering imperfect results to be more educational, (2) origin of imperfect result (a. diagnosis, b. technique, c. concept), (3) creating a hypothesis consistent with the data, and (4) the process of decision-making [5].

Like Dr. Bell, the skills of deduction and inference, the deductive reasoning, are also mandatory to plastic surgeons as well as cardiovascular surgeons. This is the ability to use general rules to find specific problems [6]. It is applying medical principles to the specific problem of the patient, as Sherlock Holmes did.

When a female patient, accompanied by her husband, appeared in my clinic with a swollen cheek and said that she had fallen down the stairs, I needed to grasp the atmosphere between them to ensure there was reasonable doubt about the possibility of assault. Deductive reasoning was needed in my observation and diagnosis.

Thinking about the above abilities that good plastic surgeons should have, I reached the conclusion that plastic surgeons, including cosmetic surgeons, should be as scientific and logical as they can be. Also, they should be humble, because the human body is a holy dwelling place for the soul.

11.3 The Artist's Creativity and the Plastic Surgeon's Creativity

Creativity is a phenomenon whereby something new and valuable is formed. Both artists and plastic surgeons need creativity [7]. Improving standards, modifying routines, and pioneering new ideas in plastic surgery require innovation through creativity, in which one's imagination sparks progress beyond known boundaries [1].

Creative processes were discussed in the late nineteenth and early twentieth centuries by the scientists Hermann von Helmholtz (1896) and Henri Poincaré, succeeded by the theorist Graham Wallas. In his book *Art of Thought* (1926), Wallas presented a five-stage model of the process underlying creative insights and illuminations:

1. Preparation (preparatory work on a problem that focuses the individual's mind on the problem and explores the problem's dimensions).
2. Incubation (where the problem is internalized into the unconscious mind and nothing appears externally to be happening).
3. Intimation (the creative person gets a "feeling" that a solution is on its way; however, this stage can be a substage).
4. Illumination or insight (where the creative idea bursts forth from its preconscious processing into conscious awareness).
5. Verification (where the idea is consciously verified, elaborated, and then applied) (Fig. 11.3).

Most arts, such as musical composition, painting, or literary work, may follow the above four—or five-stage creative process [8].

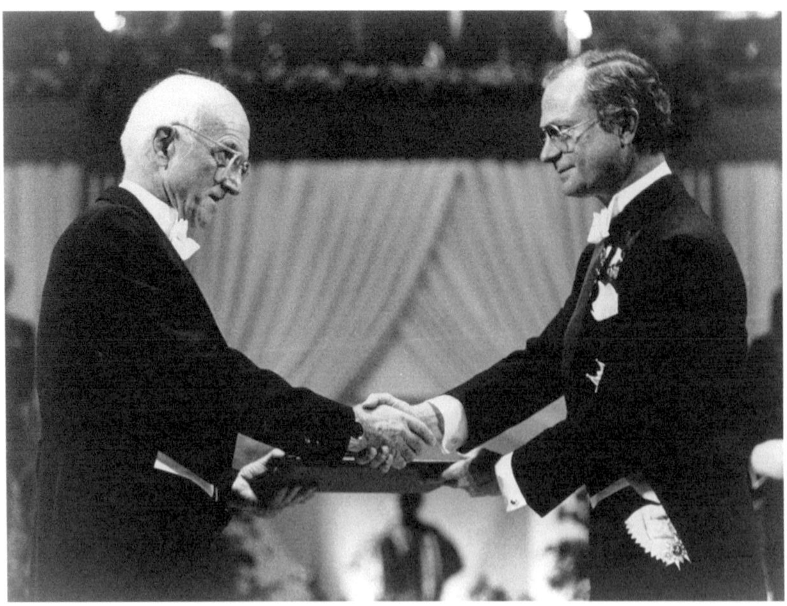

Fig. 11.3 Joseph Murray is receiving Nobel Prize from King Carl XVI Gustaf in 1990

Since a plastic surgeon is called on to make aesthetic judgements and convert them into reality, either by reshaping a part or reconstructing it to match the original, it has been proposed that creative abilities are essential to surgical problem-solving [7].

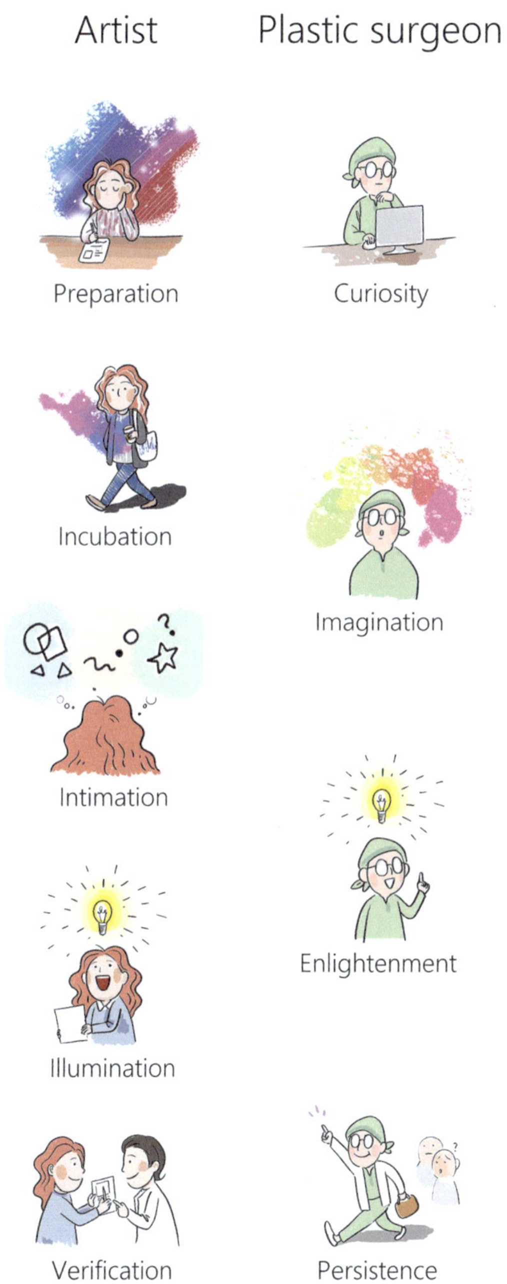

Fig. 11.4 Creative process of the artist and plastic surgeon

Januszkiewicz adapted the five-stage model to plastic surgery. His "creativity" appears similar to the concept of sudden enlightenment (sudden cultivation) in Buddhism (subitism, 頓悟頓修). However, I think otherwise. Even after reaching enlightenment, gradual practice with patience is needed (頓悟漸修).

To echo the words of Joseph Murray (Fig. 11.3), scientists should have three important stages of creativity: curiosity, imagination, and persistence (Fig. 11.4) [9]. Curiosity is an emotion related to natural inquisitive behavior such as exploration, investigation, and learning. We can have curiosity regarding a basic research question or surgical procedure. Imagination is the ability to form mental images, sensations, and concepts, in a moment when they are not perceived through sight, hearing, or the other senses. Denis Diderot (1713–1784), who edited the *Encyclopédie* (1772), believed the imagination is essential to "adorn and crown" the truth, while reason and philosophy unveil the truth [9]. Lastly, persistence is the determination to do something even though it is difficult or other people oppose it [10].

Through curiosity, imagination, and persistence over the course of the centuries, physicians and surgeons made many scientific advances, and these advances are still continuing through their patient work. On the basis of these advances, plastic surgeons have become able to translate legends into reality.

11.4 How Can Facial Deformity Stimulate the Creativity of an Artist and a Plastic Surgeon?

> To give a body and a perfect form to one's thought, this—and only this—is to be an artist.—*Jacques-Louis David (1748–1825)*

Creativity, understood as the ability to produce or use original and unusual ideas, is a phenomenon whereby something new and valuable is formed. Creativity is necessary not only for artists but also for surgeons—especially for plastic surgeons.

According to Dr. Colp, there are seven emotional factors that stimulate creativity: (1) tension, (2) personality disorder, (3) bipolar disorder, (4) observation of death, (5) physical disability or deformity, (6) sadness and dissatisfaction for the past, and (7) the Oedipus complex [11].

An example of an artist who was motivated by his physical deformity is Jacques-Louis David (1748–1825). We all know his famous painting entitled *Napoleon at the Saint-Bernard Pass.* He was a founder of the neoclassical school of art. In his death mask, we can easily see his crooked nose and markedly asymmetrical mandible, which lead us to make the diagnosis of hemifacial microsomia. The fact that both nasolabial folds are relatively intact (not erased unilaterally) excludes unilateral facial palsy (Fig. 11.5). Despite his facial deformity, which he even expressed in his self-portrait, all the portraits he made were symmetrical and never had any facial deformities. David compensated for his deformity by painting portraits that were smooth, even, and symmetrical [12].

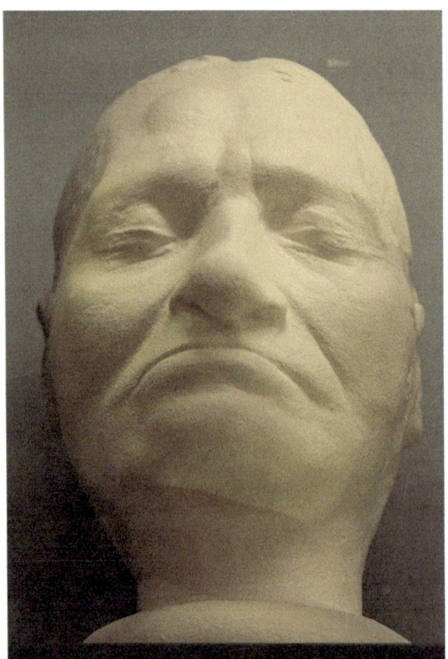

Fig. 11.5 Death mask of Jacques-Louis David (1748–1825). Available at https://commons.wikimedia.org/wiki/File:Death_mask_of_Jacques-Louis_David,_1825.JPG

From his case, we learn that feelings about bodily deformity and incompleteness can stimulate fantasies of rebirth and auto-reconstruction, generating creativity in the artist. Then, how can we plastic surgeons stimulate creativity in our operations?

Harold Gillies, the pioneering plastic surgeon, performed more than 11,000 operations for 5000 soldiers with facial injuries from 1917 to 1925. His experiences with head and facial injuries became the basis of craniofacial surgery, and his advances were also applied to congenital craniofacial malformations. Through treating severely injured faces, he accumulated surgical experiences with the face that ultimately led to the development of aesthetic surgery [13].

Much like an artist who has a deformity, a plastic surgeon is motivated by the body deformity or disability of the patients that he or she tries to improve. The more a surgeon operates, the more his or her accumulated experiences stimulate fantasies of reconstructing patients with deformities.

Most of the principles of modern facial plastic surgery were developed during the 20 years between World War I and World War II. As such, plastic surgery aims for humanity before beauty.

11.5 The Borromean Rings of Plastic Surgery: Science, Art, and Skill

Plastic surgeons are now sometimes referred to as "half artists." Surgeons are generally happy to be viewed in these terms and are eager to exploit this trend. Artists often find useful means of artistic expression from scientific fields. In this respect, science and art share a common denominator in their evolving relationship. Science is a systematic and theoretical construction of knowledge, which is acquired through measurable methods. Science consists of a body of knowledge of scientific experiments based on empiricism and methodological naturalism. Science is logical and analytical; in contrast, the arts tend to encourage intuition and imagination. Science demands predictable processes and results; the arts promote creative destruction with a tint of romanticism opposed to rationality. Over time, they have run parallel, crossed over, and separated from each other [14].

In plastic surgery, patients want to simultaneously achieve scientifically predictable results and artistic perfection. At this point, a symbol representing Trinity is coming to my mind: Borromean rings. Borromean rings or knots are 3 simple closed curves in three-dimensional space. These are topologically linked and cannot be separated from each other, but they break apart into two unknotted and unlinked loops when any one of the three is cut or removed. Thereafter, scientifically predictable results and artistic perfection compose two of the Borromean rings in plastic surgery.

A skill is a learned ability to perform an action with predictable results and good execution, often within a given amount of time, energy, or both. Plastic surgery requires personal skills as well as surgical knowledge or special technical dexterity. However, this niche surgical specialty is not very well covered in the curricula of many medical schools. Therefore, upon graduation, most junior doctors have had very limited or no exposure to common plastic surgery procedures. Recently, some courses have focused on fundamental plastic surgery skills required to perform key index operating procedures for entry into higher specialist surgical training [15]. There are also international fellowship programs teaching the essential personal skills needed in modern plastic surgery [16]. Without established personal surgical skills, it is very difficult to achieve an improved quality of life and satisfying outcomes for patients. Thereafter, surgical skill comprises the third Borromean ring.

To be an academic plastic surgeon, one must have a sound knowledge of anatomy, physiology, pathology, and pharmacology. These fields of scientific knowledge consist of a ring of plastic surgery. To be an artistic cosmetic surgeon, one must have a keen eye with an artistic viewpoint and imagination. This artistic eye comprises another ring of plastic surgery. To be a real plastic surgeon, good surgical skills for operations are needed. These skills are essential and comprise the other ring of plastic surgery.

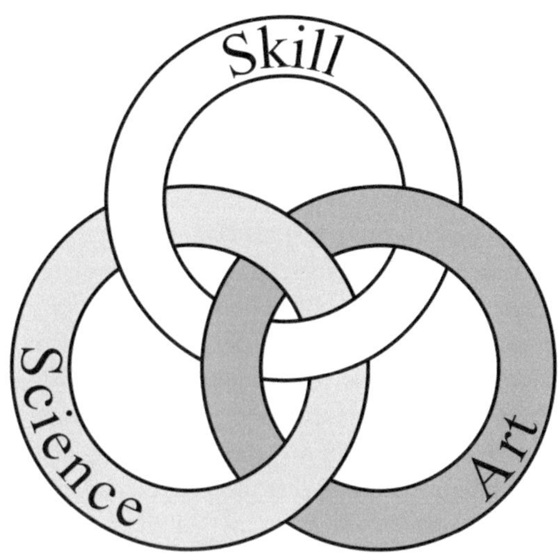

Fig. 11.6 Borromean rings of plastic surgery consisted of science, art, and skill

Good skills are taught by our teacher plastic surgeons. Dr. Converse reminds Dr. Kazanjian as a good teacher. "Imaginative and resourceful, Dr. Kazanjian taught to improvise new methods rather than follow the conventional. 'Do it just right,' he would say, meaning in his laconic way (he preferred action to talk) that each patient's problem required an individual solution. Never did I hear him denigrate a colleague's work. His kindness, warmth, and modesty are legendary [17]."

As Lacan's three registers of human experience (the symbolic, imaginary, and real) are only conceivable when considered together, plastic surgery consists of scientific knowledge (science), an artistic view (art), and surgical skill (skill) [18]. Just as Lacan's three registers are linked as in a Borromean knot of three inextricably tied rings, science, art, and skill are linked as three inseparable rings (Fig. 11.6).

11.6 The Poet-Physician's Note and the Plastic Surgeon's Note

You lethargic, waiting upon me, waiting for the fire and I attendant upon you, shaken by your beauty. Shaken by your beauty. Shaken.—*Paterson by William Carlos Williams*

I recently enjoyed watching a movie entitled "Paterson" (starring Adam Driver, directed by Jim Jarmusch). A bus driver, whose name is Paterson, works in the city of Paterson in New Jersey. During pauses, he writes poems in a notebook (Fig. 11.7). His wife, Laura, loves his poems and tries to persuade him to publish them or at least make copies. He finally promises to make copies of the poems, but their dog rips up his notebook, destroying his poems. Sad and depressed, he goes for a walk and sits down at Great Falls, his favorite site. There, a Japanese man sits beside him, and they talk about poetry after Paterson notices that the man is reading the poem *Paterson* written by William Carlos Williams. Although the driver Paterson denies it, the Japanese man thinks that Paterson himself is a poet and gives him an empty notebook as a gift. Paterson begins to write a poem in his new notebook.

After enjoying the movie "Paterson," I turned to the book-length poem *Paterson* and learned about the poet William Carlos Williams (1883–1963). He was a Puerto Rican-American poet, writer, and physician. His primary occupation was a general physician and a pediatrician; however, he was a successful poet as well as a painter. He practiced medicine by day and wrote at night.

People asked him: "Do you have time to write while continuing your treatment? You must be a superman with at least two energies." He replied: "The two are two parts of one, not each of the other. The two complement each other. When one part wears me out, the other part makes me rest" [19]. For him, medicine was a leap forward to becoming a poet, and at the same time, poetry was the driving force of his role as a doctor, as exemplified by his confession stating "I cannot practice medicine without poetry."

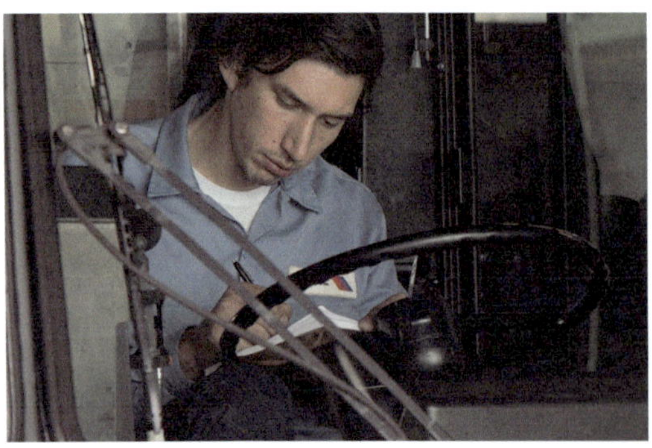

Fig. 11.7 Paterson, a bus driver writes poems in a notebook in a movie "Paterson" (starring Adam Driver, directed by Jim Jarmusch, 2016)

The poet-physician's *Autobiography* brought me to the topic of plastic surgeons' notes.

When I visited the Hunterian Museum in London, I had the chance to see some relics belonging to Thomas Pomfret Kilner (1890–1964), who established the V-Y pushback palatoplasty (Wardill-Kilner-Veau method) in 1937. The BAPRAS (British Association of Plastic, Reconstructive, and Aesthetic Surgeons) archive room of the Royal College of Surgeons had Kilner's drafts of papers, pictures of the patients he operated upon, schemas submitted to journals, and his handwritten notes. Only one drawing of palatoplasty was drawn by pencil. Interestingly, it was not made in an ordinary notebook but was drawn on the reverse side of a letter envelope from the Queen's Hotel, Birmingham. It is therefore thought that Dr. Kilner got an idea when he was staying at that hotel. Before the vivid idea went away, he sketched a schema on the nearest paper, the letter envelope [20].

Since my training period, which started 35 years ago, I have written my operative records myself or at least reviewed those that my residents make before I sign them. Alongside the official operative records, I have empty note papers upon which I write or draw to prepare for operations that I think will involve complicated procedures. Just after surgery, I fill the space with the steps of procedures I did and my regrets regarding the operation. When such operative notes are collected, they can be the basis of case reports, idea and innovation reports, case series, or even original articles.

The human brain is like molten bronze that should be poured into a mold. When inspired, ideas should be written or drawn before they disappear. This is why Dr. Williams and Dr. Kilner seized their ideas in a moment.

11.7 The Dresser and Stage Director: Scrub Nurses and Chief Residents

Recently, I enjoyed a play, entitled "The Dresser," at Jeongdong Theater in central Seoul. Song Seung-hwan, an actor who graduated from the same high school as me, played the role of a protagonist named "Sir." The very next day, I searched and watched a drama film (1983) of the same name in which Albert Finney and Tom Courtenay star as "Sir" and "Norman," respectively (Fig. 11.8).

This play, written by Ronald Harwood (1934–2020), explores the relationship between "Sir," an aging, tyrannical actor and troupe leader with a monstrous ego and delusions of grandeur, and Norman, his faithful dresser, ego-masseur, and shield from reality. The play is set in World War II, with themes of struggle and survival, emphasizing that everyone is simply struggling to survive as their world shifts and crumbles around them.

A particularly memorable scene was inside of the actor's room in the theater, where there was a desk and chair for make-up, an armchair for rest, and a hanger with many costumes. When the actor (Sir), who was wearing only underwear, raised his arms, the dresser (Norman) helped the actor put on his costume, including a triple crown.

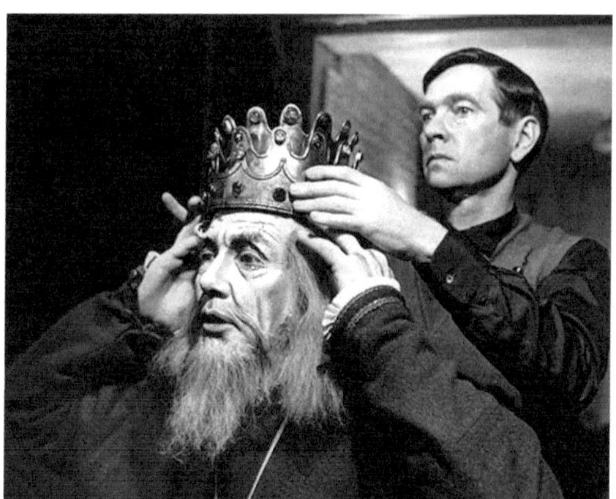

Fig. 11.8 Norman (Tom Courtenay) is putting a triple crown on "Sir" (Albert Finney) in "The Dresser" (1983)

When the actor was preparing (applying make-up and putting on a costume), the stage director (Madge) notified him of the time remaining until the opening of the curtain. When the opening was ready, the actor moved from his room to the curtain. Between the acts and intermission, the actor returned to his room and took a rest or nap on his couch, or took a bath in a tub.

In the last act of "King Lear," the entire troupe made frantic attempts to create the storm scene for Sir. However, he was not satisfied and berated them for making a noise no bigger than "farting flies."

The actor took an interest in a new actress not because she was young and pretty but because she looked lean and lighter to carry in Act V of "King Lear."

Just before his last performance as an actor, Sir talked to Madge, who had been working for him for 20 years.

Were you happy with your work? Was it worth it?

"No, I haven't been happy. Yes, it's been worth it." She replied.

Then, Sir said: "Talk about me sometimes. Actors exist only in the memory of the others. The most beautiful thing is to be remembered by somebody."

After the curtain call, Sir came back to his room, lay down on the couch, and then breathed his last breath. Only the dresser closed his eyes. In the preface of the uncompleted long-awaited autobiography, however, Sir did not mention the dresser or the stage director, who had worked for a long time.

Just as the actor plays in a theater, the surgeon works in the operating theater. Like the actor stays in the actors' room, the surgeon stays in the locker room to change clothes and rest. Usually, the chief resident or circulating nurse notifies me of the exact time I should arrive at the theater.

When the patient is anesthetized and draped, I wash my hands and open the door using my foot and then raise my arms like an actor. The scrub nurse gives me hands to fit into the aseptic surgical gown. Between operations, the surgeon returns to the locker room and takes a rest, enjoys a cup of tea, or takes a shower to remove blood from the operation.

During the important procedures of each operation, I usually need a larger visual field. Thereafter, I ask my assistants to pull the retractor tightly or the circulating nurse to adjust the lightening. As I become older, I do not berate them—instead, I say, "Thank you!"

I do not prefer pretty or young residents or physician's assistants; rather, I prefer those with strong arms and agile hands who provide me a good visual field during the operation.

I wish to be remembered by my team as a good surgeon. I sincerely hope that my pupils have been happy working with me and feel their efforts were worthwhile. As actors exist only in the memory of the audience, I believe that surgeons exist only in the postoperative results of their patients.

This play reminded me of a novel, *The Atheist's Mass*, written by Honoré de Balzac (1799–1850). He defined the glory of a surgeon [21]. "The glory of a surgeon is like that of an actor: they live only so long as they are alive, and their talent leaves no trace when they are gone. Actors and surgeons, like great singers too, like the executants who by their performance increase the power of music tenfold, are all the heroes of a moment."

As the actor passed away just after the curtain call, I would like to continue performing surgery as long as my health permits. However, unlike the character of Sir in the play, if I have a chance to write my autobiography, I certainly will dedicate it to my pupils and scrub nurses who worked with me.

11.8 Making a Narrow Path, Then a Road, through the Snow

> If they were to walk directly behind the first man, the second group would make a clearly defined but barely passable narrow path, and not a road.—*Varlam Shalamov*

This Sunday morning, we had a heavy snow in my province. Walking along the road, I was reminded of *Kolyma Tales*, written by the Russian author Varlam Shalamov (1907–1982) about labor camp life in the USSR [22]. It contains six collections of short stories, with a prologue entitled "Through the Snow."

In this preface, he explains how to make a road through the virgin snow.

"One person walks ahead, sweating, swearing, and barely moving his feet. He keeps getting stuck in the loose, deep snow. He goes far ahead, marking his path with uneven black pits" (Fig. 11.9). When totally exhausted, he selects

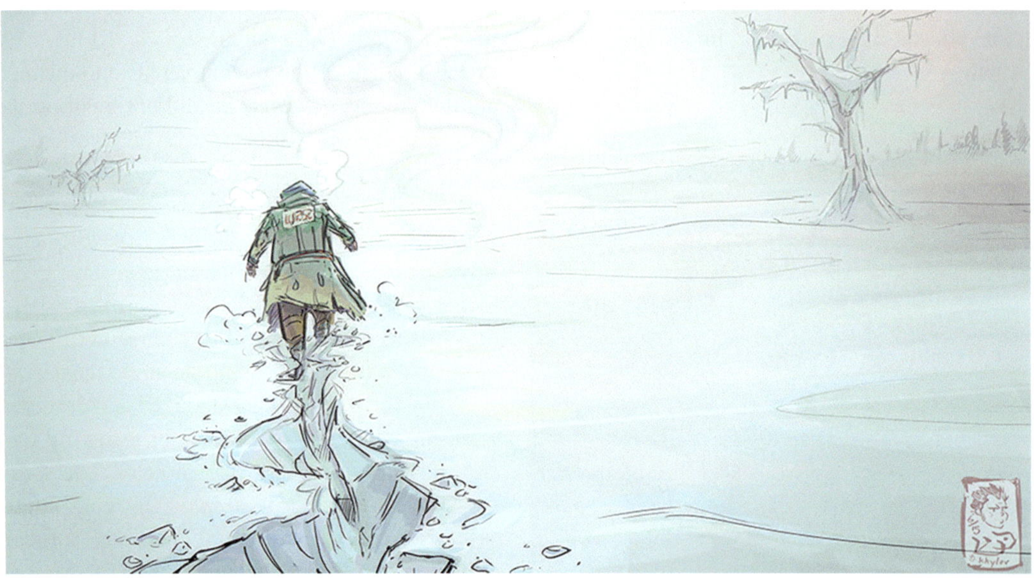

Fig. 11.9 Making a road through the virgin snow. Available at: http://2.bp.blogspot.com/-2KYjwhrJm8k/VXTbHx_X00I/AAAAAAAACxU/aQPcgH7wa6Y/s1600/khylov__kolyma_tales__shalamov__through_the_snow.jpg

points in the snow's infinity to orient himself—a cliff, a tall tree. Then, followers (5–6 men) weave along the track of the first man in a shoulder-to-shoulder scrum.

The followers walk beside the first man's path but not along it. "When they reach a predetermined spot, they turn back and tramp down the clean virgin snow which has not yet felt the foot of man." "The road is tramped down. It can be used by people, sleighs, tractors."

In plastic surgery and craniofacial surgery, conducting novel research or developing an innovative surgical method is like making a small path in the virgin snow. The first researcher works toward his purpose, carries out experiments, obtains the results, and then submits a paper. If the paper is easily accepted, he is happy. If rejected by several journals, he feels exhausted and enters a slump, as if the first man mentioned by Shalamov were to lie down on the snow and light a homemade cigarette, after which the tobacco smoke would hang suspended above the white, gleaming snow like a blue cloud. If the paper is published, a small path is made for the followers, the second group who will cite the first man's paper. However, this is not yet sufficient for the findings to be recommended to the surgeons who are readers of the journal.

When the men described by Shalamov reach a predetermined spot, "they turn back and tramp down the clean virgin snow which has not yet felt the foot of man." If the second group of roadmakers walked directly behind the first man, they would make a clearly defined but barely passable narrow path, not a road. Likewise, if the second group of authors wrote papers very similar to the first one—that is, "me-too papers"—they would hardly transform the narrow path carved out by the first paper into a road suitable for the readership of surgeons. Instead of just applying or repeating the first researcher's method, they should critique the first paper, finding its strengths and weaknesses and then modifying it if they can.

In roadmaking in the snow, the first man has the hardest task, and when he is exhausted, another man from the group of five takes his place.

When writing a paper, surgeons or researchers should not simply follow the path laid down by a previous paper; as Shalamov, a writer who spent years in the Gulag camps of the USSR, emphasized: "Each of them—even the smallest and weakest—must beat down a section of virgin snow, and not simply follow in another's footsteps."

He closed the prologue by saying "Later will come tractors and horses driven by readers, instead of authors and poets."

11.9 Aging in Mathematics and in Surgery

We can use the wisdom of the old horse.—*Guan Zhong*

Recently, I enjoyed the film entitled *A Man Who Knew Infinity*, directed by Matt Brown. It is the story of the life and academic career of the pioneer Indian mathematician, Srinivasa Ramanujan (1887–1920), and his friendship with his mentor, Professor Godfrey Harold Hardy (1877–1947).

The name of Hardy was familiar to me since I remember the Hardy–Weinberg principle, stating that allele and genotype frequencies in a population will remain constant from generation to generation in the absence of other evolutionary influences: $[(p + q)^2 = p^2 + 2pq + q^2 = 1$, where $q = 1 - p]$.

After coming home, I read Hardy's famous book, *A Mathematician's Apology,* and learned about some interesting aspects of his character. In 1896, Hardy entered Trinity College, Cambridge, where he eventually graduated.

He could not bear to look at his own reflection in a mirror. It is said that, when staying in hotels, he would cover all the mirrors with towels. He engaged in this peculiar behavior because he believed his activity and skill would decline with age and denied that he was aging.

In his book, he discussed a phrase attributed to Gauss: "Mathematics is the queen of the sciences and number theory is the queen of mathematics." He thought that mathematics is a "young man's game," meaning that anyone with a talent for mathematics should develop and use that talent while they are young, before their ability to create original mathematics starts to decline in middle age.

As a plastic surgeon who turned 60 this year, I have recently thought about aging. I recalled Dr. Harold Delf Gillies (1882–1960) (Fig. 11.10). D.r Gillies, 5 years younger than Professor Hardy, studied medicine at Gonville and Caius College, Cambridge University. Gillies suffered a slight cerebral thrombosis while undertaking a major operation at the age of 78 on the damaged leg of an 18-year-old girl.

As exemplified by Dr. Gillies, aging makes plastic surgeons more experienced and wiser than when they were young. An episode in ancient Chinese history illustrates this point: A king (Qi Huanong) and his troops embarked on a conquest in spring against a nearby nation. On their way home in winter, they lost their path. A general (Guan Zhong) said: "We can use the wisdom of the old horse." They released an old horse in front of the line of soldiers, the soldiers followed it, and they finally found their way.

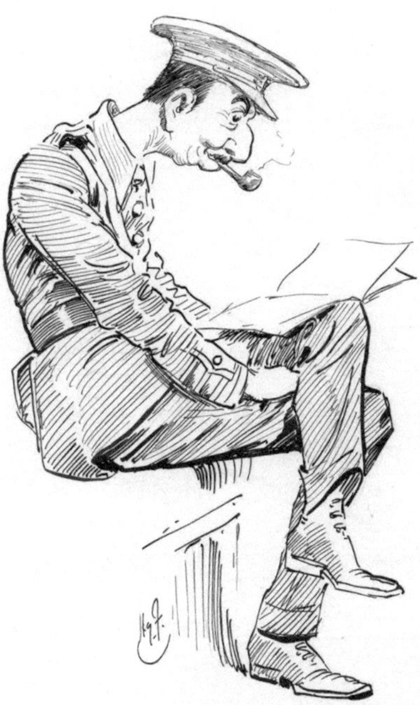

Fig. 11.10 Sir Harold Delf Gillies by Harry Furniss. Pen and ink, 1910s, 390 mm × 320 mm. Licensed from National Portrait Gallery, London

Similarly to Gauss, I think that plastic surgery is the queen of surgery, and craniofacial surgery is the queen of plastic surgery.

11.10 Bamboo Back-Scratcher

If I have seen further, it is by standing on the shoulders of giants.—*Isaac Newton (1642–1726)*

My life will be successful if someone in the future can remember me as a bamboo back-scratcher that scratched an itch.—*Kun Hwang (1957–)*

During my stay in London, I had a comfortable arrangement in my flat, since I had a washing machine and could cook easily. Free phone calls were available, and I did not feel like I was far away from my wife and my hometown.

The only discomfort was that I had nobody to scratch my back for me when it itched. I missed my bamboo back-scratcher, which I had not brought with me.

When searching references, periodicals are easy to find, but it can be difficult to find books. If the library does not have a book I am looking for, I usually order it online, but if Amazon does not have the book I need, it is similar to feeling my back itch but not being able to scratch it with my hand.

On a rainy day, I visited the British Library to look for books that were out of stock on Amazon. I walked from the King's Cross Station, famous as a location in Harry Potter, to the British Library. I was able to register as a user and find Grabb's "Cleft Lip and Palate: Surgical, Dental, and Speech Aspects" (1971), from which I copied a chapter written by James Calnan.

On my way out, there was a very large sculpture in front of the library, standing on a pedestal taller than a man. A man was wearing glasses, sitting on a square chair without a backrest, bending forward and holding a compass in his left hand, and measuring something under his feet. When I got close to the nameplate, I realized that the sculpture was "NEWTON" (1995) made by Sir Eduardo Paolozzi (1924–2005). It was written that the original painting "Newton" was created by William Blake (1757–1827). On my way back to my flat, I visited Tate Britain and saw Blake's original painting (Fig. 11.11).

A naked man sat on a rock and measured a triangle and a circle drawn on the floor using a compass. Blake expressed Isaac Newton (1642–1726) as a divine geometer. He was sitting, but leaning forward, his shoulders tilted down to his knees. It seemed that if there was someone beside him, he could easily climb onto Newton's shoulders and stand there. Seeing this painting, I remembered a saying of Newton in response those who praised him: "If I have seen further, it is by standing on the shoulders of giants." I was impressed with the creative expression of the painters and sculptors who presented a compass

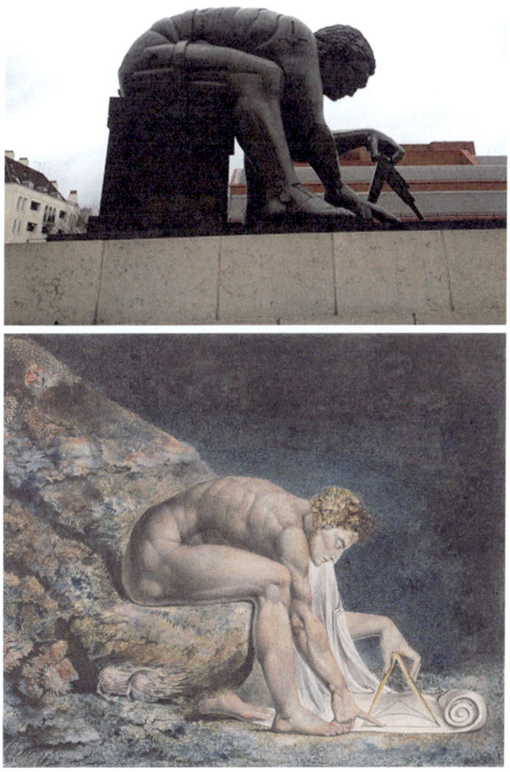

Fig. 11.11 Statue and painting of Newton. Upper: "NEWTON" by Sir Eduardo Paolozzi. Lower: "Newton" drawn by William Blake. Reproduced with permission from Tate Britain

as the symbol of this great physicist who discovered the law of gravity.

Walking out of the museum, I looked back and saw myself. What could be a symbolic object of me? What object could my fellow plastic surgeons, my students, and my children use to remember me in the distant future?

Since it was raining and chilly outside, when I came inside, I felt warm and my back became sweaty. I moved my arm behind my back and tried to scratch my back through my clothes, but I did not feel any relief. I wished I had my bamboo back-scratcher with me.

After I was trained in plastic surgery, I sought to elucidate aspects of the surgical anatomy of the human body needed for surgeons. I strove to write papers like bamboo back-scratchers that can directly reach the area that itches. However, my efforts were not enough to fully satisfy the curiosity of my fellow plastic surgeons, and fewer than 5 years remain until my retirement. Now is the time for me to bend down like Newton's body in that sculpture so that somebody can climb onto my shoulders and stand there to see further.

Will my life be successful if someone in the future can remember me as a bamboo back-scratcher that scratched an itch? (Fig. 11.11).

11.11 A Plastic Surgeon Should Be a Good Physician First

> Magic mirror in my hand, who is the fairest in the land?—*Evil Queen (Fairy tale)*

In my department, I have a weekly seminar meeting with residents, medical students in clerkship, and graduate students. The topic of the last meeting was "How much am I worth?"

The participants responded with several novel answers to this fanciful question. A resident computed his lifelong stipend, as we calculate patients' disability rating using the McBride scale. A PhD. student thought that her value could be measured only with the amount of tears her acquaintances will shed, with a price equal to that of the most expensive French cognac.

This discussion induced me to ask myself: "Am I a man of worth?" and "Am I a good plastic surgeon?"

Tips for patients about choosing a good plastic surgeon have been presented by a CNN medical news correspondent [23], as well as the American Board of Cosmetic Surgeons [24]. These tips include checking whether the plastic surgeon is board certified, checking the surgeon's record of malpractice judgments, and asking whether the surgeon has hospital privileges as part of a background check. In the United States, "Best in City X Magazine," such as "Best in Baltimore," is being judged by a survey sent to 10,000 physicians, who are being asked, "If your family member was in need of a plastic surgeon, for whom would you refer them personally?" Since all major cities in the United States have a local magazine for which votes "Best in City X," this would be the best place to start.

However, fulfilling these criteria cannot guarantee that a plastic surgeon is a "good plastic surgeon."

Patients consider a doctor to be a good doctor when they feel comfortable, safe, and human with him or her. However, from the medical perspective, good doctor is the physician or surgeon who solves the patient's problem. A good doctor is one who correctly diagnoses patients' illnesses, cures them with safe evidence-based procedures, and is honest to them. On the contrary, a poor doctor is generally credited with good intentions but inadequate knowledge or skills required for the job. The virtues needed for a good doctor are sound knowledge and competent skills to provide safety and comfort to patients while maintaining a good rapport with all around him.

Since surgeons treat people with knives and risky instruments and therefore are more frequently sued than other doctors, a good surgeon should be a good doctor with some extra skills: A good surgeon needs to learn how to operate, when to operate, and when not to operate [25]. In addition to thorough knowledge and practical skills, a good surgeon is also expected to have common sense, which enables him or her to make sound practical judgments [26].

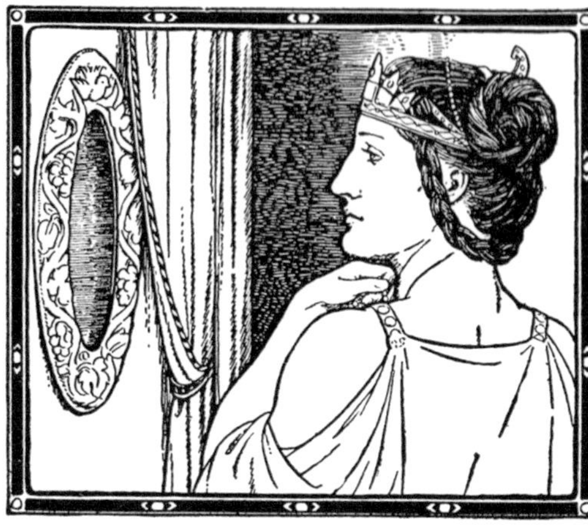

Fig. 11.12 The Evil Queen in front of the Mirror. Mirror in a 1916 illustration. Available at: https://upload.wikimedia.org/wikipedia/commons/thumb/8/8c/Illustration_at_page_201_in_Europa%27s_Fairy_Book.png/1024px-Illustration_at_page_201_in_Europa%27s_Fairy_Book.png. Accessed Jul 12, 2018

In the plastic surgery field, we sometimes meet patients who expect us to be magicians who can change them from an "ugly one" to the "fairest of them all" (Fig. 11.12). More rarely, they treat us as merchants who are selling "new faces." In this aspect, I do think that a good plastic surgeon must first be a good surgeon and that a good surgeon must first be a good doctor.

In terms of knowledge, we should understand the anatomical basis of treatment and the principles of perioperative care, including fluid and electrolyte balance. These are the values plastic surgeons must keep. Without the knowledge of anatomy and perioperative care, plastic surgeons are not different from cosmetologists. The decision of when to operate and when not to operate is essential, as well as surgical skills. Honesty and empathy for patients define the attitude of a good plastic surgeon. If artistic sense and enthusiasm are added, we might carve a "Galatea," a perfect ivory sculpture that eventually lost its hardness.

11.12 The Aging Surgeon and the Secret of Longevity

I sit down at the piano and I don't sing the opera, most of the time, until I know it.—*Plácido Domingo*

Last year, I enjoyed Verdi's Nabucco directed by James Levine and starring Plácido Domingo at the Metropolitan Opera (Fig. 11.13). In response to the audience's request for an encore, Levine gave an encore performance of the famous "Chorus of the Hebrew Slaves" of Act 3. This beautiful chorus starts as "Fly, thought, on golden wings."

Among the "Three Tenors," Luciano Pavarotti (1935–2007) passed away, and José Carreras (1946–) is not active as before. Domingo (1941–) has also had a long and beautiful career, as he himself said, but he is still active and has a beautiful voice, just as before. At the time of this performance, he was 76 years old.

I was curious how this great singer performed the "perfect aria" and how he maintained his voice in its best condition. I searched for this secret and finally found it in the following conversation among James Levine, Plácido Domingo, and Peter Gelb, the general manager of the Metropolitan Opera [27].

Levine: The art form is difficult enough. A mistake is not the end of the world…

Domingo: [To be] really, totally honest, I know exactly in my mind how to sing, but I have never been able to do it that way…though I come pretty close.

Gelb: What is, if you could say, the secret of your longevity?

Domingo: I don't know, but I think it has helped me something. Since I was a musician, always, I sit at the piano and I was preparing my operas. I wonder how many hours of coaching I have. I sit down at the piano and I don't sing the opera, most of the time, until I know it.

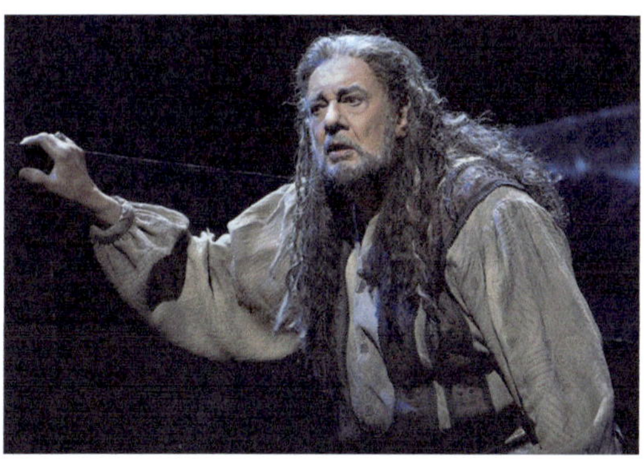

Fig. 11.13 Plácido Domingo sings an aria in Verdi's Nabucco, at New York Metropolitan Opera

Levine: He didn't have to waste voice learning it. That's a brain job, not a voice job.

As a surgeon, I have asked myself whether I carry out operations exactly as planned. Although the operations are precisely designed and usually—like Domingo—I come pretty close, I have never been able to operate in exactly the same way that I conceive of it in my mind.

I recalled that Dr. Harold Gilles continued to perform surgery until the age of 78, which led me to think about the longevity of plastic surgeons.

First, we must preserve our visual acuity, as singers spare their voice. Therefore, excessive TV watching or cellphone use should be reduced. Second, we should maintain good general health. Smoking or excess alcohol use shortens the surgeon's longevity. Lastly, the most important consideration is planning and preparing our operations. We should design our procedures carefully and make memos, schemas, or drawings while sitting at our desk, not in the operating theater. Much like opera, surgery is a brain job—not a job for the hands.

11.13 Accolade for Surgeonship

> A good plastic surgeon must first be a good surgeon, and a good surgeon must first be a good doctor.—*K. Hwang* [2]

Recently, I happened to see an accolade for knighthood while watching Season 8 of "Game of Thrones." Jaime Lannister bestows knighthood upon Brienne of Tarth, using the following words:

"In the name of the Warrior, I charge you to be brave. In the name of the Father, I charge you to be just. In the name of the Mother, I charge you to defend the innocent. Arise, Brienne of Tarth, a knight of the Seven Kingdoms."

In the medieval ages, the first step in becoming a knight was to serve as a page (a term indicating a type of servant). Seven-year-old boys were turned over to the care of the castle's lords. They were placed on an early training regimen of hunting and academic studies. Pages become assistants to older knights in battle, carrying and cleaning armor, taking care of the horses, and packing the baggage. Older pages were educated in swordsmanship, equestrianism, chivalry, warfare, and combat using wooden swords and spears. As the boys became squires at the age of 15, they continued training in combat and were allowed to have their own armor. They were required to master the prerequisite skills for knighthood while wearing armor. When squires reached the age of 21, they became eligible to be knighted.

The accolade is a ceremony to confer knighthood. Usually, the knight-elect would kneel in front of the monarch on a knighting-stool. In the ceremony, the monarch first lays the side of the sword's blade onto the accolade's right shoulder. The monarch then raises the sword gently just up over the apprentice's head and places it on his left shoulder (Fig. 11.14). The new knight then stands up, and the king or queen presents him with the insignia of his new order.

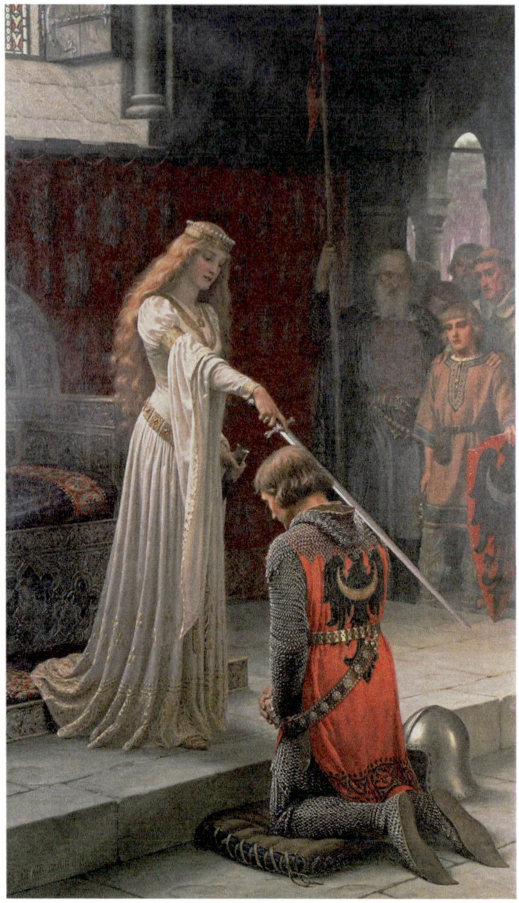

Fig. 11.14 Accolade. Edmund Blair Leighton (1901)

In March, new plastic surgeons receive their board certification from the Ministry of Health and Welfare. To become a board-certified surgeon, in the Republic of Korea, a 1-year internship and a 4-year residency are mandatory after graduating medical school and obtaining a medical license.

At the commencement of medical school, students usually take the Hippocratic Oath. Upon receiving board certification, in my department, each new surgeon takes a photograph with the training staff and junior trainees. While this is to be commended, it may not be enough for a truly memorable moment.

I propose an accolade for plastic surgeonship. I would like to prepare a knife handle with a #15 blade, tap it on the shoulders of my pupil, and then say:

"In the name of the Physician, I charge you to have medical knowledge. In the name of the Surgeon, I charge you to have surgical skill. In the name of the Teacher, I charge you to have honesty and empathy to your patients. Arise, Kun of Incheon, a plastic surgeon."

References

1. Prado A, Andrades P. Creativity in plastic surgery. Aesth Plast Surg. 2008;32:409–10.
2. Hwang K. A plastic surgeon should be a good physician first. J Craniofac Surg. 2019;30:629.
3. Kyriacou DN. Evidence-based medical decision making: deductive versus inductive logical thinking. Acad Emerg Med. 2004;11:670–1.
4. Rothman KJ, Rothman KJ. 2. Causal inference in epidemiology. In: Modern Epidemiology. 1st ed. Boston: Little, Brown & Co; 1986. p. 7–22.
5. Spencer FC. Deductive reasoning in the lifelong continuing education of a cardiovascular surgeon. Arch Surg. 1976;111:1177–83.
6. Patel VL, Arocha JF, Zhang J, Holyoak K. Thinking and reasoning in medicine. In: Cambridge handbook of thinking and reasoning. Cambridge: Cambridge University Press; 2005. p. 1–34.
7. Januszkiewicz JS. The hidden art in plastic surgery. Plast Reconstr Surg. 2002;109:2463–70.

8. Edwards B. Drawing on the artist within. New York: Touchstone; 1987. p. 2–9.
9. Hwang K. How to write a scientific paper: three tips to remember. Arch Plast Surg. 2012;39:77.
10. Hwang K. Goddess of imagination. J Craniofac Surg. 2017;28:857.
11. Colp R. Psychiatry and creative process. In: Kaplan HI, Freedman AM, Sadock BJ, editors. Comprehensive textbook of psychiatry. 3rd ed. Baltimore: Williams & Wilkins; 1980. p. 3112.
12. Niederland WG. Psychoanalytic approaches to artistic creativity. Psychoanal Q. 1976;45:185–212.
13. Hwang K. Trench coats, Cushing, and Gillies. Arch Craniofac Surg. 2018;19:83–4.
14. Choi J. Cosmetic surgery: is it science or art? Arch Plast Surg. 2015;42:672–4.
15. Teklay S, Dhillon D. Course review: mid Yorkshire plastic surgery course-essential plastic surgery skills for junior doctors. Ann Plast Surg. 2021;87(4):e25–6.
16. Abdelhakim M, Soto Diez C, Huang C, et al. Plastic surgery fellowship at Nippon medical school hospital: an integrative approach to modern plastic surgery education. Plast Reconstr Surg Glob Open. 2021;9:e3367.
17. Converse JM, Varaztad H. Kazanjian. In: Converse JM, editor. Kazanjian & Converse's surgical treatment of facial injuries, vol. 1. 3rd ed; 1974. p. IX.
18. Eyers T. Lacan and the concept of the real. Hampshire: Plagrave Macmillan; 2012. p. 17.
19. Williams WC. The autobiography of William Carlos Williams. New York: W. W. Norton & Company; 1951.
20. Hwang K. Meet Dr Kilner at the Hunterian museum. J Craniofac Surg. 2017;28:1402–3.
21. Hwang K. Trauma surgeons: heroes of a moment. J Trauma Inj. 2021;34:79–80.
22. Kolyma SK, Tales. London. UK: Penguin Books Ltd; 1994. p. 3–4.
23. Cohen E. Five tips for picking a good plastic surgeon. http://edition.cnn.com/2007/HEALTH/11/22/ep.cosmetic.surgery/. Accessed 22 Nov 2007.
24. American Board of Cosmetic Surgeons. Choosing a cosmetic surgeon. https://www.americanboard-cosmeticsurgery.org/patient-resources/choosing-a-cosmetic-surgeon/. Assessed 25 Feb 2018.
25. Ghanem AN. Good doctor, what makes a good surgeon? BMJ. 2018;324:1533.
26. Akopov AL, Artioukh DY. Good surgeon: a search for meaning. Turk J Surg. 2017;33:49–50.
27. Metropolitan Opera. James Levine, Plácido Domingo, and Peter Gelb in Conversation. https://www.youtube.com/watch?v=QmnagKbhXGY. Assessed 16 Dec 2017.

MIX
Papier aus verantwortungsvollen Quellen
Paper from responsible sources
FSC® C105338

If you have any concerns about our products,
you can contact us on
ProductSafety@springernature.com

In case Publisher is established outside the EU,
the EU authorized representative is:
Springer Nature Customer Service Center GmbH
Europaplatz 3, 69115 Heidelberg, Germany

Printed by Libri Plureos GmbH
in Hamburg, Germany